AF439909

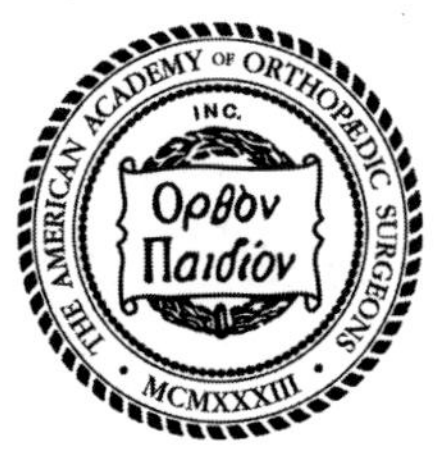

American Academy of Orthopaedic Surgeons

Pathophysiology of Orthopaedic Diseases

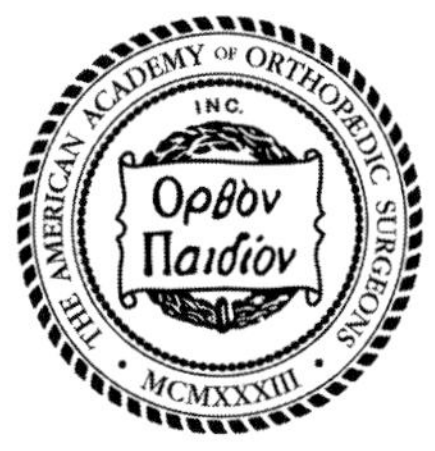

American Academy of Orthopaedic Surgeons

Pathophysiology of Orthopaedic Diseases

Henry J. Mankin, MD

Published 2006 by the
American Academy of Orthopaedic Surgeons
6300 North River Road
Rosemont, IL 60018

Copyright © 2006
by the American Academy of Orthopaedic Surgeons

The material presented in *Pathophysiology of Orthopaedic Diseases* has been made available by the American Academy of Orthopaedic Surgeons for educational purposes only. This material is not intended to present the only, or necessarily best, methods or procedures for the medical situations discussed, but rather is intended to represent an approach, view, statement, or opinion of the author(s) or producer(s), which may be helpful to others who face similar situations.

Some drugs or medical devices demonstrated in Academy courses or described in Academy print or electronic publications have not been cleared by the Food and Drug Administration (FDA) or have been cleared for specific uses only. The FDA has stated that it is the responsibility of the physician to determine the FDA clearance status of each drug or device he or she wishes to use in clinical practice.

Furthermore, any statements about commercial products are solely the opinion(s) of the author(s) and do not represent an Academy endorsement or evaluation of these products. These statements may not be used in advertising or for any commercial purpose.

ISBN 10: 0-89203-416-5
ISBN 13: 978-0-89203-416-1

Printed in the USA

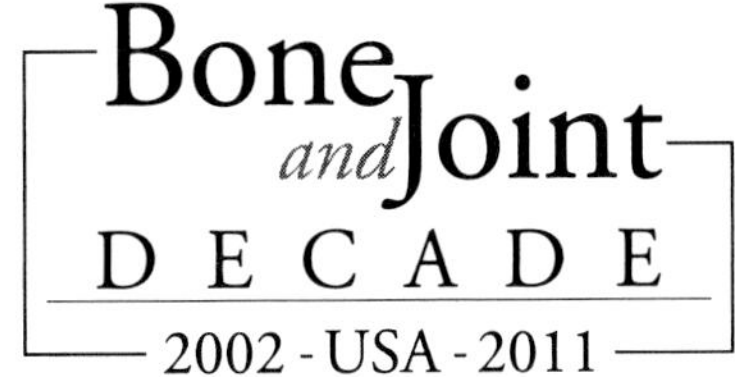

Table of Contents

Foreword

Dr. Henry Mankin has had an extraordinary career in orthopaedics, and his contributions to both clinical knowledge and basic science are truly remarkable. His book *Pathophysiology of Orthopaedic Diseases* is a valuable resource for residents and all orthopaedic surgeons and represents a lifetime of work devoted to understanding the pathophysiology of disease. It is a wonderful example of Dr. Mankin's commitment to teaching residents, fellows, and colleagues.

This book pays special tribute to Henry L. Jaffe, MD, who was Chief of Pathology and Director of the Laboratories at the Hospital for Joint Diseases when Dr. Mankin worked as a resident there. When Dr. Mankin returned later in his career as Chief of Orthopaedics at the Hospital for Joint Diseases, Dr. Jaffe had retired, but remained as a consultant and teacher while completing his classic book *Metabolic, Degenerative and Inflammatory Diseases of Bones and Joints.* By writing a current book about basic principles of specific orthopaedic diseases, as did Dr. Jaffe in1972, Dr. Mankin pays personal tribute to Dr. Jaffe. In it Dr. Mankin records citations of Dr. Jaffe's publications in 13 of the 24 disease-specific chapters and to his own publications in 14 of the diseases discussed. Dr. Mankin also uses the first chapter to inform the orthopaedic community about the valuable collection of pathologic material that Dr. Jaffe collected throughout his career, including Jakob Erdheim's collection, and willed to Dr. Mankin. He also refers to the Crawford Campbell collection and to his own—all to be included as the "Jaffe-Erdheim-Campbell-Mankin" collection.

Just as Dr. Jaffe was an expert in the orthopaedic diseases and their pathophysiology that he wrote about in his textbook, so too is Dr. Mankin an expert in the pathophysiology of the many orthopaedic diseases he writes about in his book. He has authored publications on many of the diseases included, has for years given a popular AAOS Instructional Course Lecture at the Academy's Annual Meeting in "Metabolic Bone Disease," has been a leader in research on articular cartilage and the biology of allografts, and has lectured all over the world on most topics in this book. As Dr. Springfield stated in the dedication of the fourth edition of the *Orthopaedic Journal* at Harvard Medical School: "He (Dr. Mankin) is the master of the lecture. He makes metabolic bone disease interesting, a feat unparalleled in medical education. Those who hear his lecture on cartilage sit on the edge of their seats to catch each word. His visual effects, often having the audience participate while he demonstrates a point, are all original and help the student of any age understand better." Although the reader will not be able to hear and see Dr. Mankin in action at the podium, this book will "help the student of any age understand better" the pathophysiology of orthopaedic diseases.

Each chapter, with some variation, details the history, incidence, biologic cause, genetic characteristics, clinical features, laboratory diagnosis, imaging findings, histologic features, and management of orthopaedic diseases. Treatment is discussed in the broadest scope, focusing on medical treatments with orthopaedic surgical treatment described in general terms only. The reader will need to seek other sources for details of orthopaedic surgical treatments. After one reads this book, however, it will be obvious why additional volumes by Dr. Mankin will be desired and expected.

James H. Herndon, MD

Preface

At my age, writing a book such as this is heavy labor...but for me it became a labor of love! I enjoyed reading about these diseases, reviewing the literature, learning about the history, and adding pictures of important aspects to improve the readers' understanding of the disorders. It has, in fact, been a joy to produce it and see it published.

I really cannot define why I chose the subjects I did, except perhaps because they have all fascinated me over a lifetime of study and teaching. Some of the diseases are not seen very often anymore but are fascinating, and in many ways, they're really the origin of our specialty. These are the disorders that taught orthopaedic surgeons in ancient days to develop special techniques for diagnosis and treatment and especially to plan new operations to deal with some very complex problems.

The question that arises is why I did it at all...at my age and stage of life. The answer is probably best related to my life in medicine, research, and especially education. I loved treating over 9,000 patients and, even more, caring for them and in many cases restoring them to reasonably good health. I did all I could to be a competent investigator in fields such as cartilage, osteoarthritis, bone grafting, genetic disorders, tumors, etc, and maintained a good laboratory with very good friends for many years. Some of the disorders in this book were included in our research agendas. But education was the greatest joy of my many years in orthopaedics and medicine. I became a teacher to perhaps 600 residents, 100 fellows, and a lot of medical students over these many years. I loved teaching them and, perhaps more important, learning from them. They not only taught me aspects of orthopaedics and orthopaedic science but they taught me how to teach—and that was my greatest joy.

I have many people to thank for inspiring me and helping me create this book. The group at the Academy, especially Marilyn Fox, have been wonderful in helping me to put it together. Sharon O'Brien provided excellent copyediting and good editorial advice. I am really grateful! In my life in research, I wish to include as my partners my research team going back to Antra Zarins, Louis Lippiello, Ben Treadwell, and most recently Christine Towle, Gertrud Fondren, and Carol Trahan, who has been my angel with the Jaffe collection. The list includes my colleagues over the years in orthopaedic medicine; I can literally list hundreds, but have to single out Joseph Milgram, Emanuel Kaplan, Albert Ferguson, Thomas Brower, Richard Smith, Augustus White, Clement Sledge, Mark Gebhardt, Dempsey Springfield, and most recently Francis Hornicek and Kevin Raskin. My true mentor and teacher and inspiration, however, was Henry Jaffe, who started me on the road to science and knowledge but especially on the long happy road of education.

Finally, I must express my greatest appreciation to Carole Mankin, my bride of 53 years who as a librarian helped me with the references, read and corrected each chapter, and most importantly dearly loved and supported me. She not only gave me the greatest life that anyone could ever have, but she also produced and nurtured and inspired three wonderful children and three sweet grandchildren who make both of us very, very proud. They represent our immortality; all of them are teachers and care for their students. Carole and the children are the real patrons of my life and are the stimulus for me to write this book, such as it is, and I dedicate it to them.

Henry J. Mankin, MD

Chapter 1

Henry Jaffe and His Legacy

Henry L. Jaffe, MD (Figure 1) was an extraordinary person who contributed perhaps more than anyone else to our knowledge of musculoskeletal pathology. Born in New York City in 1896, he completed his undergraduate study at New York University and went on to earn his doctorate in medicine there in 1920. He served two internships—one at Bellevue Hospital in surgery and a second at Montefiore Hospital in medicine. Despite these early interests, he became fascinated with pathology and became a student and colleague of David Marine, an illustrious chief of pathology at the Montefiore Hospital during the early part of the 20th century. Based on his remarkable work, in 1922 Dr. Jaffe was appointed assistant pathologist at Montefiore, where he quickly established a reputation for the intensity of his commitment and his extraordinary discoveries. In 1925, Jaffe accepted the position of Chief of Pathology and Director of the Laboratories at the Hospital for Joint Diseases (HJD), an institution devoted to the care of patients with orthopaedic disorders. He held that post for almost four decades until his retirement in 1964, but then stayed on as a consultant, teacher, and writer until he completed his second major volume on bone pathology in 1972.

During his tenure at the HJD, Henry Jaffe taught medical students, residents, and fellows in orthopaedics and pathology—not only at HJD, but also at Columbia Presbyterian Hospital, New York Medical College, and Albert Einstein College of Medicine. His lectures were legendary, and remarkable for the spectacular material he presented without the benefit of today's visual display technologies. He became a renowned consultant in bone, joint, and soft-tissue pathology. Colleagues from all over the world sent him cases, asking for his opinion regarding not only the diagnosis, but also what the patients might expect and how such a disorder may best be treated. Dr. Jaffe included the imaging and pathologic material for all the patients for whom he gave an opinion in what become a vast collection of connective pathology.

Working with a group of associates including Aaron Bodansky, Arthur Ginzler, Sheldon Jacobson, John Blair, Louis Lichtenstein, Thomas Horowitz, and Golden Selin, Jaffe contributed an outstanding body of knowledge to medical science. His areas of interest included endocrine pathology, skeletal development, and bone and soft-tissue diseases. He wrote over 130 original articles in the field of pathology and authored two books, both of which remain major reference sources for information on bone disease. *Tumors and Tumorous Conditions of the Bones and Joints*[1] was published by Lea and Febiger in 1958; a second volume, *Metabolic, Degenerative and Inflammatory Diseases of Bones and Joints*,[2] was published in 1972. Material from both these volumes is still widely quoted today; many authors find the descriptions and illustrations for these diseases unparalleled in current literature.

Jaffe and his associates were responsible for describing an array of clinical entities. His early studies included aspects of the biologic nature of hyperparathyroidism, rickets, and renal osteodystrophy.[3-7] He and Aaron Bodansky defined the role of alkaline phosphatase activity in a number of disorders, including rickets, hyperparathyroidism and Paget's disease.[3,8] In subsequent decades, Jaffe and Louis Lichtenstein collaborated over a 13-year period to describe or clarify the nature of tumorous disorders of bone, including unicameral bone cyst,[9] aneurysmal bone cyst,[10] osteoblastoma,[11] osteoid osteoma,[12,13] giant cell tumor of bone,[14-16] eosinophilic granuloma,[17,18] pigmented villonodular synovitis,[19] chondroblastoma,[20] nonossifying fibroma,[21] fibrous dysplasia,[22] chondromyxoid fibroma,[23] hereditary exostosis,[24] juxtacortical chondroma,[25] chondrosarcoma,[26] osteosarcoma,[27] myeloma,[28] and lymphoma.[29] In addition, Louis Lichtenstein incorporated Henry Jaffe's material into a book published in 1952;[30] this volume expanded on these and other entities, including fibrous dysplasia,

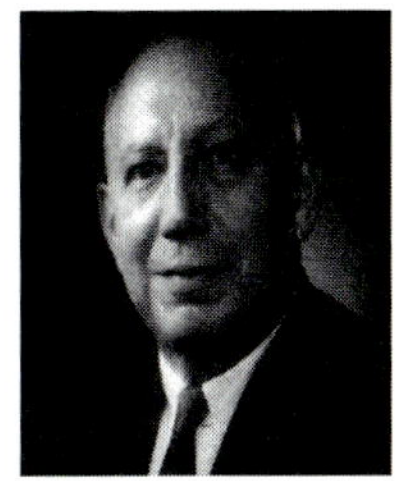

Figure 1
Dr. Henry L. Jaffe—a gifted pathologist, superb educator, and great collector.

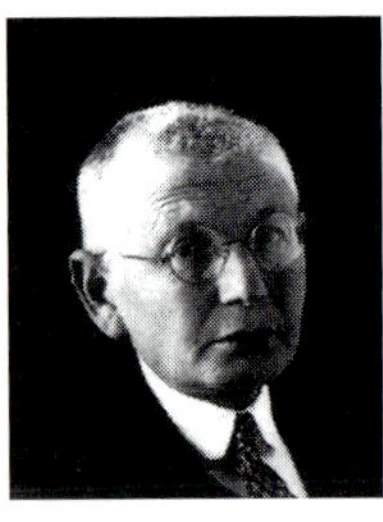

Figure 2
Dr. Jakob Erd-
heim, renowned
Viennese
pathologist.

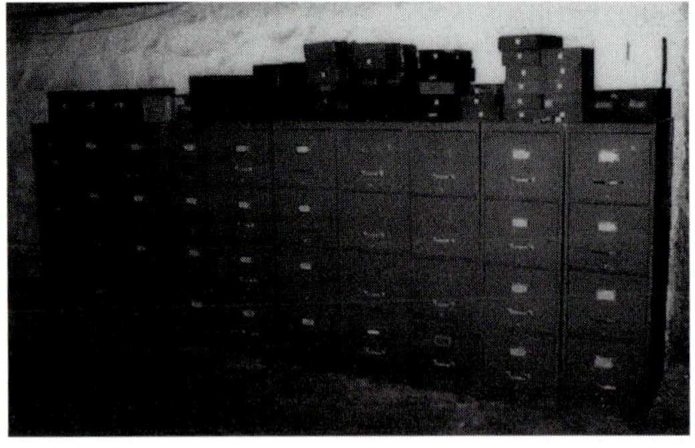

Figure 3
The Jaffe collection in Dr. Mankin's basement.

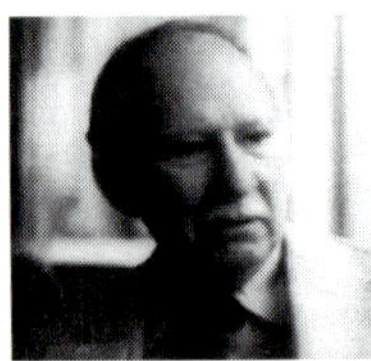

Figure 4
Dr. Crawford
Campbell contrib-
uted hundreds of
radiographic im-
ages of tumors.

histiocytosis, and tumors such as chondrosarcoma, osteosarcoma, Ewing's tumors, and myeloma.

Henry Jaffe's skill and extraordinary commitment to education and patient care did not go unnoticed by his colleagues. In 1953, he became an Honorary Member of the Royal Society of Medicine of England and of the British Orthopaedic Association. In 1957, New York University granted him a Distinguished Service Award; he was named an Honorary Member of the American Orthopaedic Association in 1960 and earned similar status with the American Academy of Orthopaedic Surgeons in 1969. His reputation within the pathology community was equally distinguished. He was elected to and maintained memberships in the College of American Pathologists, the American Society of Experimental Pathologists, the Society of Experimental Biology and Medicine, and the International Academy of Pathology.

Perhaps Dr. Jaffe's most extraordinary contribution, which has lived on after him, is the collection of pathologic material that he acquired throughout his career. The material originally consisted of pathology for patients treated at HJD as well as examinations of tissue obtained at autopsy. However, Dr. Jaffe expanded the collection to include beautifully recorded information from an enormous number of his consultations, cases sent to him from all over the world. Some of this material, particularly that used for his educational efforts, was given to Ralph Marcove. On the basis of his Jaffe collection, Marcove coauthored a book with Myron Arlen in 1992 entitled *Atlas of Bone Pathology with Clinical and Radiographic Correlations*.[31] Another excellent two-volume work that used the Jaffe pathology collec-

tion as a major source was developed by James Milgram in 1990.[32]

Although Henry Jaffe maintained a close association with many pathologists and clinicians during his career, he held Jakob Erdheim (1874-1937) of Vienna (Figure 2) in particularly high regard. Erdheim was a superb clinical pathologist, a world famous educator, and a major collector of pathologic material for patients with bone and soft-tissue disorders. Shortly before he was killed by the Nazis during the Anschluss in Vienna in 1937; he sent his collection of pathologic material to Henry Jaffe. He wrapped all the pathology slides he had collected over many years in a rug and sent them to Jaffe through several trusted individuals. Jaffe revered the Erdheim collection, keeping it separate from his own material but periodically using it for education or pathologic description of disease.

When Jaffe died in 1979, he willed his own collection and the Erdheim collection to me. The material, housed in filing cabinets and slide trays, was originally sent to Newport, Rhode Island, where the Boston Orthopaedic Course was held annually from 1979 to 1993. The material was stored and maintained by Howard Browne, MD, who was the administrator for the course. When the course was moved to Boston in 1993, the collection was sent to Massachusetts General Hospital. The new administrative staff who joined the hospital in 1998 required more space and were planning to send the collection to a storage facility, but the Orthopaedic Oncology Service intervened and had it all delivered to the basement of my home in Brookline, where it currently resides today (Figure 3). Surrounding the Jaffe-Erdheim collection is the Crawford Campbell collection of hundreds of radiographic images of patients with tumors. Crawford (Figure 4) was a dear friend and associate of mine, and also willed his collection to me. In addition, I have a personal collection of thousands of 2 × 2 photographic slides that my colleagues and I have acquired over the past 40 years. These cases are not only in slide trays, but are also registered in a computer file, allowing access to them by patient name, age, or gender; diagnosis; Musculoskeletal Tumor Society stage; anatomic site; or treatment.

The Jaffe collection includes over 3000 cases; each one is in a brown envelope with the patient's name, diagnosis, referring physician, and a Jaffe number, which relates to a series of filing cards contained in boxes. Using the Jaffe system, developed well before everday use of computers, patients can be easily located by name, diagnosis, or Jaffe number. The file cards are also used for the Erdheim collection, and a similar system exists for the Crawford Campbell collection; accordingly, large amounts of pathologic material can be accessed with relative ease. Each brown envelope contains the imaging studies, usually in the form of radiographs but occasionally specimen photographs, and hematoxylin- and eosin-stained slides of different relative magnification ranging from $10\times$ to $400\times$. In addition, many of the cases include typed pathology reports and letters to the referring physicians, all signed by Dr. Jaffe. Documents are also available for many of the Erdheim materials, but these are written in German.

Jaffe included material on a number of metabolic bone disorders, including hyperparathyroidism, rickets, renal osteodystrophy, and osteoporosis. He also had a collection of material on infectious diseases such as syphilis, tuberculosis, and osteomyelitis. His collections of cases of eosinophilic granuloma, Paget's disease, fibrous dysplasia, Gaucher disease, neurofibromatosis, and mucopolysaccharidoses are extraordinary. He also included large numbers of patients with various forms of arthritis, including both rheumatoid and osteoarthritis, and uncommon lesions such as those associated with sarcoidosis or Reiter's syndrome. Fracture healing and osteonecrosis are also included in his material. The tumor cases comprise much of his material, as well as Erdheim's and Campbell's. All forms of benign tumors—eg, giant cell tumor, enchondroma, osteocartilaginous exostosis, chondroblastoma, chondromyxoid fibroma, nonossifying fibroma, osteoid osteoma, osteoblastoma, and unicameral and aneurysmal bone cysts—are included. Malignant bone and soft tissues make up another large component of the collections. There are many central and parosteal osteosarcomas, chondrosarcomas, Ewing's sarcomas, adamantinomas, myelomas, chordomas, lymphomas, fibrosarcomas, liposarcomas, and neurofibrosarcomas, as well as metastatic carcinomas. Although some of the material was obtained as biopsies or surgical specimens, a sizeable amount of Jaffe and Erdheim material appears to be from very extensive autopsies. The spinal tissue obtained in this manner is particularly illustrative of many disorders, especially metabolic diseases, myeloma, tuberculosis, and metastatic carcinoma.

Just what is the value of the Jaffe-Erdheim-Campbell-Mankin collection? In this modern day of genetic diagnostic tools and sophisticated systems for biologic measurement of cytokines, antibodies, reactive agents, and abnormal tissue structures, the material in the collections may seem to be arcane. The collections are of value for study and diagnosis of entities that are diagnosed by visual observation of pathologic material or imaging studies. The material on hyperparathyroidism does not define the nature of the genetic abnormalities that may be present. Those specimens in the collections that describe diseases such as osteopetrosis, osteogenesis imperfecta, vitamin D-resistant rickets, mucopolysaccharidoses, and Gaucher disease do not provide any indication of the genetic errors, the abnormal elements present in the tissues, or for that matter current approaches to treatment.

The true beauty of the system is the opportunity to learn about the nature, appearance, and clinical behavior of an array of orthopaedic diseases and abnormalities. This knowledge should stimulate comparable review and investigation of disease characteristics and diagnostic features of more recently evolved diseases.

The Jaffe collection is a spectacular addition to our base of knowledge and our capacity to teach and to learn.

References

1. Jaffe HL: *Tumors and Tumorous Conditions of the Bones and Joints*. Philadelphia, PA, Lea and Febiger, 1958.
2. Jaffe HL: *Metabolic, Degenerative and Inflammatory Diseases of Bones and Joints*. Philadelphia, PA, Lea and Febiger, 1972.
3. Jaffe HL, Bodansky A, Blair JE: The sites of decalcification and of bone lesions in experimental hyperparathyroidism. *Arch Pathol* 1931;12:715-728.
4. Jaffe HL, Bodansky A, Blair JE: Fibrous osteodystrophy (osteitis fibrosa) in experimental hyperpar-

athyroidism of guinea pigs. *Arch Pathol* 1931;12:207-228.

5. Jaffe HL: Hyperparathyroidism (Recklinghausen's disease of bone). *Arch Pathol* 1933;16:63-112.

6. Jaffe HL: Hyperparathyroidism and its relationship to diseases of bone. *Bull N Y Acad Med* 1934;10:539-552.

7. Jaffe HL: Hyperparathyroidism. *Bull N Y Acad Med* 1940;16:291-311.

8. Bodansky A, Jaffe HL: Phosphatase studies: III. Serum phosphatase in diseases of bone. *Arch Intern Med* 1934;54:88-110.

9. Jaffe HL, Lichtenstein L: Solitary unicameral bone cyst with emphasis on the roentgen picture, the pathologic picture and the pathogenesis. *Arch Surg* 1945;46:1004-1025.

10. Jaffe HL: Aneurysmal bone cyst. *Bull Hosp Joint Dis* 1950;11:3-13.

11. Jaffe HL: Benign osteoblastoma. *Bull Hosp Joint Dis* 1956;17:141-151.

12. Jaffe HL: Osteoid osteoma. *Arch Surg* 1935;31:709-728.

13. Jaffe HL, Lichtenstein L: Osteoid osteoma. *J Bone Joint Surg* 1940;22:645-682.

14. Jaffe HL, Lichtenstein L, Portis RB: Giant cell tumor of bone: Its pathologic appearance, grading, supposed variants and treatment. *Arch Pathol* 1940;30:933-1031.

15. Jaffe HL: Giant cell tumor of bone: Problems of differential diagnosis. *Bull Hosp Joint Dis* 1944;5:84-95.

16. Jaffe HL: Giant-cell tumour (osteoclastoma) of bone: Its pathologic delimitation and the inherent clinical implications. *Ann R Coll Surg Engl* 1953;13:343-355.

17. Lichtenstein L, Jaffe HL: Eosinophilic granuloma of bone—with report of a case. *Am J Pathol* 1940;16:595-604.

18. Jaffe HL, Lichtenstein L: Eosinophilic granuloma of bone: A condition affecting one, several or many bones, but apparently limited to the skeleton, and representing the mildest clinical expression of the peculiar inflammatory histiocytosis also underlying Letterer Siwe disease and Schüller Christian disease. *Arch Pathol* 1944;37:99-118.

19. Jaffe HL, Selin G: Tumors of bones and joints. *Bull N Y Acad Med* 1951;27:165-174.

20. Jaffe HL, Lichtenstein L: Benign chondroblastoma of bone: A re-interpretation of the so-called calcifying or chondromatous giant cell tumor. *Am J Pathol* 1942;18:969-991.

21. Jaffe HL, Lichtenstein L: Non-osteogenic fibroma of bone. *Am J Pathol* 1942;18:205-221.

22. Lichtenstein L, Jaffe HL: Fibrous dysplasia of bone. *Arch Pathol* 1942;33:777-816.

23. Jaffe HL, Lichtenstein L: Chondromyxoid tumor of bone: A distinctive benign tumor likely to be mistaken especially for chondrosarcoma. *Arch Pathol* 1948;45:541-551.

24. Jaffe HL: Hereditary multiple exostosis. *Arch Pathol* 1943;36:335-357.

25. Jaffe HL: Juxtacortical chondroma. *Bull Hosp Joint Dis* 1956;17:20-29.

26. Lichtenstein L, Jaffe HL: Chondrosarcoma of bone. *Am J Pathol* 1943;19:552-589.

27. Jaffe HL: Osteogenic sarcoma of bone. *Clin Orthop Relat Res* 1956;38:27-40.

28. Lichtenstein L, Jaffe HL: Multiple myeloma. *Arch Pathol* 1947;44:207-246.

29. Jaffe HL: Skeletal manifestations of leukemia and malignant lymphoma. *Bull Hosp Joint Dis* 1952;13:217-238.

30. Lichtenstein L: *Bone Tumors*. St Louis, MO, CV Mosby, 1952.

31. Marcove RC, Arlen M: *Atlas of Bone Pathology with Clinical and Radiographic Correlations*. Philadelphia, PA, JB Lippincott, 1992.

32. Milgram JW: *Radiologic and Histologic Pathology of Nontumorous Diseases of Bones and Joints*. Northbrook, IL, Northbrook Publishing Company, Inc, 1990.

Chapter 2

Tuberculosis of Bones and Joints

How nice it would be if there were no longer a compelling reason to write this chapter or to even comment historically about one of mankind's oldest and most deadly scourges, tuberculosis. If this chapter had been introduced 30 years ago, it would have been regarded purely as an historical treatise. Today, however, tuberculosis has not only returned, but in some cases in a very distressingly resistant form that suggests that the "white plague" is upon us again and the "red king" has returned. More people now have tuberculosis than any other disease; it remains the world's leading cause of infectious disease.[1] An estimated eight million new cases of tuberculosis occur annually, and as many as two million people will die of the disease each year.[1,2] The disease is one of urban societies—in those cities where human immunodeficiency virus (HIV) is prominent, the disease is now being diagnosed with great frequency.[1-4] Because the world now has a large population of immunologically incompetent individuals, an actively infected person can rapidly transmit the disease with a single cough to a large number of passengers on an airplane or to those in a crowded theater or church.[5] Furthermore, the organism is no longer as easily treated with drugs that were once effective in eliminating the disease and saving patient lives. Some strains of the mycobacterium have now developed resistance to isonicotinic hydrazide, streptomycin, pyrazinamide, rifampin, and the other agents that in the past were quite effective—not always in curing patients, but certainly reducing their capacity to infect others.[2] Although the purpose of this chapter is to review the history and the biologic, clinical, and treatment systems for the disease, the chapter is also intended to serve as a warning that we are now dealing with an increasing problem in disease control and management.

History of the Red King

Tuberculosis is the oldest recognized disease of humans. Egyptian mummies bear evidence of infections with *Mycobacterium tuberculosis*,[6,7] called by some the red king based on the red color of the organism on Ziehl-Nielsen staining.[8-10] The disease was found in the remains of prehistoric humans in Italy,[11] ancient pre-Columbian Iroquois Indians,[12] and in many other archeological sites.[13] The disease was recognized in biblical times, as Deuteronomy 28:22 reads "The Lord shall smite thee with a consumption and with a fever and with an inflammation and they shall pursue thee until they perish." The ancient terms for the disease—phthisis, consumption, white death, or white plague (to distinguish it from the bubonic "black" plague)—correctly implied that, without treatment, the disorder consumed the patient, was easily transmissible and had a high death rate.[2]

In view of the easy transmissibility of the disease by coughing, it is quite remarkable that people in urban communities survived at all, but amazingly they did. The survivors appeared to have an inherent immunity, possibly on a genetic basis, which they transmitted to their children. Accordingly, the frequency of tuberculous disease varies among populations based on their duration of urbanization. Nevertheless, vast numbers of patients contracted the disease, suffered with it (in many cases for years), and died.[2,7,14-16] Sir William Osler remarked "Everyone in the end has a touch of tuberculosis," and Alexandre Dumas said "It was the fashion to suffer from chest complaints. Everybody was consumptive, poets especially—it was good form to spit blood after each emotion and to die before reaching the age of thirty." The disease did not respect wealth, or literary or musical accomplishment. Many famous people died of the disease (Table 1); some, like John Keats and

Table 1	Sampling of Famous People Who Died of Tuberculosis	
Hopalong Cassidy	Anton Chekov
Cardinal Richelieu	Anne Brontë
Thomas Wolfe	Vivien Leigh
Bela Bartok	Frederic Chopin
George Orwell	John Keats
Friedrich von Schiller	Sir Walter Scott
Charlotte Brontë	Nicola Paganini
Robert Louis Stevenson	Christy Mathewson
Eugene O'Neill	Henry David Thoreau
John Harvard	Earnest Dawson
Edgar Allen Poe	Emily Brontë
Branwell Brontë	Franz Kafka
Eleanor Roosevelt	Percy Bysshe Shelley
D.H. Lawrence	Aubrey Beardsley

Aubrey Beardsley, succumbed as early as 25 years of age.

There was no recognized treatment in the early days. George Bodington, a British physician, noted that people in rural areas had a lower incidence of tuberculosis than those in cities and recommended open air treatment in an isolated environment.[2] This was the beginning of the sanatorium concept—the only way to treat tuberculosis was proposed to be isolation, sunlight, fresh mountain air, and bed rest. As a result, hundreds of sanatoria were established all over the world; the most famous was in Davos, Switzerland. Edward Livingstone Trudeau, who had the disease but survived, established a city filled with sanatoria near Saranac Lake in upstate New York where such greats as the poet Adelaide Crapsey, the baseball pitcher Christy Mathewson, the composer Bela Bartok, and the poet and author Robert Louis Stevenson were treated.[17] Sanatoria sprang up in many major cities and mountain sites—Firland in Seattle; Royal Hospital in Stanmore, England; Sea View on Long Island; Bellevue and Blackwell's Island in New York City; Provincetown in Massachusetts; Oakwood in Chicago; Jewish Hospital in Denver; Leech Farm in Pittsburgh, and many more.[2,16] Some of these are now hotels or hospitals, but can still be distinguished by the large porches that were an essential part of the treatment. People suffering with the disease spent months and sometimes years lying on the porches in the sun, hoping that the disease would become sufficiently modified to prevent death from pulmonary bleeding (John Keats and the Brontë family), secondary miliary disease (Eleanor Roosevelt), brain involvement (Thomas Wolfe), or just wasting away (Vivian Leigh and many others). The art and literature communities recognized the disease as well. Charlotte Brontë wrote *Wuthering Heights* in 1847 to commemorate the loss of her brother Branwell to tuberculosis;[18] she died of the same disease in 1858. In Charles Dickens' *David Copperfield* (1849), Little Blossom died gracefully of tuberculosis.[19] Verdi's opera "La Traviata" (1853) was a tribute to Alphonsine Plessis, who died of the disease. Mimi, the heroine of Puccini's "La Boheme" (1896), also succumbed to tuberculosis. In the preface to his book of poems, *Underwoods* (1887), Robert Louis Stevenson[20] thanked his physicians for the care of his diseased lungs—yet he still died of the disease 7 years later. Edgar Allen Poe wrote his beautiful and heart-rending poem "Annabel Lee" to commemorate the death of his beloved wife Virginia from tuberculosis. He wrote "That was the reason (as all men know in this kingdom by the sea) that the wind came out of the cloud, chilling and killing my Annabel Lee." Shortly after the poem was published in 1849, Poe himself died of the disease. Perhaps the two most famous literary contributions about tuberculosis, however, were *The Magic Mountain* by Thomas Mann,[21] whose wife was a patient at Davos for many years, and George Bernard Shaw's play "The Doctor's Dilemma,"[22] in which the central figure dies of tuberculosis on stage in the last act.

The disease not only was present universally, but had a language all its own that included such terms as miasma, night sweats, primary complex, Ghon tubercle, consumptive cough, cold abscess, scrofula, spina ventosa, tuberculoma, tuberculous meningitis, kissing sequestrae, Pott's disease, and Pott's paraplegia.[2,14,23,24]

A monumental discovery was made in 1908, when Robert Koch microscopically identified the tubercle bacillus and related it to the pulmonary and peripheral disease of patients.[25] The organism was difficult to identify with standard stains, but was bright red using the Ziehl-Nielsen staining technique—hence the name the red king.[2,8,9,16] Although this finding allowed scientists to

---

Primary Disease

Pulmonary inhalation of bacteria→Ghon tubercle + mediastinal node→**Stable disease**
(tuberculin-positive primary complex)

Disseminated primary→widespread miliary disease→ death?

Reinfection or Secondary Tuberculosis   **Unstable disease**

Mild to moderate pulmonary disease; renal, pleuritic or other lesions; or bone and joint disease (especially spine). In the face of lowered immune competence, may go on to miliary disease and death.

Figure 1
Natural history of tuberculosis.

---

try to develop treatment protocols to kill the bacteria and such agents as Prontosil were introduced, none were very effective against the mycobacterium.[2,26] In 1943, Selman Waksman, an emigrant from the Ukraine with a PhD in soil biology, and his coworkers Oswald Avery and Albert Schatz[2,26-28] discovered that a material obtained from a fungus, *Streptomyces griseus*, could kill the mycobacterium. This milestone changed the world for tuberculosis patients; in fact, the discoverers of the drug now known as streptomycin were awarded a Nobel Prize in 1952. With the subsequent introduction of isonicotinic hydrazide, para-aminosalicylic acid, rifampin, ethambutol, pyrazinamide, and other drugs,[28-30] patients could now be treated effectively, becoming less likely to die or infect others. The result was the relative disappearance of the virulent and infectious forms of pulmonary disease in the cities of the civilized world. Sanatoria either closed or became general hospitals, psychiatric institutions, or hotels.[17] Far less material appeared in the world literature and tuberculosis seemed, like other scourges such as smallpox and poliomyelitis, to be eliminated as a threat to mankind.[2,14,15,28,30]

Unfortunately, the advent of HIV infection and other immune deficiency states resulted in a sharp increase in the rate of tuberculosis infections in major cities.[2-5,15,31-39] In addition, the red king developed its own modification of gene structure so that in some cases, it no longer responded to the drugs that had so beautifully controlled it in the past.[3,15,39,40] Physicians and managed care organizations have to take part of the blame for this, because they reduced the length of time of administration (thus the cost) of the drugs that controlled the disease, thus allowing the organism to develop some forms of immunity.[31,33]

Natural History of Tuberculosis

The events that occur with tuberculous infections are shown in Figure 1. Some patients, especially children, develop tuberculosis as a result of gastrointestinal infection (based in part on infection with the less common avian and bovine forms of mycobacteria).[8,41] Occasionally, one encounters pleurisy, cutaneous lesions, peritonitis, cerebral lesions, cervical-nodal disease (scrofula), or uveitis as the presenting findings for tuberculosis.[2,14,42,43] The pulmonary infection caused by inhalation of the bacteria, however, remains the most common form of the disease.[10,43] The mycobacteria, which are transmitted from infected sputum during coughing, enter the lung and produce an infectious nodular granulomatous process that enlarges as the bacteria reproduce and also spread via lymphatics to the mediastinal lymph nodes.[3,8,9] The localized infectious area, which is visible on radiographic imaging, is called the Ghon tubercle; the tubercle together with the infected sentinal mediastinal nodes are known as the primary com-

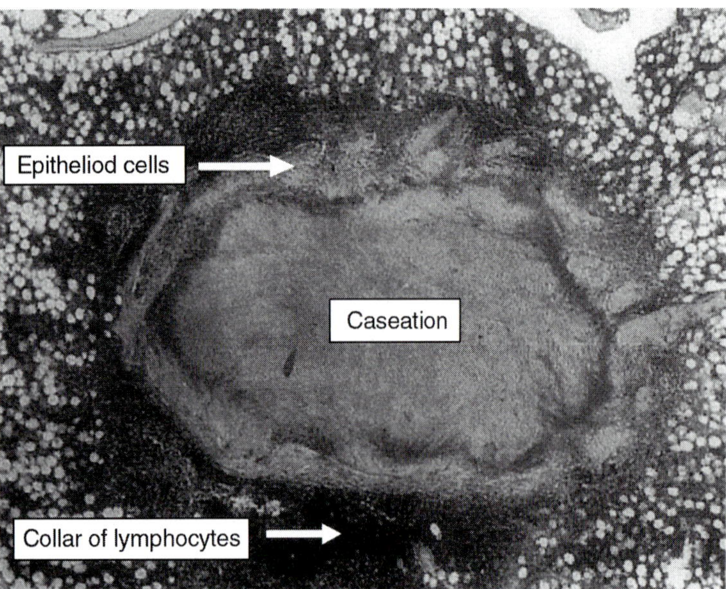

Figure 2

Histologic image of a tuberculous granuloma, showing is central caseation, a surrounding zone of epitheliod cells, and then a collar of lymphocytes. Hematoxylin and eosin × 20.

plex.[2,8,9,14,24] For most patients with competent immune systems, the disease is controlled by the macrophagic cells of the reticuloendothelial system and becomes dormant and less infectious.[33] At this point, and in many cases as a badge of successful control of the disease, the patient becomes tuberculin skin-test positive, a condition that persists in most healthy individuals for the rest of their lives.[8,14,33,44,45] The tuberculin positivity represents an immune response to the disease and is likely a characteristic of controlled disease. Tuberculin positivity may be modified by diffuse illness, sarcoidosis, and most recently by alteration in the immune system such as that occurring with HIV infection.[9,38,46-48] Some patients whose immune systems fail to protect them develop "disseminated primary disease," often with miliary spread to pleura, peritoneum, bones, and brain; this can result in rapid death.[2,4,30,39] Most of these patients are impaired by chronic illness that affects the immune response.

The second form of infection is known as reinfection, or secondary tuberculosis. Tuberculin-positive patients who are partially immunized against the disease may develop reinfection tuberculosis, which is milder than disseminated primary (far fewer acute disasters) but may affect many organ systems.[2,3,9,14,24,49] The principal location of the disease is still the lung and as a result of the progress to secondary state, the patients develop consumptive pulmonary disease with multiple granulomatous deposits in the lung, more often apical in location.[2,50] Although kidney disease or even brain lesions may develop, the joints and the bones are more frequent sites for secondary disease.[24] Patients who have secondary tuberculosis with lung lesions become fatigued, febrile, and chronically ill (miasma). They lose weight, become pale, have night sweats, and develop a productive cough often with hemoptysis (consumption).[2] These individuals represent the leading source of transmittal of the disease. They are not always sick enough to seek care or be hospitalized, yet their productive cough, which contains the mycobacteria, is dangerously contagious. A large percentage of these patients would once have been isolated in sanatoria and after several years restored to reasonably good health and allowed to return to a productive life.[17] Unfortunately, even with the sanatorium treatment, if these patients' immune systems of control diminished, they frequently developed miliary disease and died.[2,17,24] More recently, with the aid of drugs such as isoniazide, rifampin, streptomycin, and pyrazinamide, some patients were able to rapidly feel well and renew their lives.[2,14,31,51] Even with such restoration, however, many of the patients retained stigmata of the disease and a psychological depression created by the prolonged period of chronic illness.[2]

Histology

The histology of the mycobacterial focus in the lung or other sites is characterized by the presence of a highly specific structure called a tuberculous granuloma, often multiple in number and occupying a large part of the tissue structure (Figure 2).[9,10,14,25,38,52] The central portion of the single granuloma often shows necrotic tissue, which does not accept a stain and is "cheese-like" in appearance, hence the use of the descriptive terms "caseation" or "caseous necrosis."[9,24] Surrounding this region is a string of large altered monocytes, which have an epithelial appearance and are called epitheliod cells. These cells and the caseation site are the places where the bacteria may be identified,

8

usually by the Ziehl-Nielsen stain.[9] Surrounding the caseous and epitheliod components of the granuloma is an irregular collar of lymphocytes that are in turn surrounded by a collection of fibrocytes known as the fibrous capsule. The fibrous capsule separates the granuloma from adjacent such lesions, and in most cases many such structures are closely arranged. One of the most distinctive features of the tuberculoma is the frequent presence of a highly characteristic large multinucleate giant cell with centrifugal distribution of the nuclei. This cell is known as the Langhans giant cell; although some other disorders have similar cells, the giant cell is highly characteristic and almost diagnostic for tuberculosis[9,24] (Figure 3).

Tuberculous granulomas have the capacity to increase in number and, based on the fibrous capsules, produce scarring in lung fields and other organs. The organisms and the granulomatous tissues also can invade tissue such as bone, kidney, liver, or bowel and produce an inflammatory response. Of particular interest is the remarkable feature that, although the granulomas may arise in synovial tissues of the joints and produce extensive masses there, they have very limited capacity to invade or destroy articular cartilage.[23]

Bone and Joint Tuberculosis

Prior to the development and use of antibiotic agents, tuberculosis of bone was common and quite disabling. Today, bone disease that does not involve an adjacent joint is rare in the United States but still exists in many other countries. In the US and Canada, bone tuberculosis can still be seen among Indian and Eskimo populations.[10,23,38,40,42,50,53-55] Other types of mycobacterium may affect the lungs but more often affect the soft tissues and especially the bone. These include *Mycobacterium kansasii, M avium, M fortuitum,* and *M marinum;* many of these occur in patients with chronic illness, especially diabetes mellitus.[10,41,44]

The tuberculous tumors of bone and joint include:

- *Tuberculoma of bone.* An enlargement of the bone, often in midshaft, usually with some cortical destruction and occasionally a soft-tissue mass.[9,14,24,38,40,42,44,50] The bone is weak and subject to fracture.[24]

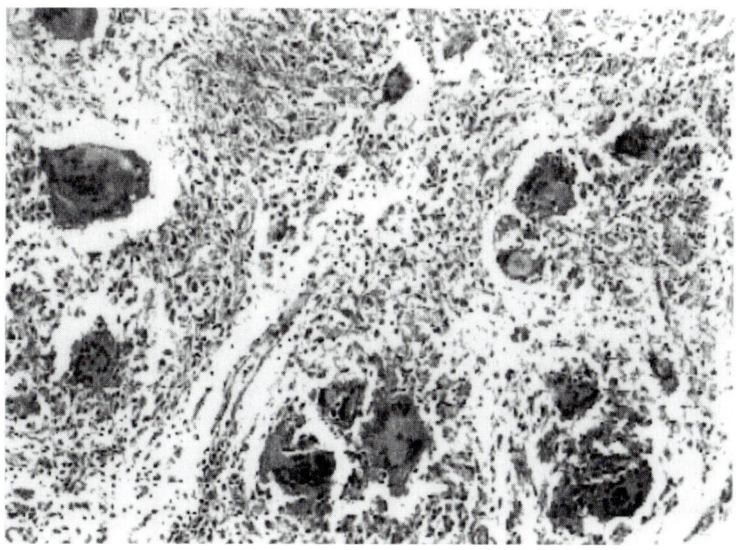

Figure 3

Langhans giant cells are characteristic for tuberculosis but may be confused with giant cell lesions seen in other disorders. Hematoxylin and eosin × 40.

- *Tuberculous osteomyelitis.* A destructive lesion of bone, whether in the peripheral skeleton or in the spine, that may produce a soft-tissue mass; this mass, particularly in the spine, is known as a cold abscess.[9,17,24,38,52,54,56] These infection sites are less destructive and even far less productive than standard bacterial osteomyelitis, producing some osteopenia in the adjacent bony segments.[9,24]
- *Spina ventosa.* A destructive and productive change in the shaft of a metacarpal or phalanx, which causes considerable pain and local soft-tissue swelling.[10,24,50,57,58]
- *Pott's disease.* Tuberculosis of the spine accounts for 50% of all cases of bone tuberculosis. Changes are slow to appear on imaging, and patients may not show destructive lesions for 6 to 8 months after the onset of back pain.[16,24,59,60] A destructive lesion that usually occurs starts in the anterior portion of a vertebra and then involves an adjacent segment, often in the lower thoracic and adjacent upper lumbar region.[9,24,59,60] Fairly profound osteopenia may be the earliest sign, along with progressive narrowing of the disk space and subsequent increasing kyphosis and scoliosis[24,38,56] (Figure 4). A soft-tissue abscess is frequently

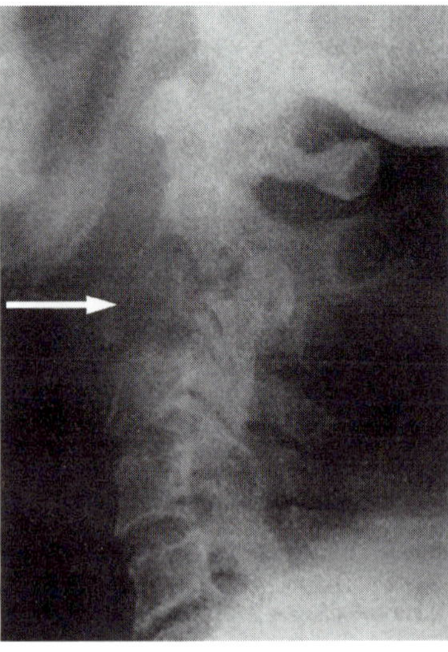
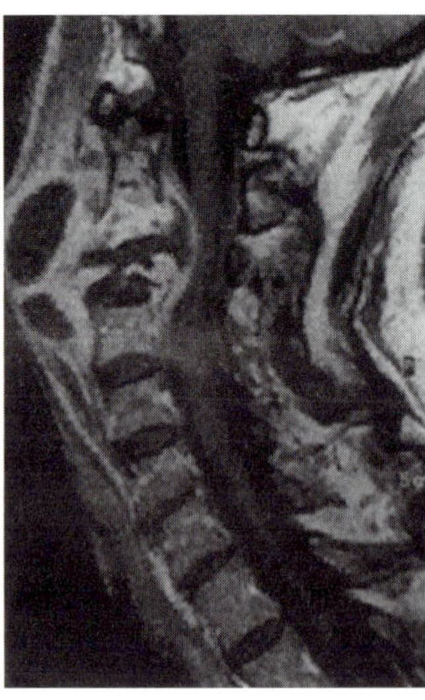

Figure 4
Imaging study of tuberculosis of the spine (Pott's disease). Note the destructive changes in the two adjacent vertebral segments and the extension into the canal, which for this patient resulted in a slow progressive quadriplegia.

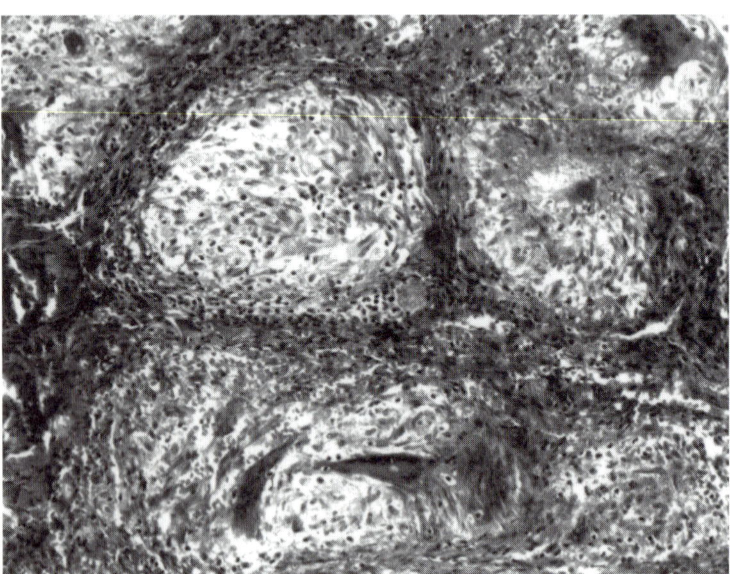

Figure 5
Histologic appearance of tuberculous granulomas occurring in the synovium of an infected joint. Hematoxylin and eosin × 30.

present; this may track along and down the iliopsoas muscle to present as a cold abscess below the inguinal ligament.[9,24,61] These abscesses may also extend along the iliac brim to present as large soft-tissue masses near the anterior-superior iliac spine or directly through the back in the paravertebral musculature. Pott's paraplegia is an effect of the abscess formation in the vertebral canal pressing on the dura.[62] Because tuberculous infection and inflammatory change usually cannot transgress the dural sleeve, the paraplegia represents the collection of a cold abscess, which presses on the dura externally but does not directly affect the spinal cord.[9,24,63] Thus patients who have had pressure on the canal for long periods may recover after treatment with antituberculous medication and especially surgical procedures, which relieve the pressure.[64]

- *Tuberculosis of joints.* The most common orthopaedic presentation of the disease in the US, tuberculosis of joints occurs most frequently in the hip or knee but can occur in any synovial-lined articulation.[1,24,49,61,65-67] The entity begins with a synovial focus of disease that usually shows all the histologic features of the disorder, including caseation, epitheliod cells, lymphocytes, fibrosis, and Langhans giant cells[9,53] (Figure 5). The disease progresses rapidly in many cases and the entire synovium becomes involved, causing significant swelling of the joint without increased warmth. One of the most striking features at this point is a marked juxta-articular osteopenia, which resembles the changes seen in rheumatoid arthritis but is markedly different from the bony sclerosis seen in osteoarthritis.[8,50,68] (Figure 6). As noted above, articular cartilage ordinarily resists the granulomatous invasion but the bone does not; the result is juxta-articular osseous destruction. The abscesses break through the juxta-articular cortices, eventually (on the basis of impaction-type fractures) breaking through the cartilage from the bony side to produce a "tuberculous sequestrum," which is easily distinguished from an osteomyelitic sequestrum by the severe osteopenia that is present in the tuberculous bone.[14,24,53,69] Frequently the sequestrae are located on both sides of the joint and come in contact with complete fracture; they are then known as "kissing sequestrae," a unique finding in tuberculosis of joints.[24] Eventually the joint collapses and the cartilaginous surface is destroyed.[9,24] Hip disease

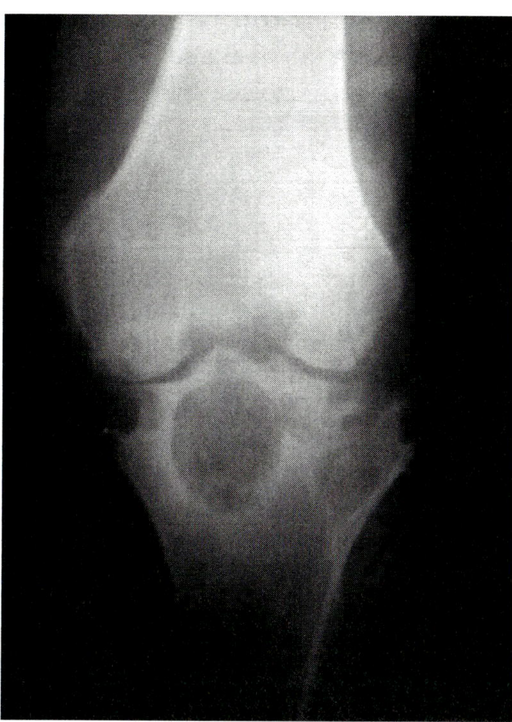

Figure 6

Radiograph of the knee joint of a patient with chronic tuberculosis. The narrowing and the destructive lesions at the joint margins are evident in addition to a cyst-like lesion in the tibial bone adjacent to the joint.

may be associated with cold abscesses; in some cases the disorder is more prominent around the trochanter, with only minimal changes in the hip.[65,66,70] Tuberculosis of the knee is more common than hip disease and is often quite destructive.[9,24,38,61,71,72] It appears to be more prevalent in children than in adults, and is slightly more common initially on the medial side. The patients show enlarged joints, often limited in motion and later severely painful.[1,24,66] If untreated, the abscess may erode through the skin and form a tuberculous ulceration. Lesions of the foot are also difficult to diagnose, chiefly because the entire foot may show swelling and tenderness even when the site of the infection is in the tibiotalar or talonavicular joints.[9,24,50,58,73-75] *M marinum* may penetrate the skin as a result of a laceration caused by the spine of the spiny sea urchin; this will show histologic characteristics of standard tuberculosis in most cases but will not create tubercu-

lin positivity in most cases.[10] Elbows and shoulders are less commonly involved, but the lesion can be very destructive. Tuberculous lesions of the digits in the hand and feet are usually osseous rather than arthritic in origin.[9,50,57,73] The only site in which tuberculous joint disease usually shows an increased density on imaging is the sacroiliac joint.[63]

Diagnosis of Tuberculosis

The most important aspect in diagnosis of tuberculous disease today is for the physician to even consider the disease, and to be aware of its possible presence as a cause of unusual symptoms.[15,36,48] Tuberculosis had become a rarely encountered disease until recently. However, it is becoming much more common today, particularly in large urban communities or disadvantaged countries.[1-3,14,15,32,34,36,37,40,42-44] Physicians should be suspicious of patients with a chronic cough, night sweats, easy fatigability, spine or joint pain, and a low-grade fever.[1,31,48,50,53,69] Chest radiographs may reveal a tuberculous infiltrate,[50] and a tuberculin skin test may be helpful. Once the purified protein-derivative tuberculin test or even the old tuberculin test become positive, they usually remain so for the life of the patient unless the patient has a reduced immune response, HIV infection, or sarcoidosis.[2] Highly accurate serologic tests are available to detect mycobacterium infection in patients with reduced immune response; these may be of considerable value in establishing the diagnosis.[1,3,46-48,76,77] They include specific antigen detection by enzyme-linked immunosorbent assay tests, analysis of DNA sequence by probes and polymerase chain reaction, and demonstration of tuberculostearic acid by chromatography and mass spectrometry.[2,46-48,76,77]

Imaging studies can be very helpful in diagnosis. Although plain radiography is useful in showing joint destruction, computed tomography (CT) may reveal more joint damage and also show the small islands of bone destruction that occur with tuberculous sequestrae.[50,53,54,57,68,69,75,78] Calcification my also be present in cold abscesses and are visualized best with CT. The chest CT is very helpful in showing pulmonary involvement (particularly the Ghon tubercle and the primary complex), which is usually present for the life of the patient. New pulmonary disease associated with secondary tuberculosis is seen best in the apices. Magnetic resonance imaging is quite valuable, particularly for diagnosing patients with Pott's disease and Pott's paraplegia, and is frequently helpful in assessing the degree of structural loss in joints.[57,60,79]

Treatment of Tuberculosis

The antimicrobial treatment of the disorder, clearly best handled by someone interested and experienced in infectious disease, currently includes an array of antituberculous medication that usually should be continued for a year (often more) to ensure that the disease is under control.[2,8,10,14,28,31] Some of the problems over the past several years have been related to premature withdrawal of medication. This has allowed the organisms to stay alive and develop resistance to the various agents that, had medication been continued, would have cured the disease. Multiple agents are available for the treatment of tuberculosis.[29,31,38,51] Isoniazid is currently the best choice of the single agents but has some side effects of peripheral neuritis, which may be relatively easily controlled by administration of vitamin B6. Rifampin is another good choice with minimal side effects. Streptomycin continues to be an effective agent that can cure the patient with limited side effects; however, renal disease may occur. Pyrazinamide is an excellent antituberculous drug but carries a high risk of hepatitis. Ethambutol may also be used. The addition of some second-line drugs may be necessary in treating resistant strains of tuberculous organism; these drugs include para-aminosalicylic acid, ethionamide, cycloserine, capreomycin, kanamycin, amikacin, thiacetazone, and rifabutin.

Surgical treatment of the chest lesions has dominated the history of this disease and includes such procedures as artificial pneumothorax, which was helpful in dealing with life-threatening hemoptysis, and thoracoplasty to gain control over apical active tuberculosis.[15] Spinal disease was al-

ways a problem and remains so today. Opening up the canal and draining the abscesses is a valuable treatment for patients with Pott's paraplegia, and most recently adding bone graft to fuse the spine and correct deformity has been shown to be very helpful.[24,56,59,60,62-64,79] Evacuation of cold abscesses is sometimes useful.[24,72] Surgery for bone disease is useful in preventing or treating fractures, and polymethylmethacrylate can be introduced into destructive sites to prevent collapse. Surgery for joint disease is clearly feasible; arthroscopic washout of knees and total joint replacements are sensible and reasonable, but should be postponed until the antituberculous drugs have had a chance to take effect on the disease.[38,52,65,66,70-74] Physicians have always been at high risk in their exposure to patients with active tuberculosis, thus all precautions should be taken (including masks, gloves, and isolation protocol).[3,5,36,37,40,44]

Summary and Conclusions

There is no doubt that medicine has made enormous strides in the management of patients with tuberculosis since the early days of high infection and incidence of death. The white plague is no longer a major factor in the health of the majority of individuals in North America and much of Europe. Sadly, other parts of the world continue to experience high rates of disease and an alarming death rate; recent reports from South America, Africa, Russia, India, and even Japan are frightening. The susceptibility of patients with AIDS to tuberculous infection represents a serious threat in major cities in the US, and the development of resistant strains of mycobacteria is terrifying. Vaccine development and immunotherapy are currently under study in a number of centers. One of the most promising approaches being investigated is infection of the tubercle bacillus with plasmids that may render it less virulent or more susceptible to certain drugs. Nevertheless, despite our attempts to wipe out mankind's ancient enemy, the red king still lives and continues to thrive despite our best efforts.

References

1. Babhulkar S: Editorial comment. *Clin Orthop Relat Res* 2002;398:2-3.
2. Ryan F: *The Forgotten Plague: How the Battle Against Tuberculosis was Won—and Lost*. Boston, MA, Little Brown and Company, 1992.
3. Hall S: The return of tuberculosis in a new more

menacing form, in *The Race Against Lethal Microbes*. Chevy Chase, MD, The Howard Hughes Institute, 2000, pp 6-21.

4. Zumla A, Malon P, Henderson J, Grange JM: Impact of HIV infection on tuberculosis. *Postgrad Med J* 2000;76:259-268.

5. Mensen ME: Risk of infection with Mycobacterium tuberculosis in travelers to areas of high tuberculosis epidemicity. *Lancet* 2000;356:461-465.

6. Cave AJE: The evidence for the incidence of tuberculosis in ancient Egypt. *Br J Tuberc Dis Chest* 1939;33:142-152.

7. Zimmerman MR: Pulmonary and osseous tuberculosis in an Egyptian mummy. *Bull N Y Acad Med* 1979;55:604-608.

8. Barnes DS: Historical perspectives on the etiology of tuberculosis. *Microbes Infect* 2000;2:431-440.

9. Jaffe HL: Tuberculosis of bones and joints, in *Metabolic, Degenerative and Inflammatory Diseases of Bones and Joints*. Philadelphia, PA, Lea and Febiger, 1972, pp 952-1004.

10. Meier JL, Beekmann SE: Mycobacterial and fungal infections of bone and joints. *Curr Opin Rheumatol* 1995;7:329-336.

11. Formicola V, Milanesi Q, Scarsini C: Evidence of spinal tuberculosis at the beginning of the fourth millennium BC from Arene Candide Cave (Liguria, Italy). *Am J Phys Anthropol* 1987;72:1-6.

12. Pfeiffer S: Paleopathology in an Iroquoian ossuary, with special reference to tuberculosis. *Am J Phys Anthropol* 1984;65:181-189.

13. Manchester K: Tuberculosis and leprosy in antiquity: An interpretation. *Med Hist* 1984;28:162-173.

14. Dubos RJ, Dubos J: *The White Plague: Tuberculosis, Man and Society*. London, England, Victor Gollanz Ltd, 1953.

15. Frieden TR, Lerner SH, Rutherford BR: Lessons from the 1800s: Tuberculosis control in the new millennium. *Lancet* 2000;355:1088-1092.

16. Peltier LH: *Orthopaedics: A History and Iconography*. San Francisco, CA, Norman Publishing Co, 1993, pp 149-160.

17. Taylor R: *Saranac: America's Magic Mountain*. Boston, MA, Houghton Mifflin Company, 1986.

18. Bronte E: *Wuthering Heights* (1847) Oxford, England, Oxford World Classics, 1999.

19. Dickens C: *David Copperfield* (1849). New York, NY, Penguin Classics, 1997.

20. Stevenson RL: *A Child's Garden of Verses and Underwoods (1887)*. New York, NY, Current Literature Publishing Company, 1906.

21. Mann T: *The Magic Mountain*. New York, NY, Knopf Publishers, 1924.

22. Shaw GB: *The Doctor's Dilemma: A Play*. New York, NY, Penguin New York, 1946.

23. Babhulkar S, Pande S: Unusual manifestations of osteoarticular tuberculosis. *Clin Orthop Relat Res* 2002;398:114-120.

24. Steindler A: *Post-graduate Lectures on Orthopedic Diagnosis and Indications: Tuberculosis of the Skeletal System*. Springfield IL, Charles C. Thomas, 1952, vol 3.

25. Koch R: Die aetiologie der Tuberuculose. *Berline Klinisch Wochenschrift* 1882;19:221-230.

26. Feldman WH: Streptomycin: Some historical aspects of its development. *Am Rev Tuberc* 1954;69:859-868.

27. Waksman SA: Antibiotics and tuberculosis. *JAMA* 1947;135:478-485.

28. Waksman SA: *The Conquest of Tuberculosis*. Cambridge University Press, 1964.

29. Shembekar A, Babhulkar S: Chemotherapy of osteoarticular tuberculosis. *Clin Orthop Relat Res* 2002;398:20-28.

30. Williams H: *Requiem for a Great Killer*. London, England, Health Horizon, 1973.

31. Bleed D, Dye C, Raviglione MC: Dynamics and control of the global tuberculosis epidemic. *Curr Opin Pulm Med* 2000;6:174-179.

32. Bloch AB, Cauthen GM, Onorato IM, et al: Nationwide survey of drug-resistant tuberculosis in the United States. *JAMA* 1994;271:665-671.

33. Flynn JL, Ernst JD: Immune responses in tuberculosis. *Curr Opin Immunol* 2000;12:432-436.

34. Hadley M, Maher D: Community involvement in tuberculosis control: Lessons from other health care programmes. *Int J Tuberc Lung Dis* 2000;4:401-408.

35. Jellis JE: Human immunodeficiency virus and osteoarticular tuberculosis. *Clin Orthop Relat Res* 2002;398:27-31.

36. Beckhurst C, Evans S, MacFarlane AP, Packe GE: Factors influencing the distribution of tuberculosis cases in an inner London borough. *Commun Dis Public Health* 2000;3:28-31.

37. Moss AR, Hahn JA, Tulsky JP, Daley CL, Small PM, Hopewell PC: Tuberculosis in the homeless. *Am J Respir Crit Care Med* 2000;162:460-464.

38. Watts H, Lifeso RM: Current concepts review: Tuberculosis of bones and joints. *J Bone Joint Surg Am* 1996;78:288-298.

39. Woods GL: Generalized tuberculosis in the acquired immunodeficiency syndrome. *Arch Pathol Lab Med* 2000;124:1267-1274.

40. Ruiz G, Garcia Rodriquez J, Guerri ML, Gonzalez A: Osteoarticular tuberculosis in a general hospital during the last decade. *Clin Microbiol Infect* 2003;9:919-923.

41. Dankner WM, Davis CE: Microbacterium bovis as a significant cause of tuberculosis in children residing along the United States-Mexican border in the Baja California region. *Pediatrics* 2000;105:E79.

42. Hwang S, Simsar A, Waisman J, Moreira AL: Extrapulmonary tuberculosis as a mimicker of neoplasia. *Diagn Cytopathol* 2004;30:82-87.

43. Kafetzis DA: Extra-pulmonary tuberculosis in children. *Arch Dis Child* 2000;83:342-346.

44. Crump JA, Reller LB: Two decades of disseminated tuberculosis at a university medical center: The expanding role of mycobacterial blood culture. *Clin Infect Dis* 2003;37:1037-1043.

45. Donald PR: Childhood tuberculosis. *Curr Opin Pulm Med* 2000;6:187-192.

46. Portillo-Gomez L, Morris SL, Panduro A: Rapid and efficient detection of extra-pulmonary Mycobacterium tuberculosis by PCR analysis. *Int J Tuberc Lung Dis* 2000;4:361-370.

47. Pottumarthy S, Wells VC, Morris AJ: A comparison of seven tests for serological diagnosis of tuberculosis. *J Clin Microbiol* 2000;38:2227-2231.

48. Wisnivesky JP, Kaplan J, Henschke C, McGinn TG, Crystal RG: Evaluation of clinical parameters to predict Mycobacterium tuberculosis in inpatients. *Arch Intern Med* 2000;160:2471-2476.

49. Aboudola S, Sienko A, Carey RB, Johnson S: Tuberculous tenosynovitis. *Hum Pathol* 2004;35:1044-1046.

50. Harisinghani MG, McLoud TC, Shepard JA, Ko JP, Shroff MM, Mueller PR: Tuberculosis from head to

toe. *Radiographics* 2000;20:449-470.

51. Iseman MD: Treatment of multidrug-resistant tuberculosis. *N Engl J Med* 1993;329:784-791.

52. Vohra R, Kang JS, Dogra S, Saggar RR, Sharma R: Tuberculous osteomyelitis. *J Bone Joint Surg Br* 1997;79:562-566.

53. Apley AG, Solomon L: *Apley's System of Orthopaedics and Fractures*. Oxford, England, Butterworth, Heinemann Ltd, 1993, pp 47-54.

54. Sharma P: MRI features of tuberculous osteomyelitis. *Skeletal Radiol* 2003;32:279-285.

55. Wardle N, Ashwood N, Pearse M: Orthopaedic manifestations of tuberculosis. *Hosp Med* 2004;65:228-233.

56. Tuli SM: Severe kyphotic deformity in tuberculosis of the spine. *Int Orthop* 1995;19:327-331.

57. Hsu CY, Lu HC, Shih TT: Tuberculous infection of the wrist: MRI features. *AJR Am J Roentgenol* 2004;183:623-628.

58. Sawlani V, Chandra T, Mishra RN, et al: MRI features of tuberculosis of peripheral joints. *Clin Radiol* 2003;58:755-762.

59. Hodgson AR, Skinsnes OK, Leong JCY: The pathogenesis of Pott's paraplegia. *J Bone Joint Surg Am* 1967;49:1147-1156.

60. Lifeso RM, Weaver P, Harder EH: Tuberculous spondylitis in adults. *J Bone Joint Surg Am* 1985;67:1405-1413.

61. Hoffman EB, Allin J, Campbell JA, Leisegang FM: Tuberculosis of the knee. *Clin Orthop Relat Res* 2002;398:100-107.

62. Moon MS, Ha KY, Sun DH, et al: Pott's paraplegia. *Clin Orthop Relat Res* 1996;323:122-128.

63. Moon MS, Moon YW, Moon JL, et al: Conservative treatment of tuberculosis of the lumbar and lumbosacral spine. *Clin Orthop Relat Res* 2002;398:40-49.

64. Hibbs R: Treatment of vertebral tuberculosis by the spine fusion operation: A report of 286 cases. *J Bone Joint Surg* 1928;10:805-815.

65. Babhulkar S, Pande S: Tuberculosis of the hip. *Clin Orthop Relat Res* 2002;398:93-99.

66. Crespo M, Pigrau C, Flores X, et al: Tuberculous trochanteric bursitis: Report of 5 cases and literature review. *Scand J Infect Dis* 2004;36:552-558.

67. Silber JS, Whitfield SBV, Anbari K, et al: Insidious destruction of the hip by Mycobacterium tuberculosis and why early diagnosis is critical. *J Arthroplasty* 2000;15:392-397.

68. Griffith JF, Kumta SM, Leung PC, et al: Imaging of musculoskeletal tuberculosis: A new look at an old disease. *Clin Orthop Relat Res* 2002;398:32-39.

69. De Vuyst D, Vanhoenacker F, Gielen J, et al: Imaging features of musculoskeletal tuberculosis. *Eur Radiol* 2003;13:1809-1819.

70. Campbell JAB, Hoffman EB: Tuberculosis of the hip in children. *J Bone Joint Surg Br* 1995;77:319-326.

71. Kerri O, Martini M: Tuberculosis of the knee. *Int Orthop* 1985;9:153-157.

72. Lee AS, Campbell JAB, Hoffman EB: Tuberculosis of the knee in children. *J Bone Joint Surg Br* 1995;77:313-318.

73. Dhillon MS, Nagi ON: Tuberculosis of the foot and ankle. *Clin Orthop Relat Res* 2002;398:107-113.

74. Tuli SM: General principles of osteoarticular tuberculosis. *Clin Orthop Relat Res* 2002;398:11-19.

75. Zacharia TT, Shah JR, Patkar D, et al: MRI in ankle tuberculosis: Review of 14 cases. *Australas Radiol* 2003;47:11-16.

76. Greenwood CM, Fujiwara TM, Boothroyd LJ, et al: Linkage of tuberculosis to chromosome 2q35 loci including NRAMP1 in a large aboriginal Canadian family. *Am J Hum Genet* 2000;67:405-416.

77. Warnon S, Zammatteo N, Alexandre I, Hans C, Remacle J: Colorimetric detection of the tuberculosis complex using cyclic probe technology and hybridization in microplates. *Biotechniques* 2000;28:1152-1156.

78. Leigh Moore S, Rafii M: Advanced imaging of tuberculous arthritis. *Semin Musculoskelet Radiol* 2003;7:143-153.

79. Pande KC, Babhulkar SS: Atypical spinal tuberculosis. *Clin Orthop Relat Res* 2002;398:67-74.

Chapter 3

Syphilis and Its Effect on Bones and Joints

Syphilis, an infection with *Treponema pallidum*, was the most frequently encountered venereal disease in the world until approximately 40 years ago; it was considered a form of plague, with hundreds of thousands of cases occurring annually.[1-4] Due to heightened awareness of the nature of the disease, the sensitivity of the organism to penicillin, testing of prospective mothers prior to delivery of their children, and the use of protective devices during sexual activities, the disease is now much less common in the US and many other countries.[3-9] Because of human immunodeficiency virus (HIV) infections, there appears to be a recent rise in the frequency of luetic infections; it still represents a problem for sexually active individuals, particularly males, with some 17,000 cases reported annually to the US Centers for Disease Control and Prevention.[10]

Syphilis occurs in stages. In the primary stage, the organism is passed from an infected person to another and causes a lesional site, usually on the sexual organ.[3,4,10,11] In the secondary form, the disease disseminates to skin and other organ systems and remains highly infectious.[3,4,10,11] In a latent form, the patient remains asymptomatic but a tertiary form may occur sometimes years after the secondary disease, affecting the skin and soft tissues early and the neurologic and cardiac system, as well as the bones and joints, later in the course.[2-4,10,12-17] A fourth form of the disease, congenital syphilis, was at one time a terrible affliction; the fetus was infected by in utero transmission of the maternal spirochetal disease.[2,8,18-24] Many of the children died early in the course or became deformed or neurologically impaired and developed significant osseous abnormalities.[16,19,24-32]

The History and Language of Syphilis

Although attempts have been made to determine if Egyptian mummies or bones from archaeologic sites in other countries had evidence of syphilitic infection, there are no consistent findings to support the presence of the disease in these ancient populations.[15,33] Some of the bone changes seen were probably due to leprosy, which may have some resemblance to the changes seen in tertiary or congenital syphilis. The most consistent reports support the concept that the disease, present in the Western Hemisphere, was brought back to Europe by Columbus and his sailors in the 15th century to cause a plague-like infectious state that persisted for centuries.[1,2,15,34-36] Several investigators have found evidence of syphilitic changes in the skulls of Pueblo Indians and in primitive bony parts from Peru, Argentina, and Mexico.[2,15,35-37] Because syphilis is transmitted as a venereal infection and no antibiotics or protective devices were available, the disease spread throughout Europe and the Far East without any limiting systems.[1,7,15,38]

T pallidum was identified by Schaudinn and Hoffman in 1905.[39] The organism and, to some extent, the disease resemble other treponemal disorders such as yaws and pinta.[3,4,11,15] Physicians who treated the disorder during the early period quickly identified the various components of the disease. Although they could not effectively treat the patients, they could diagnose it and suggest that the affected individuals avoid sexual contact. Syphilis is a disease that can affect anyone. Many famous individuals were reported to have been infected, including Al Capone, King Charles VIII of France, Randolph Churchill, Paul Gaugin, Vincent Van Gogh, King Henry VIII of England, Adolf Hitler, Toulouse Lautrec, Napolean, Eduard Manet, Friedrich Nietzche, Franz Schubert, Robert Schumann, William Shakespeare, and Oscar Wilde.

The descriptive presentations of syphilis soon provided an entire terminology that remains unique to the disease. Among the terms in the language of syphilis are:

- *Chancre:* In primary disease, the acute, relatively painless inflammatory

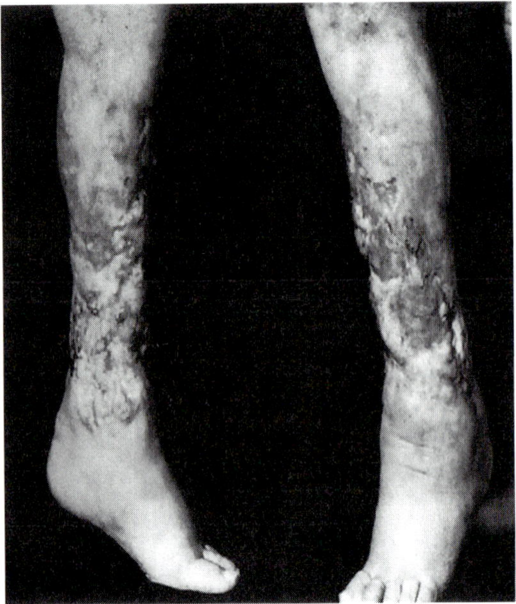

Figure 1
Condyloma lata in a male with secondary syphilis. Lesions are often painful.

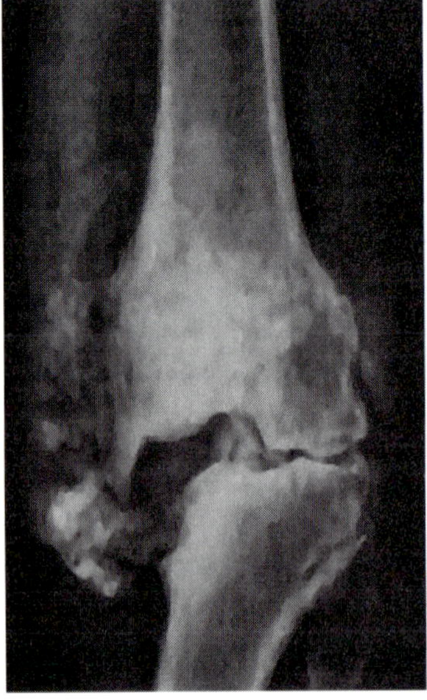
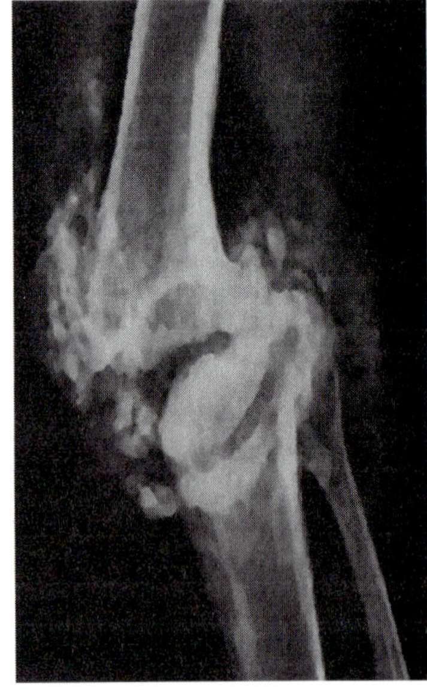

Figure 2
Tertiary syphilis may result in tabes dorsalis, which can cause Charcot's arthropathy. The joints are destroyed and unstable. Although poorly functional, the joints are not necessarily very painful.

granulomatous lesion usually located on the sexual organ.[3,4,10,11]

- *Bubo:* An infected lymph node in the region of the chancre.[3,10]
- *Condyloma lata:* A painful, destructive granulomatous skin lesion seen in many sites in patients with secondary syphilis, sometimes associated with irregular "moth-eaten" alopecia[2-4,10] (Figure 1).
- *Gumma:* A markedly deforming, relatively pain-free granulomatous soft-tissue swelling seen in patients with tertiary disease or in children with congenital disease.[2-4,10,16,22,40]
- *Babinski syndrome:* Cardiovascular disease in patients with tertiary syphilis.[41]
- *General paresis:* Severe mental impairment seen in patients with tertiary syphilis.[2,3,10]
- *Tabes dorsalis:* Spinal disease affecting both the cord and peripheral nerves in patients with tertiary syphilis.[14,17,42]
- *Romberg's sign:* Proprioceptive loss characterized by ataxia and inability to maintain a standing posture with the eyes shut. The syndrome is related to spinal cord injury seen in tabes dorsalis.[2,3]
- *Charcot's joints:* Severe destructive changes seen in the joints of patients

with tabes dorsalis who have lost sensation but retain motor function[2,14,17,42-48] (Figure 2).

- *Wimberger's tibial lesions:* Osteomyelitic foci in the medial upper ends of the tibiae in patients with congenital syphilis[20,23,28-31,40,49,50] (Figure 3).
- *Parrot's nodes:* Nodules and lytic areas in the skulls of infants with congenital syphilis.[51]
- *Rhagades:* Granulomatous nodules at the corners of the mouth in children with congenital disease.[4]
- *Snuffles:* Thick whitish discharge from the nose of infants with congenital syphilis.[4,52]
- *Hutchinson's incisors and mulberry molars:* Multiple teeth abnormalities with increased space between the incisors and marked alterations in the structure of the molars in older children with congenital syphilis[2,4,22,29,53] (Figure 4).
- *Saddle nose:* Flattening alteration of the midportion of the nose in children with congenital syphilis.[4,22,25,27,29,40]
- *Argyll-Robertson pupil:* Small and irregular pupil that reacts to accommodation but not to light. Present in congenital and occasionally in tertiary disease.[54]

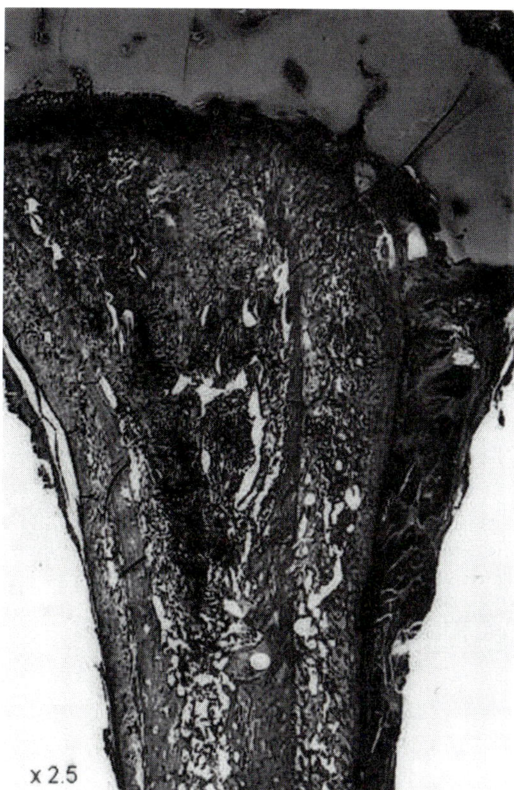

x 2.5

Figure 3
Wimberger's joint destruction in the tibia occurs in children with congenital disease. It may be the result of treponema infection and resembles a septic process with considerable periosteal inflammation. Hematoxylin and eosin × 40.

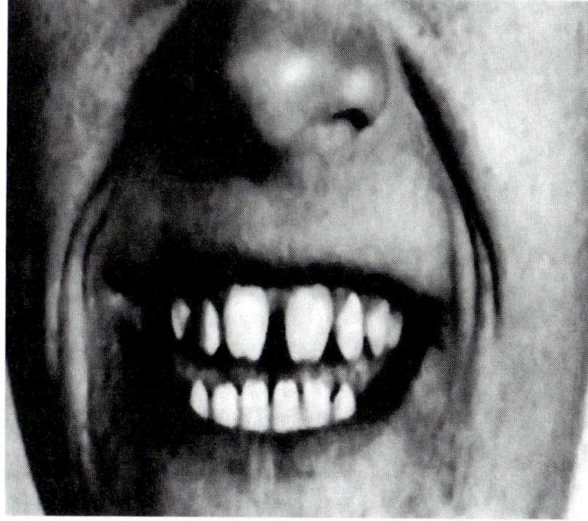

Figure 4
Hutchinson's incisors occur in patients with congenital syphilis. The space between the incisors is characteristic.

- *Clutton's joints:* Marked swelling of the knees with sterile effusions, usually painless and generally seen in congenital disease.[55]
- *Saber shins:* Smooth, painless prominences of the anterior surfaces of the tibiae seen in patients with congenital syphilis.[2]

Although protocols for the treatment of syphilis started before the turn of the century, the only three agents thought to be even modestly successful (bismuth, mercury, and salvarsan) all had significant side effects.[3,7,15] No really effective system was developed until 1928, when Sir Alexander Fleming discovered penicillin. Introduced for the treatment of syphilis in 1936, penicillin proved to be highly successful in killing the organism and, for primary and some secondary forms, completely eliminating the disease.[3,4,7,10,11,21] Penicillin and some of its modifications are still the principal agents used to treat patients with primary and secondary disease, and sometimes children with congenital disease.[3,4,8,10,21,26,56]

The Pathophysiology of Syphilis

Syphilis is caused by infection with *T pallidum*, a thin helical organism measuring approximately 0.15 by 25 or more microns.[3,4,18,21] On cross-section, the organism shows an outer sheath, periplasmic flagella, and a peptidoglycan layer. The organism is labile and cannot survive drying or exposure to disinfectants. *T pallidum* is solely a human pathogen; transmission occurs by penetration of the spirochete through mucosal membranes or abrasive defects on epithelial surfaces.[3,4,18,21] The focal lesions are an endarteritis and periarteritis that produce a chancre in primary disease; this is characterized by the presence of the organism surrounded by abundant mononuclear lymphocytes and macrophages in a fibrous capsule.[2] The lesions generally occur in relation to the site of sexual contact and may appear approximately 3 weeks after exposure, often accompanied by an adjacent inflamed lymph node (bubo).[3,4,10]

The lesions of secondary syphilis are highly variable, but the most frequent are mucocutaneous lesions known as condylomata lata.[3,4,10] These skin defects are macular, reddish-brown, and sometimes pustular, annular, or scaling. They contain the spirochetes and are infectious with contact. The lesions in the scalp may cause a secondary irregular alopecia.[2-4,10]

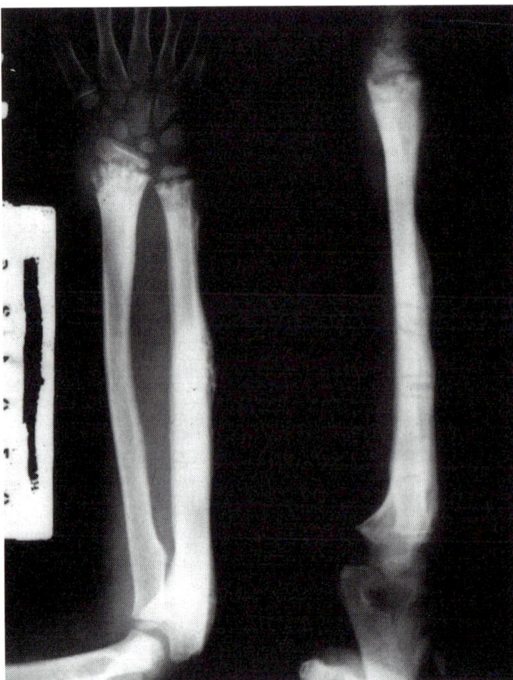

Figure 5
Pseudo-osteomyelitis of the radius and ulna in a child with congenital syphilis.

Early tertiary syphilis is primarily characterized by the gumma, which has a center of necrotic tissue with a rubbery texture and often a fibrous capsule.[2-4,16] Treponemas are ordinarily not present in gummas, in the lesions associated with cardiac disease in early tertiary syphilis, or in the nervous system lesions in late disease.[3,4] The neurologic disorders are characterized by obliterative endarteritis causing cell death and cerebral atrophy in the brain (paresis) and damage to the posterior aspect of the spinal cord, resulting in a loss of deep sensation but with retention of motor power (tabes dorsalis).[3,4,11,15,41] The spinal cord problem frequently results in Charcot's arthropathy.[2,17,43,44,46]

In congenital syphilis, the spirochetes are transmitted through the maternal placenta and infect the fetus.[10,21,25,40,57] The problems that occur are related principally to the effect of the granulomatous lesions on growth and body structure. Hence rhagades,[26] snuffles,[25] Hutchinson's incisors,[53] mulberry molars,[40] Argyll-Robertson pupils,[54] blindness,[21] saddle nose,[21] Clutton's joints,[55] saber shins,[2] gummatous deposits,[20,40] and Parrot's calvarial lesions[51] all result from the actions and effects of the spirochetes on the growing tissue. Of particular

interest are the findings in the skeleton, which may result in marked alterations in growth and structure.[2,23,24,27-32,52,58,59]

Diagnosis of Syphilis

Immunofluorescence staining of mucocutaneous lesions demonstrates the spirochete in primary, secondary, and early congenital disease. Serologic screening tests for syphilis include the Venereal Disease Research Laboratory (VDRL) and Rapid Plasma Reagin (RPR) tests, both of which turn positive 1 to 2 weeks after chancre formation.[3,6,9,10] A fluorescent treponemal antibody absorption test is useful in diagnosis of secondary or latent cases. In addition, *T pallidum* hemagglutination and particle agglutination tests can be conducted, as well as the treponemal enzyme immunoassay, when the VDRL or RPR tests do not seem reliably positive.[6,9]

Bone Lesions in Patients With Syphilis

Acquired primary or secondary syphilis does not usually present with changes in the bones. Occasionally, in patients with extensive secondary disease, a periostitis may be the cause of pain in the tibiae, femora, or ulnae; in radiographic studies, this may present as irregular cortical bone destructive lesions with adjacent productive processes that resemble superficial osteomyelitis[2,60] (Figure 5). These lesions are often painful and contain a great number of spirochetes. An even rarer type of process may occur in relation to the synovium of the knee or elbow, which may produce joint swelling, local heat, and tenderness.[2,60] Both of these inflammatory processes usually respond to penicillin. If the periosteal lesions cause sufficient cortical erosion, fractures are not uncommon and may require surgical treatment along with antibiotic therapy.[60]

Congenital Syphilis and Bone Lesions

The number of patients with congenital syphilis in the US today is now quite small, thanks to the important contribution of Thomas Parran, who introduced the proposal that each state require serologic testing of women for syphilis early in their pregnancy.[7,8,56,57] Women who test positive are given penicillin or other antibiotics in sufficient quantities so that the spirochetes are less likely to infect the fetus.[8,56,57]

In congenital syphilis, when the fetus becomes infected by fluid from the maternal placenta, the spirochetes are distributed into the bones by the fetal blood stream and multiply perivascularly. They enter the marrow of the bones and are present at the sites of endochondral ossification, particularly in the metaphyseal regions.[2,21,23,28,52] After birth, the number of spirochetes in the bones are markedly decreased and the changes seen are difficult to define as being related to syphilis, even at the time of cultures or autopsy studies for infants who have had severe infections. The bone changes seen in the very young infant with congenital syphilis include osteochondritis, diaphyseal osteomyelitis, and (considerably later) gummatous periostitis. The osteochondritis usually begins to appear at approximately the fifth fetal month and consists of widening of the zone of provisional calcification along with irregularity and accentuation of serrations.[2,52,58,59] With continued disease, the osteochondral zone becomes wider and results in loosening of the connection between the epiphysis and metaphysis, which leads to an epiphyseal separation. This may be present at multiple sites, but is most common in the distal femora and proximal tibiae.[2,52,58,59] The result of these changes in the surviving infant is shortening of the affected extremities and sometimes extraordinary deformities when healing occurs.[27,52,61]

Diaphyseal osteomyelitis (Wimberger's disease) occurs later in the course, usually at the time of birth or within the first year.[23,25,50,52,61] The disease consists of an active periostitis associated with sometimes irregular cortical erosions (Figure 3). These are most commonly located in the upper ends of both tibiae and are often symmetrical in appearance. They are quite inflammatory in character, and the appearance on radiographs or in tissue samples resemble a surface osteomyelitis.[2,19,26,27,52] Spirochetes have been found in the cambium layer of the overlying periosteum and are presumed to be responsible for the disease.[2,3]

Even later in the course of congenital syphilis, after 1 or more years, gummatous lesions may appear and produce swelling of the soft tissues over bony sites, resulting in periosteal changes in the bones.[61] These are usually asymmetrical and may not contain large numbers of spirochetes. Other features of congenital syphilis that are generally seen at 7 years of age or later are Clutton's joints and saber shins. Clutton's joints are characterized by painless swelling of the knee joints, which are not inflamed and contain fluid without spirochetes.[2,55,62] The synovium contains many macrophages and lymphocytes. Saber shins are represented by a thickening of the cortices and anterior bowing of the middle and lower parts of the tibiae.[2] The lesions are painless and are present throughout the life of the patient.

Other findings present in untreated older patients with congenital syphilis include dactylitis[2] and productive and destructive lesions in the bony calvarium (Parrot's nodes).[51] In addition, the patients may show irregularity of the structure of the nasal bones (saddle nose), the teeth (Hutchinson's incisors and mulberry molars), and the mandibles and maxillae, all of which result in sometimes remarkable facial deformities.[2,4,22,25,27-32,49,53] These changes often occur in association with either Argyll-Robertson pupils or blindness.[54]

Tertiary Syphilis and Bone Lesions

Tertiary syphilis may not appear for decades following primary and secondary disease. In some patients whose primary disease was inadequately treated or ignored, the patient and physician may have no reason to suspect syphilis as the cause of the symptoms. The principal disorders are cardiovascular problems, consisting primarily of large vessel disease (usually aortitis).[2-4,10] Aortic dilatation and a tambour quality of the sound of aortic closure are often present, and usually occur above the abdominal aorta.[10] Iritis is frequent and is usually associated with pain and dimness of vision. The pupil is often fixed, based on adhesions of the iris to the anterior lens and patients may become blind.[10] Gummatous disease is common in patients with tertiary syphilis.[10,16] Lesions, ranging in size from microscopic to enormous, may be attached to bones, skin, mouth, or abdominal organs.

Neural tertiary syphilis presents in two forms. Generalized paresis is characterized by widespread parenchymal damage that results in personality disorders, decreased memory, altered orientation, illusions, delusions, and hallucinations associated with hyperactive reflexes and often very poor vision or blindness.[2-4,10] The second form of the disease, known as tabes dorsalis, results from demyelinization of the posterior columns of the spinal cord and damage to the dorsal roots and dorsal root ganglions.[2,12,13,44,45] The patient becomes unsteady, particularly when the eyes remain closed (Romberg's sign), and may develop bone disease consisting of neuropathic arthropathy of Charcot.[2,12,13,44] These lesions principally affect the knees and hips, and less commonly the spine, shoulders, and ankles.[13,14,17,46-48,63] Characteristically the joint becomes swollen and distorted in shape and movement; sometimes synovial tissue may erode through the skin[17] or result in fractures[64] (Figure 2). The synovium almost always contains small segments of bone and cartilage from the damaged joint.[2,17,42,47] Charcot's arthropathy may also occur in patients with diabetes, spinal lesions, Riley-Day syndrome, and congenital insensitivity to pain.[44,45]

Treatment of Syphilis

Most organisms become resistant to antibiotics, particularly in the face of HIV infections. This in part explains the recent resurgence of diseases such as tuberculosis, hepatitis, resistant staphylococcus, and chlamydia. This does not appear to be true for *T pallidum*, however, which remains sensitive to penicillin.[10] Most patients with primary or second-

ary syphilis can be treated effectively with 2.4 million units of benzathine penicillin G in a single dose. Latent disease is most frequently treated with three doses of crystalline penicillin for approximately 3 weeks. For patients who are allergic to penicillin, doxycycline and erythromycin both have been shown to inhibit the growth of the spirochetes, but less effectively than penicillin.[3,10]

Dealing with the multiple deformities and disabilities that result from congenital and tertiary syphilis is sometimes very difficult and complex. Both the congenital patients and particularly the patients with tertiary disease may have life-threatening cardiac, visceral, and neural diseases that may not respond to penicllin or even various forms of supportive care.

Is syphilis now a disease of the past? In the US, it is clearly far less common than it was before the use of penicillin, the increased awareness of the dangers associated with intercourse, and the introduction of prophylactic measures such as condoms and Parran's testing of pregnant women. The problem lies with other countries that are far less supportive of these measures. Many of the new syphilis patients in the US are recent arrivals from disadvantaged countries, who are far less knowledgeable of the problems that the disease may cause. Health agencies and physicians in this country have a responsibility to educate these individuals, defining the disease and introducing prophylactic and treatment protocols.

References

1. Cripps DJ, Curtis AC: Syphilis maligna praecox: Syphilis of the great epidemic. An historical review. *Arch Intern Med* 1967;119:411-418.

2. Jaffe HL: Syphilis of bones and joints, in Jaffe HL (ed): *Metabolic, Degenerative and Inflammatory Diseases of Bones and Joints*. Philadelphia, PA, Lea and Febiger, 1972, pp 907-952.

3. Lukehart SA, Holmes KK: Syphilis, in Isselbacher KJ, Brauwald E, Wilson JD, Martin JB, Fauci AS, Kaspar DL (eds): *Harrison's Principles of Internal Medicine*, ed 13. New York, NY, McGraw Hill, 1994, pp 726-737.

4. Olansky S, Thomas EW: *Syphilis: Modern Diagnosis and Management*. Washington, DC, US Department of Health, Education, and Welfare, Public Health Service, 1961.

5. Bowell P, Mayne K, Puckett A, Entwistle C, Selkon J: Serological screening tests for syphilis in pregnancy: Results of a five year study (1983-87) in the Oxford region. *J Clin Pathol* 1989;42:1281-1284.

6. Farnes SW, Setness PA: Serologic tests for syphilis. *Postgrad Med* 1990;87:37-41.

7. Parran T: *Shadow on the Land—Syphilis*. New York,

NY, Reynal and Hitchcock Inc, 1967.

8. Slatkin MH, Nelson CT: Syphilis in pregnancy: Serologic diagnosis and treatment. *Clin Obstet Gynecol* 1959;2:658-673.

9. Wicher K, Horowitz HW, Wicher V: Laboratory methods of diagnosis of syphilis for the beginning of the third millennium. *Microbes Infect* 1999;1:1035-1049.

10. Centers for Disease Control: 1989 sexually transmitted disease treatment guidelines. *MMWR Morb Mortal Wkly Rep* 1989;38(suppl 8):1-43.

11. Stokes JA, Beerman H, Ingraham NR Jr: *Modern Clinical Syphilology*, ed 3. Philadelphia, PA, Saunders, 1945.

12. Eichenholtz SN: *Charcot Joints*. Springfield, IL, Charles C. Thomas, 1966.

13. Johns D: Syphilitic disorders of the spine. *J Bone Joint Surg Br* 1970;52:724-731.

14. Pomeranz MM, Rothberg AS: A review of 58 cases of tabetic arthropathy. *Am J Syph* 1941;25:103-119.

15. Pusey WA: *The History and Epidemiology of Syphilis*. Springfield, IL, Charles C. Thomas, 1933.

16. Rocha N, Horta M, Sanches M, et al: Syphylitic gumma-cutaneous tertiary syphilis. *J Eur Acad Dermatol Venereol* 2004;18:517-518.

17. Steindler A: The tabetic arthopathies. *JAMA* 1931;96:250-256.

18. Brown WJ, Moore MB Jr: Congenital syphilis in the United States. *Clin Pediatr (Phila)* 1963;2:220-222.

19. Drucker MG, Mankin HJ: Congenital syphilis in 1970: A case report. *Bull Hosp Joint Dis* 1970;31:132-140.

20. Fiumara NJ, Lessell S: Manifestations of late congenital syphilis: An analysis of 271 patients. *Arch Dermatol* 1970;102:78-83.

21. Krugman S, Katz SL: *Infectious Diseases of Children.* St. Louis, MO, CV Mosby, 1981.

22. McDonald R: Congenital syphilis has many faces. *Clin Pediatr (Phila)* 1970;9:110-114.

23. McLean S: Roentgenographic and pathologic aspects of congenital osseous syphilis. *Am J Dis Child* 1931;31:130-152.

24. Saxoni F, Lapaanis P, Pantelakis SN: Congenital syphilis: A description of 18 cases and re-examination of an old but ever-present disease. *Clin Pediatr (Phila)* 1967;6:687-691.

25. Cremin BJ, Fisher RM: The lesions of congenital syphilis. *Br J Radiol* 1970;43:333-341.

26. Ewing CI, Roberts C, Davidson DC, Arya OP: Early congenital syphilis still occurs. *Arch Dis Child* 1985;60:1128-1133.

27. Hira SK, Bhat GJ, Patel JB, et al: Early congenital syphilis: Clinico-radiologic features in 202 patients. *Sex Transm Dis* 1985;12:177-183.

28. Rasool M, Govender S: The skeletal manifestations of congenital syphilis: A review of 197 cases. *J Bone Joint Surg Br* 1989;71:752-755.

29. Russo PE, Shryock LF: Bone lesion of congenital syphilis in infants and adolescents: Report of 46 cases. *Radiology* 1945;44:477-484.

30. Sachdev M, Bery K, Chawla S: Osseous manifestations in congenital syphilis: A study of 55 cases. *Clin Radiol* 1982;33:319-323.

31. Solomon A, Rosen E: Focal osseous lesions in congenital lues. *Pediatr Radiol* 1978;7:36-79.

32. Wilkinson RH, Heller RM: Congenital syphilis: Resurgence of an old problem. *Pediatrics* 1971;47:27-30.

33. Smith GE, Dawson WR: *Egyptian Mummies.* London, England, Allen and Unwin, 1924.

34. Hudson EH: Christopher Columbus and the history of syphilis. *Acta Trop* 1968;25:1-16.

35. Rothschild BM, Calderon FL, Coppa A, Rothschild CA: First European exposure to syphilis: The Dominican Republic at the time of Columbian contact. *Clin Infect Dis* 2000;31:936-941.

36. Tello JC, Williams HU: An ancient syphilitic skull from Paracas in Peru. *Ann Med Hist* 1930;2:515-519.

37. Hooton EA: *The Indians of Pecos Pueblo: A Study of Their Skeletal Remains.* New Haven, CT, Yale University Press, 1930.

38. Mansilla J, Pijoan CM: Brief communication: A case of congenital syphilis during the colonial period. *Am J Phys Anthropol* 1995;97:187-195.

39. Schaudinn R, Hoffman E: Uber spirochatenbefunde in lymphdrusenshaft syphilitischer. *Dtsch Med Wschschr* 1905;31:711-720.

40. Fleming TC, Bardenstein MB: Congenital syphilis. *J Bone Joint Surg Am* 1971;53:1648-1651.

41. Babinski J: Des troubles pupillaires dans les aneurisme de l'aorte. *Bull Soc Hop Paris* 1901;18:1121-1124.

42. Potts WJ: The pathology of Charcot joints. *Ann Surg* 1927;86:596-606.

43. Charcot JM: Sur quelques arthropathies qui paraissant dependre d'une lesion du cerveau on de la moelle epiniere. *Arch Physio Norm Et Pathol* 1868;1:161-178.

44. Delano PJ: The pathogenesis of Charcot's joint. *AJR Am J Roentgenol* 1946;56:189-200.

45. Jones EA, Manaster BJ, May DA, Disler DG: Neuropathic osteoarthropathy: Diagnostic dilemmas and differential diagnosis. *Radiographics* 2000;20:S279-S293.

46. Key JA: Clinical observations on tabetic arthropathies (Charcot's joints). *Am J Syph* 1932;16:429-446.

47. Storey G: Charcot joints. *Br J Vener Dis* 1964;40:109-116.

48. Taylor HL: Charcot joints as initial or early symptom in tabes dorsalis. *J Am Med Assn* 1913;61:1784-1788.

49. Horodniceanu C, Grunebaum M, Volovitz B, Nitzan M: Unusual bone involvement in congenital syphilis mimicking the battered child syndrome. *Pediatr Radiol* 1978;7:232-234.

50. Wimberger H: Klinisch-radiologische diagnostik ven rachitis, skorbut und lues congenita in kindesalter. *Ergebn Inn Med Kinderh* 1925;28:264-270.

51. Parrot JM: Lesions du crane, causes par le syphilis hereditaire. *Progr Med (Paris)* 1879;7:268-269.

52. Oppenheimer EH, Hardy JB: Congenital syphilis in the new born infant: Clinical and pathological observations in recent cases. *Johns Hopkins Med J* 1971;129:63-82.

53. Hutchinson J: Report of the effects of infantile syphilis in marring the development of the teeth. *Tr Path Soc London* 1858;9:449-455.

54. Robertson A: On an interesting series of eye-symptoms in a case of spinal disease with remarks on the action of belladonna on the iris etc. *Edinburgh Med J* 1868;14:696-708.

55. Clutton HH: Symmetrical synovitis of the knee in hereditary syphilis. *Lancet* 1886;1:391-393.

56. Nelson NA, Struve VR: Prevention of congenital syphilis by treatment of syphilis in pregnancy. *JAMA* 1956;161:869-672.

57. Fiumara NJ, Fleming WL, Downing JG, Good FL: The incidence of prenatal syphilis at the Boston City Hospital. *N Engl J Med* 1952;247:48-52.

58. Coblentz DR, Cimini R, McKity VG, Rosen R: Roentgenographic diagnosis of congenital syphilis in the newborn. *JAMA* 1970;221:1061-1064.

59. Levin TL, Schulman M, Zieba P, Goldman HS: Absence of lower extremity ossification centers in term infants with congenital syphilis. *J Perinatol* 1994;14:106-109.

60. McGladdery H: Osteolytic bone syphilis. *J Bone Joint Surg Br* 1950;32:226-229.

61. Ghadouane M, Benjelloun BS, Elharim-Roudies L, et al: Skeletal lesions in early congenital syphilis (a review of 86 cases). *Rev Rhum Engl Ed* 1995;62:433-437.

62. Borella L, Goobar JE, Clark GM: Synovitis of the knee joints in late congenital syphilis: Clutton's joints. *JAMA* 1962;180:190-192.

63. Moran SM, Mohr JA: Syphilis and axial arthropathy. *South Med J* 1983;76:1032-1035.

64. Johnson JTH: Neuropathic fractures and joint injuries: Pathogenesis and rationale of prevention and treatment. *J Bone Joint Surg Am* 1967;49:1-30.

Chapter 4

Anterior Poliomyelitis

Nature and History

Some of the most extraordinary deformities and disabilities in orthopaedic history were produced by infantile paralysis, which later became known as anterior poliomyelitis. Although recognized in ancient Egypt,[1] the clinical characteristics of the disease were first described in 1788 by Underwood,[2] who defined it as a form of paralysis affecting young children and more commonly occurring in the lower extremities. In 1840, Jacob Heine further defined the disease as occurring in relation to the spinal cord.[3] Later that century, Jean Marie Charcot performed an autopsy on a patient with poliomyelitis who had died of tuberculosis and discovered damage to the structure of the anterior horns of the gray matter in the spinal cord.[4] In 1890, Medin[5] defined the infectious nature of the disease based on a study of a Scandinavian epidemic in which a large number of patients became paralyzed. Based on these contributions, the syndrome of poliomyelitis became known as Heine-Medin disease.[6]

In the early part of the 20th century, several investigators classified the disease as contagious and suspected the existence of a specific infectious agent. In a 1908 report on cases treated at Children's Hospital in Boston[7] and a subsequent book,[8] Robert Lovett clearly defined the paralytic changes that were present in the patients seen at Children's Hospital. Based on his studies of these 635 patients, he proposed that rest, bracing, and moderate exercise could be of value in reducing deformity and disability.[7,8] It was not until the 1930s, however, that the virus origin was identified.[6,9] Based on the remarkable studies of Enders and coworkers,[10,11] the causative agent was isolated and discovered to be an RNA enterovirus of the picornovirus family with three serotypes, all of which can cause human infection.

The initial infection rate in urban communities was high. Epidemics occurred in the US as early as 1905, with a large percentage of the patients developing paralysis.[6,9,12] More recently, even without vaccination, autoimmunity to all three forms of the virus has been discovered; although many exposed patients have complaints of fever, chills, headache, and malaise, a considerably smaller percentage (particularly adults) develop motor paralysis.[6,9,12-14] The last great epidemic occurred in 1952. Some 21,000 patients developed paralysis, but many more had the disease without motor loss.[6,9,13-15]

The three types of small virus particles known to be the causative agent for this entity are transmitted to other patients by oral exposure to the viruses from infected patient's urine, bowel contents, and occasionally sputum.[7,14] Patients afflicted with the disease have an incubation period of 3 to 35 days, followed by a 3- to 4-day period of fever, chills, malaise, headache, coryza, and limb pain.[6,9,12,15-18] In some patients, this syndrome terminates after 3 to 4 weeks and the patients fully recover.[6,9,19] However, anywhere from 4% to 50% of the patients (particularly the young), experience a neurologic syndrome that can sometimes be severe.[15-18]

Although the principal site of disease involvement is in the central nervous system, initially other systems are involved. An increased number of lymphocytes in the serum are noted, and a small number of patients develop a myocarditis that can be fatal.[9,13,17] The neurologic process that occurs affects the motor neurons in the anterior horn of the spinal cord or the brain stem and causes damage to the cell and ultimately cell death and destruction with a striking lymphocyte inflammatory ingrowth; after 3 to 4 weeks, scarring of the site occurs.[6,9,12,16,20] The changes take place most frequently in the anterior horn motor cells, which are more susceptible to the virus than those of other sites or the cerebral cortex; however, changes have been noted in the spinal cord, the medulla, the pons, the midbrain, and even the cerebellum.[9,13] Ultimately, as a result of the changes, there is a loss of motor function; this can occur in a portion of a muscle or, more commonly, an entire muscular component. Initially, the patients complain of muscle pain and ten-

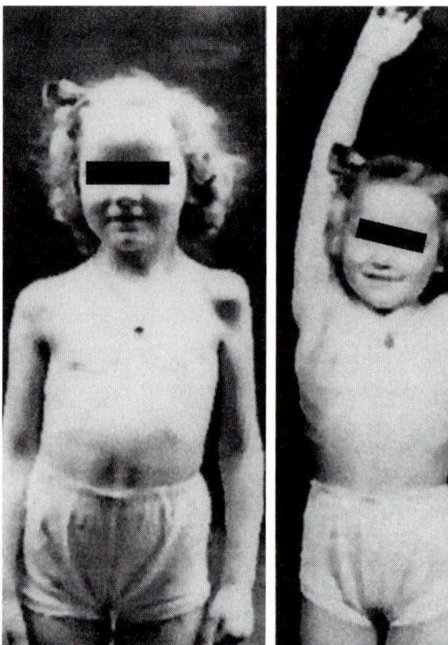

Figure 1
A 7-year-old child with poliomyelitis that has resulted in a loss of shoulder abductor power. Note the atrophy of the deltoid area.

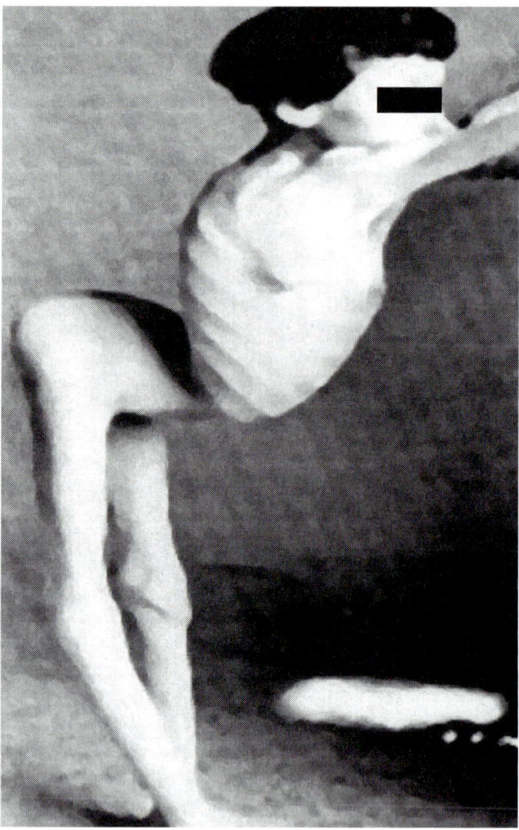

Figure 2
A 17-year-old patient with severe scoliosis and deformity of the lower extremities. There is really no way to treat this problem, either surgically or with bracing. He was never able to walk.

derness with moderate spasm, and then a progressive loss of motor function without any sensory loss.[9,12,16,17,21] The patient may at first have some degree of sympathetic malfunction and some coldness to the extremity sites, but these findings subside as the inflammatory components diminish. Over time (often a matter of 3 to 4 weeks although sometimes longer), the patient may be left without pain or inflammatory findings yet with a profound and often complete flaccid paralysis in one or several muscles including, at times, the bladder, bowel, or diaphragm.[6,9,12,13,16-18,21]

The most frequently affected muscular system is in the lower extremity in very young children, and in the upper extremity or spine in older individuals.[9,12,13,16,21] In some older individuals, the muscles of the chest wall from the second thoracic site down and the diaphragm become paralyzed (known as bulbar polio), frequently causing the patients to have severe respiratory impairment and an early demise. Initially, the muscular weakness may improve somewhat; however, after a period of several months, affected persons are paralyzed for life. Depending on their age and the site of the motor loss, they may develop sometimes quite striking and disabling deformities, ex-

tremity shortening, scoliosis, and functional loss.[6,7,9,16,17,21-26]

As noted by both Medin[5] and Lovett,[8] the disease was by most standards an epidemic. The disease was transmitted more frequently in the summer months, particularly in relation to infection from contaminated water in swimming pools. Because other viral diseases may also produce neurologic complaints, at least initially, they should be considered as a possible cause, particularly of muscle pain and tenderness. These diseases include Guillain-Barré syndrome, California encephalitis, and West Nile virus infection.[6,9,12,13,27,28]

Many famous people had polio, but perhaps the most famous was Franklin Delano Roosevelt, who developed his disease in 1921 and spent the remainder of his life in a wheelchair, including his tenure as President of the US from 1933 to 1945.[29] To further research in caring for patients with poliomyelitis, the Roosevelts established the

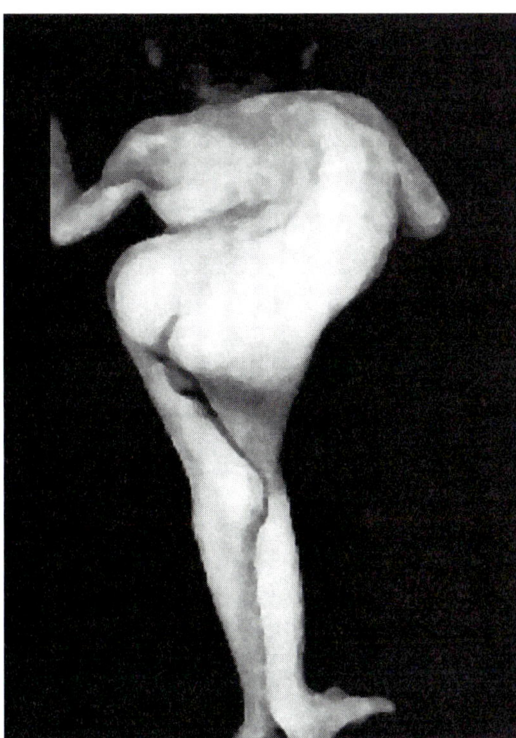

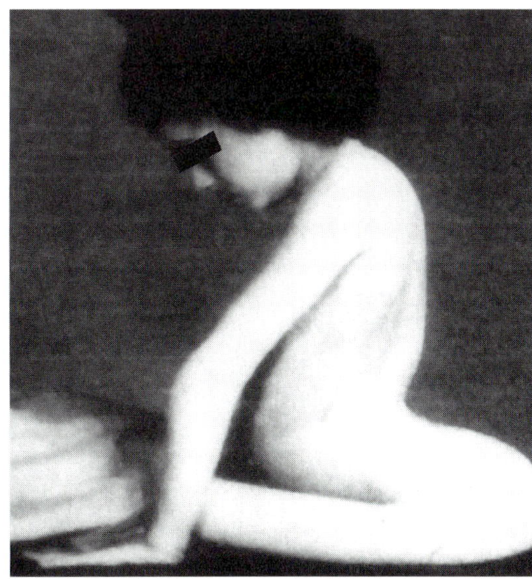

Figure 4
A 7-year-old girl with severe scoliosis and lower extremity paralysis. She is unlikely to ever ambulate, even with braces.

Figure 3
A 12-year-old child with very severe scoliosis and paralysis of the costal muscles. The patient not only cannot walk or stand, but also has respiratory difficulty.

Georgia Warm Springs Foundation; this organization not only provided a site for physiotherapy for patients with poliomyelitis, but became an important contributor to our understanding and treatment of the disease.[13]

Clinical Findings

The findings in patients with anterior poliomyelitis may vary considerably. Early in the course, the patients are quite ill. They are frequently febrile, with elevated white counts; a spinal fluid analysis may show increased numbers of lymphocytes and increased concentrations of protein.[9,12,13,18] Muscles are initially painful, tender to pressure, and resistant to movement. If the patient does not recover from this early course (approximately 50% do, without progressive neurologic loss), one of several muscles become progressively weaker; with time, the tenderness over the site diminishes and flaccidity occurs. Depending on the site and the number of muscles that are affected, the patient may develop very minor problems with little disability or limitation of function.[12,18] Much more likely for many of the patients, they can become severely affected and clinically functionally impaired.[12,17,18,21] Thus patients with a weakness of a part of the quadriceps musculature are limited in their ability to extend against resistance, but can often walk without difficulty if they have a mild degree of hyperextension. Similarly, patients whose gastrocnemius musculature is affected may lose their ability to plantar flex their foot, but can often manage with only a shoe correction and limited additional support.

However, some quite severe alterations can occur that cause the patients difficulty with ambulation and function. Loss of the function in the dorsiflexors of the foot may result in not only motor weakness, but often shortening and a sometimes troublesome valgus deformity.[12,16] Similar changes in the upper extremity lead to weakness in the shoulder, scapula, elbow, wrist, and hands, along with shortening and sometimes striking deformities[16,30-32] (Figure 1). Weakness of the abdominal musculature sometimes causes deformity, and the most severely affected patients are those with lumbar or thoracic musculature weakness, which leads to scoliosis[12,13,22,24,25] (Figure 2). One of the more common findings is a very severe lordosis, which makes it difficult for the patient to ambulate (Figures 3 and 4).

Perhaps the most distressing effect of anterior poliomyelitis is the weakness of the thoracic musculature and diaphragm, which sometimes causes severe respiratory impairment. Patients with this problem found it difficult to breathe, and were often required to spend many hours of the day in an "iron lung" in order to maintain their oxygen saturation and respiratory function.[6,12,13,16,17,22,24] Their clinical course was limited by respiratory disease and pulmonary infection, often resulting in central nervous system disease and an early demise.

Clinical Management

The historical approaches to the management of these disorders included rest, bracing, an exercise and physiotherapy program, an iron lung for pulmonary disease, and an array of surgical procedures to lessen the disabilities and improve motor function.

- *Rest.* When the patient was first struck by the disease, it seemed appropriate to be maintained in a sedentary state, receive anti-inflammatory agents and adequate concentrations of fluids, and hopefully recover without motor loss or alteration in limb structure. This treatment protocol was established before the turn of the 20th century, and physicians believed that it would be successful in preventing progress of the disease and reducing deformity.[3,7,26,33,34] One of the advocates of this approach was Robert W. Lovett, who became Chairman of the Harvard Infantile Paralysis Commission in the early 1920s; the Commission was charged with organizing care in hospital settings as well as follow-up care and nutrition for the Boston residents who became ill with the disease.[35,36]
- *Bracing.* As a major addition to the treatment protocol for rest, many patients were placed into an array of braces that prevented movement in the limbs and spine and also, in theory, limited deformity.[7,8,12,13,16,35] The braces included short below-knee braces for foot and ankle deformities and above-knee braces, sometimes including the hip, for patients with disabilities affecting the upper parts of their lower extremities and pelvis. Braces were also devised to compensate for the some-

times severe lordosis and scoliosis, and were commonly employed to prevent progressive deformity.
- *Physiotherapy.* The treatment of poliomyelitis patients with exercises, local heat, massage, and physical manipulation became a major component of patient management. Although the protocols were initially suggested by Lovett,[7,8] they were enthusiastically endorsed by an important contributor to poliomyelitic patient care, Sister Elizabeth Kenny. Sister Kenny was a World War I nurse from Australia who became fascinated by the problems of patients with polio; she developed a series of protocols for patient management, at times to the distress and concern of the caring physicians.[33,35,37,38] Sister Kenny's efforts were a major factor in the development of the clinical specialty of physiotherapy, and many hospitals developed specialized centers for the purpose of treating patients with poliomyelitis. When polio disappeared from the US, these facilities became therapeutic centers for the management of patients with disabilities. These protocols undoubtedly represented the most clinically valuable components of treatment in the early days—indeed, even after surgical procedures were introduced.
- *Surgical procedures.* Once it became apparent that the disease was continuous and the crippling progressive, many orthopaedic surgeons became more involved in the care of patients with poliomyelitis. Many famous surgeons of the late 19th and early 20th centuries contributed to the development of procedures and protocols for the management of the disabled patients. In 1881, Nicoladoni[39] suggested that the peroneus could be used to compensate for a paralyzed gastrocnemius. Allesandro Codavilla[40] proposed in 1905 that tendons and muscles could be lengthened to reduce deformity. Fritz Lange[36] of Munich described methods of anchoring elongated tendons using nonresorbable sutures in 1903, and Konrad Biesalski and Leo Mayer[41] authored a text that become one of the leading sources of methods and approaches to dealing with shortened and distorted tendons.

In 1895, Joel Goldthwaite described a number of tendon transplant procedures;[42] Royal Whitman[43] and Sir Robert Jones[44] enlarged and refined the protocols in 1901 and 1911, respectively. Many contributors in both Europe and the US defined new methods of tendon transfer for paralyzed muscles in both the lower and upper extremities.[13,19,25,43,45-49] Notable contributions included a report by Colonna for the paralyzed hamstrings,[22] a proposal for paralyzed hips by Dickson,[50] an approach to problems in the lower extremity weakness by Dunn,[51] and some special protocols for foot paralysis by Hoke.[46] Arthur Legg proposed a technique for transfer of the tensor fascia femoris for a weakened gluteus in 1923.[52] Two of the greatest contributors to the technology of polio treatment were Leo Mayer, who devised and reported on a series of lower extremity tendon transfers,[20,30] and Arthur Steindler, who contributed systems for treatment of elbow, shoulder, and even hand paralyses.[18,32,53-55] Steindler wrote books addressing the nature of the paralytic condition,[18] the rehabilitation of the polio patient,[55] and a description of surgical procedures and end results.[32] In addition, a number of surgeons described techniques for correcting bone deformities and lengthening short limbs or shortening long ones by epiphysiodesis and surgical shortening and stabilization, including Vittorio Putti, one of the leading figures at the Istituto Rizzoli in Bologna who in 1921 proposed a technique for lengthening the short femur.[56] Paul Harrington,[57] Russell Hibbs,[58] J.I.P. James,[24] and other surgeons described the need and technology for early treatment of scoliosis in patients with poliomyelitis; many used the Harrington instrumentation[57] to at least partially correct severe and debilitating deformities.

Development of a Vaccine

In 1946, John Enders and his coworkers at the Children's Hospital in Boston isolated the virus that caused poliomyelitis; this great discovery earned them a Nobel Prize in 1954.[10,11] However, the major break-throughs came from two other individuals—Jonas Salk of the University of Pittsburgh, who in the early 1950s developed an inactivated injectable vaccine against the organisms,[59-61] and Albert Sabin of the University of Cincinnati, who a few years later developed an attenuated live vaccine that could be taken orally.[62,63] Both agents served to prevent the occurrence of the disease. What a spectacular pair of discoveries! In a short period of time, poliomyelitis, which once caused extraordinary crippling and disability and sometimes death in many young people in the US every year, virtually disappeared.[6,9,12-15] Hospitals that had ward and outpatient services filled with paralyzed patients, and floors in which patients in iron lungs filled the rooms, now closed their special units. The physiotherapy programs in many hospitals became involved in caring for patients with arthritis, trauma, stroke, and other disabling diseases; indeed, a new specialty—physiatry—was created.

However, the vaccines are underutilized in many countries where there is limited support for health care. Some countries have a high incidence of polio and still experience epidemics; not only do they have thousands of patients with disability, but they also have a high death rate from poliomyelitis.[6,9,14,63,64] These countries include India, Pakistan, Nigeria, Sudan, Afghanistan, and Niger.[1,15,64] One would hope that the governments of these countries will adopt use of the vaccine as prevention for the disease and eventually completely wipe out this scourge from the world.

Postpolio Syndrome

In recent years a syndrome characterized by slowly progressive decrease in limb strength has been described in patients who had poliomyelitis as children. The nature and cause of this disorder remain obscure, and the chemical and histologic studies do not support the concept that the disease in the nervous system is activated.[6,9,14,65] Because the syndrome occurs as late as 20 to 30 years after the primary disease, one hypothesis is that it represents another form of motor weakness, possibly also viral in origin, which more actively affects the damaged muscles. Still another possibility is that the postpolio syndrome may be caused by further damage to the already partially injured anterior horn cells, which became more active at the time of the demise of the cells that caused the paralysis.[9] The syndrome not only affects the damaged musculature, but in some cases other sites that were considered to be reasonably normal at the time of the primary disease.[6,65] The syndrome is characterized by a slow progression of muscle atrophy and weakness, often associated with fasciculations. Muscle biopsy is not very revealing and the most difficult differential is from amyotrophic lateral sclerosis or possibly other viral diseases such as West Nile fever, both of which often rapidly progress,[9,27-29] while the postpolio syndrome stays relatively constant.[9,65] The prognosis for the syndrome appears to be reasonably good in that it is only slowly progressive and ceases to increase or extend to other sites over time.

References

1. Hamada G, Rida A: Orthopaedics and orthopaedic diseases in ancient and modern Egypt. *Clin Orthop Relat Res* 1972;89:253-268.

2. Underwood M: *A Treatise on the Diseases of Children*, ed 2. London, England, J Mathews, 1788, pp 53-57.

3. Heine J: *Beobachtungen uber Laihmungszustande der Untern Extremitaten und Deren Behandlung.* Stuttgart, Germany, Kohler, 1840.

4. Charcot JM, Joffroy A: Cas de paralysie infantile spinale avec lesions des cornes anterieures de la substance grise de la moelle epiniere. *Arch Physiol Norm Path* 1870;3:134-152.

5. Medin O: En epidemi af infantil paralysi. *Hygiea* 1890;52:657-658.

6. Paul A: *A History of Poliomyelitis*. New Haven, CT, Yale University Press, 1971.

7. Lovett RW, Lucas WD: Infantile paralysis: A study of 635 cases from the Children's Hospital, Boston with special reference to treatment. *JAMA* 1908;60:1677-1683.

8. Lovett RW: *The Treatment of Infantile Paralysis.* Philadelphia, PA, Blakiston Son and Company, 1917.

9. Rowland LP: Viral infections of the nervous system: Syndrome of acute anterior poliomyelitis, in Rowland LP (ed): *Merritt's Neurology*, ed 10. Philadelphia, PA, Lippincott William and Wilkins, 2000, pp 136-137.

10. Robbins FC, Enders JF, Weller TH, Florentino GL: Studies on the cultivation of poliomyelitis viruses in tissue culture: V. The direct isolation and serologic identification of virus strains in tissue culture from patients with non-paralytic and paralytic poliomyelitis. *Am J Hyg* 1951;54:286-293.

11. Robbins FC, Weller TH, Enders JF: Studies on the cultivation of poliomyelitis viruses in tissue culture: II. The propagation of the poliomyelitis viruses in roller-tube cultures of various human tissues. *J Immunol* 1952;69:673-694.

12. Ferguson AB: *Orthopaedic Surgery in Infancy and Childhood*, ed 2. Baltimore, MD, Williams and Wilkins Company 1963, 570-592.

13. Peltier LF: *Orthopedics: A History and Iconography.* San Francisco, CA, Norman Publishing Company, 1993, pp 168-194.

14. Strebel PM, Sutter RW, Cochi SL, et al: Epidemiology of poliomyelitis in the United States: One decade after the last reported case of indigenous wild virus-associated disease. *Clin Infect Dis* 1992;14:568-579.

15. Sutter RW, Prevots DR, Cochi SL: Poliovirus vaccines: Progress toward global poliomyelitis eradication and changing routine immunization recommendations in the United States. *Pediatr Clin North Am* 2000;47:287-308.

16. Mitchell JI: The residual paralysis and deformity of anterior poliomyelitis. *J Bone Joint Surg* 1925;7:619-629.

17. Sharrard WJW: Muscle paralysis in poliomyelitis. *Br J Surg* 1957;44:471-480.

18. Steindler A: *Postgraduate Lectures on Orthopaedics Diagnosis and Indications: Paralytic Disabilities.* Springfield IL, Charles C. Thomas 1951, Vol IIA, pp 1-60.

19. Brooks DM, Seddon HJ: Pectoral transplantation for paralysis of the flexors of the elbow. *J Bone Joint Surg Br* 1959;41:36-43.

20. Mayer L: Transplantation of the trapezius for paralysis of the abductors of the arm. *J Bone Joint Surg* 1927;9:412-420.

21. Sharrard WJW: The distribution of permanent paralysis in the lower limb in poliomyelitis: A clinical and pathological study. *J Bone Joint Surg Br* 1957;37:540-558.

22. Colonna PC: Hamstring transplantation for quadriceps paralysis. *J Bone Joint Surg* 1923;21:472-479.

23. Elzinga E, Key JA: Paralytic dislocations of the hip in poliomyelitis. *J Bone Joint Surg* 1932;11:867-881.

24. James JIP: Paralytic scoliosis. *J Bone Joint Surg Br* 1956;38:660-685.

25. Reidy JA, Broderick TF Jr, Barr JS: Tendon transplantations in the lower extremity: A review of the results in poliomyelitis. I: Tendon transplantation about the foot and ankle. *J Bone Joint Surg Am* 1952;34:900-908.

26. Somerville EW: Paralytic dislocation of the hip. *J Bone Joint Surg Br* 1959;41:279-288.

27. Al-Shekhlee A, Katirji B: Electrodiagnostic features of acute paralytic poliomyelitis associated with West Nile virus infection. *Muscle Nerve* 2004;29:376-380.

28. Jeha LE, Suka CA, Lederman RJ, et al: West Nile virus infection: A new acute paralytic illness. *Neurology* 2003;61:55-59.

29. Goldman AS, Schmalstieg EJ, Freeman DH Jr, Goldman DA, Schmalstieg FC Jr: What was the cause of Franklin Delano Roosevelt's paralytic illness? *J Med Biogr* 2003;11:232-240.

30. Mayer L, Green W: Experiences with the Steindler flexorplasty at the elbow. *J Bone Joint Surg* 1954;36A:775-789.

31. Segal A, Seddon HJ, Brooks DM: Treatment of paralysis of the flexors of the elbow. *J Bone Joint Surg* 1959;41B:44-50.

32. Steindler A: *Orthopedic Operations: Indications, Tech-

niques and End Results. Oxford, England, Blackwell Scientific Publishing Ltd, 1947.

33. Cohn V: *Sister Kenny: The Woman Who Challenged The Doctors.* Minneapolis, MN, University of Minnesota Press, 1975.

34. Lange F: The orthopedic treatment of spinal paralysis. *Arch Pediatr* 1910;8:837-848.

35. Kenny E: *The Treatment of Infantile Paralysis in the Acute Stage.* Minneapolis, MN, Bruce Publishing Company, 1941.

36. Lange F: Die schnenverpflanzumg. *Zeit Orthop Chir* 1903;12:16-44.

37. McCarroll HR, Crego CH: An evaluation of physiotherapy in the early treatment of anterior poliomyelitis. *J Bone Joint Surg* 1941;23:851-861.

38. Pohl JF, Kenny E: *The Kenny Concept of Infantile Paralysis and its Treatment.* St. Paul, MN, Bruce Publications, 1943.

39. Nicoladoni C: Nachtrag zum pes calcaneus und zur transplantation der peronealsehnen. *Arch Klin Chir* 1881;27:660-666.

40. Codavilla A: On the means of lengthening in the lower limbs, the muscles and tissues which are shortened through deformity. *Am J Orthop Surg* 1905;11:353-369.

41. Biesalski K, Mayer L: *Die Physiolgische Sehenverpflanzung.* Berlin, Germany, Julius Springer, 1916.

42. Goldthwaite JE: Tendon transplantation in the treatment of paralytic deformities. *Trans Amer Orthop Assoc* 1895;8:20-30.

43. Whitman R: The operative treatment of paralytic talipes of the calcaneus type. *Am J Med Sci* 1901;122:593-601.

44. Jones R: Certain operative procedures in paralysis of children. *BMJ* 1911;2:1520-1524.

45. Hoffa A: The final results in tendon transplantation. *Am J Orthop Surg* 1904;2:34-37.

46. Hoke M: An operation for stabilizing paralytic feet. *J Orth Surg* 1921;3:494-507.

47. Peabody CW: Tendon transplantation: An end result study. *J Bone Joint Surg* 1938;20:193-205.

48. Schwartzmann JR, Crego CH: Hamstring tendon transplantation for the relief of quadriceps femoris paralysis in residual poliomyelitis. *J Bone Joint Surg* 1941;30A:541-549.

49. Yount CC: An operation to improve function in quadriceps paralysis. *J Bone Joint Surg* 1938;20:314-319.

50. Dickson FD: An operation for stabilizing paralytic hips: A preliminary report. *J Bone Joint Surg* 1927;9:1-7.

51. Dunn N: Reconstructive surgery in paralytic deformities of the leg. *J Bone Joint Surg* 1930;11:299-308.

52. Legg AT: Transplantation of tensor fasciae femoris in cases of weakened gluteus medius. *JAMA* 1923;23:242-244.

53. Steindler A: *The Rehabilitation of the Paralyzed Patient.* New York, NY, Appleton Century Crofts, Inc, 1925.

54. Steindler A: The treatment of the flail ankle: Pan-astragaloid arthrodesis. *J Bone Joint Surg* 1923;5:284-294.

55. Steindler A: Operative treatment of paralytic conditions of the upper extremity. *J Orthop Surg (Hong Kong)* 1919;21:608-624.

56. Putti V: The operative lengthening of the femur. *JAMA* 1921;77:934-935.

57. Harrington PR: Treatment of scoliosis: Correction and internal fixation by spine instrumentation. *J Bone Joint Surg Am* 1962;44:591-610.

58. Hibbs RA: The treatment of deformities of the spine caused by poliomyelitis. *JAMA* 1917;69:787-791.

59. Salk JE: Studies in human subjects on active immunization against poliomyelitis: I. A preliminary report of experiments in progress. *JAMA* 1953;151:1081-1098.

60. Salk JE: Immunization against poliomyelitis. *Pediatr Clin North Am* 1953;1:49-51.

61. Salk JE: Recent studies on immunization against poliomyelitis. *Pediatrics* 1953;12:471-482.

62. Sabin AB: Oral poliovirus vaccine: History of its development and prospects for eradication of poliomyelitis. *JAMA* 1965;194:872-876.

63. Sabin AB: Poliomyelitis vaccination: Evaluation and direction in continuing application. *Am J Clin Pathol* 1978;70(1 suppl):136-140.

64. Centers for Disease Control and Prevention (CDC): Progress for global eradication of poliomyelitis, January 2003-2004. *MMWR Morb Mortal Wkly Rep* 2004;53:532-535.

65. Dalakas MC, Elder G, Hallett M, et al: A long term follow-up of patients with post-poliomyelitis neuromuscular symptoms. *N Engl J Med* 1986;314:959-963.

Chapter 5

Hematogenous Osteomyelitis

Spontaneously occurring infection of a bone is an ancient disorder. Aside from fractures, it was probably the most common cause of pain and disability in the osseous system. Recognition of the various disease syndromes, improved culture techniques, and most of all the discovery of penicillin and other antibiotics have markedly diminished the frequency and the severity of hematogenous osteomyelitis. Instead, traumatic or surgically induced osteomyelitis has now in large measure replaced the hematogenous disorder as the principal cause of bone infection. Hematogenous disease still represents the major model of the process. Today, for some children and, to a lesser extent, adults the diagnosis and treatment remain problematic.

History of Hematogenous Osteomyelitis

The history of hematogenous osteomyelitis is quite fascinating—in terms of description of the various forms of the disease, identification of the complications, introduction of treatment protocols, and now the marked decline in frequency of the disorder. Characteristic changes have been described in the study of fossil bones.[1] The clinical syndrome in patients was described by several physicians in times long past, who indicated that probing the site and causing drainage could relieve the pain and reduce the extent of the damage.[2-5] The disease was described in detail in 1773 by William Bromfield[6] and subsequently in 1831 by Nathan Smith;[7] both defined some of the unique features such as the bone abscess, the presence of septic necrosis, and the involucrum arising from the periosteum. Shortly thereafter, Benjamin Collins Brodie[8] described a form of the disease with an extensive collection of purulent tissue and fluid but with less bone reaction, which subsequently became known as a Brodie's abscess. The name for the disease, osteomyelitis, was introduced in the middle 19th century by Nelaton[9] and Chassaignac.[10] Becker[11] described the organism most commonly found in patients with osteomyelitis, which was subsequently determined to be *Staphylococcus aureus*. Carl Garre[12] supported this finding and also described a special form of the disease characterized by dense bone surrounding the abscess, which is now known as sclerosing osteomyelitis of Garre. By the 1920s, the organisms were well identified; Starr's article[13] and Wilensky's classic text[14] clearly defined the disease and the problems in management. Several authors described surgical techniques, including saucerization of the infection site; they hoped that eliminating the dead bone would allow blood vessels to enter the site and help to eliminate the disease.[15-17] Through the magnificent efforts of Alexander Fleming, Earnest Chain, and Howard Florey in the 1940s, however, penicillin was discovered; the world of infection and even that of osteomyelitis changed radically.[18,19] Although there have been challenges in recent years with changes in the organisms and the need for other antibiotics and different surgery, hematogenous osteomyelitis is no longer the devastating problem that it once was.

Biology and Histology

Hematogenous osteomyelitis is a bacterial disease in which the organisms are implanted in the bone through vascular channels and then proceed to proliferate and cause highly characteristic changes in the bone structure.[20-25] Osteomyelitis adheres to "Phemister's "Law," which states that the highest rate of occurrence of the disorder is in the most rapidly growing part of the longest bone in the body—hence the distal femur. The next most frequent occurrence is, by definition, the proximal tibia, followed by the proximal femur, proximal humerus, and distal radius in that order.

The pathogenesis of the disease is not completely understood, but is believed to occur in relation to arterial and venous blood flow. The arterial flow is highest in the sites adjacent to the epiphyses, but this region is also the site of slower venous flow because of the size of the bone and the metaphyseal structure.[25,26] Partial venous obstruction may occur in the small veins at the site of subchondral bone formation beneath the epiphysis in the child, or in the same site even after epiphyses are closed in the adult. Furthermore, at least for the distal femur and proximal tibia, it is the most frequent site of trauma. Whatever the cause,

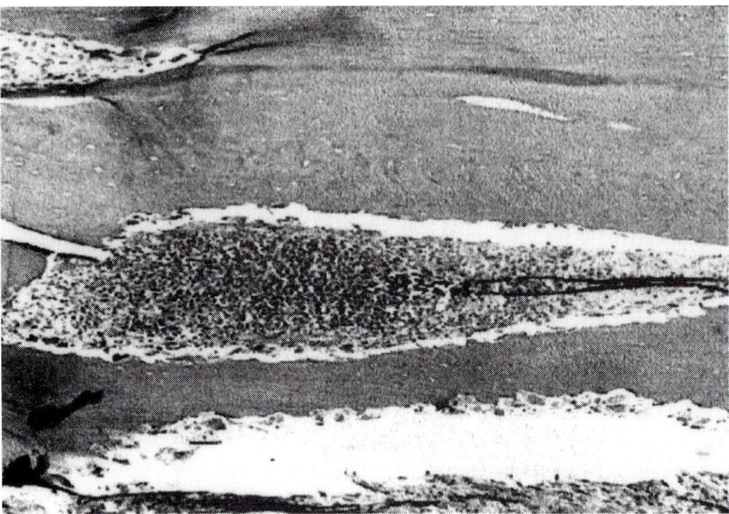

Figure 1
Histologic picture of an intraosseous osteomyelitic focus and resultant osteonecrosis in the adjacent bone. Hematoxylin and eosin × 40.

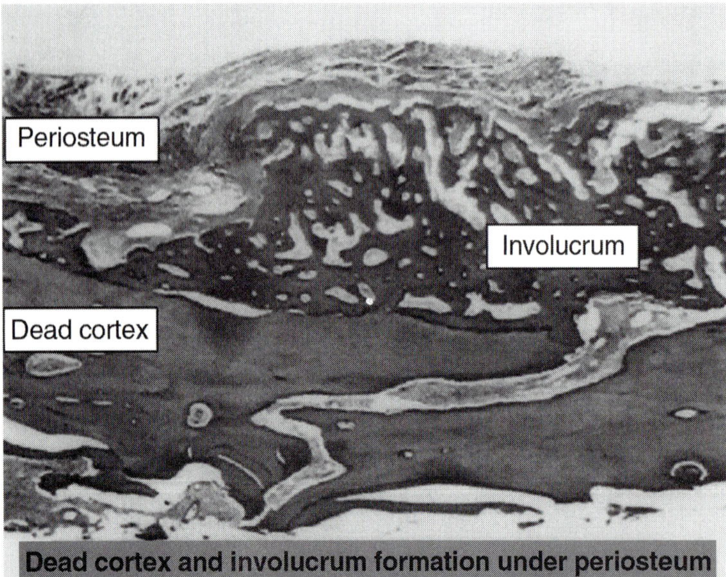

Figure 2
Bone formation occurring in the periosteal involucrum of an osteomyelitic focus that has broken out of the osteonecrotic cortex. Hematoxylin and eosin × 20.

the bacteria that have entered the body (usually through the oral cavity) and are circulating in the blood stream end their voyage in the partially obstructed veins and begin to divide. With division, the organisms not only produce further venous and arterial obstruction, but also produce toxic substances that cause localized tissue death and further obstructive damage to the bones' vascular supply; this then results in the condition known as septic necrosis of bone[22,23] (Figure 1). The bone is damaged by the organisms and their toxic materials, and is partially destroyed. The bacterial fluid then tracks through to and destroys the cortex to form a fistulous tract to the periosteal sleeve. The periosteum is pushed away from the bone and periosteal new bone appears at the site and ultimately surrounds the bone (Figure 2). The three characteristics of this process are described in Latin, and have been termed the osteomyelitis Latin lesson. The osteonecrotic segment is known as a sequestrum; the defects in the bone and cortex are described as cloacae; and the subperiosteal bone around the cortex is defined as the involucrum.[22,23,27]

Most patients today with hematogenous osteomyelitis are children.[22-24,28,29] The disease has become rare in adults unless they have some systemic disorder that puts them at greater risk for infectious disease.[22,23,25,27] Systemic conditions that render patients more susceptible include malnutrition, renal failure, alcohol abuse, immune deficiency, human immunodeficiency virus (HIV) infection, chronic hypoxia, malignancy, diabetes mellitus, steroid therapy, and tobacco abuse. In addition, local factors that may increase the likelihood of osteomyelitis include lymphadenitis, venous stasis, vascular compromise, chronic deforming arthritis, scarring, and radiation exposure. Most osteomyelitic processes in adults are currently related to trauma, surgical procedures, skin loss, insertion of allografts, and total joint procedures.[22,30-33]

Classification of Osteomyelitis

Two systems have been proposed for the classification of hematogenous and other types of osteomyelitis. The first, published in 1970, was developed by Waldvogel and associates,[25] who defined the disease as either acute or chronic. The second scheme,

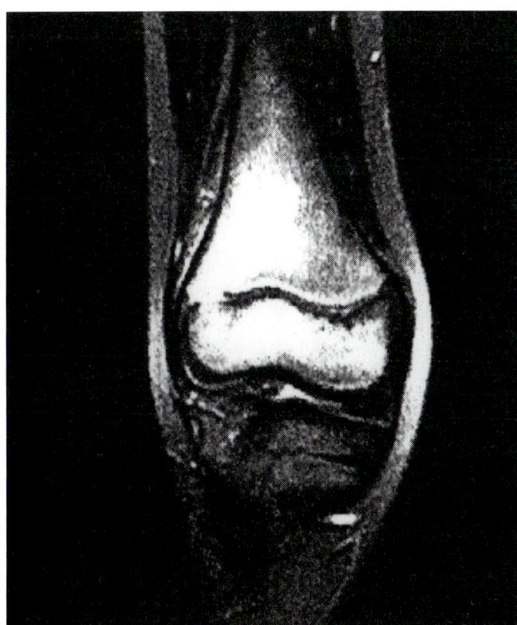

Figure 3
Early acute osteomyelitis is often not visible on standard radiography, but MRI may disclose an extraordinary degree of osseous edema.

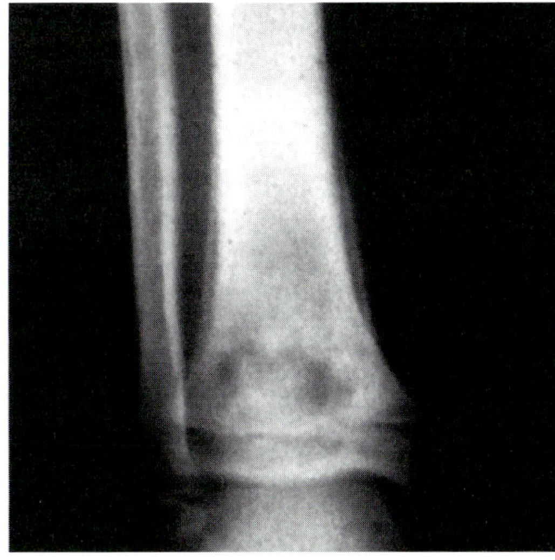

Figure 4
Subacute disease usually shows the destructive focus within the bone and the presence of subperiosteal involucrum.

published by Cierny, Mader, and Penninck,[27] consisted of four stages: medullary disease (stage 1), in which the infection is confined to the medullary cavity; cortical disease (stage 2), in which the lesion is located in the cortex and remains superficial; localized disease (stage 3), in which both the cortex and the medullary cavity are involved; and diffuse disease (stage 4), in which the infection involves the entire thickness of the bone with loss of stability and nonunion.

Physical Findings, Laboratory Tests, and Imaging Studies

Early osteomyelitis is predictably associated with pain and tenderness over the affected part. In children, modest swelling may be present that gradually increases, and the skin over the site often becomes erythematous.[23,24,29,34,35] The patient may have a fever, leukocytosis, a rapid sedimentation rate, and increased C-reactive protein.[36] Adults with early osteomyelitis may be only vaguely symptomatic for months and have a low-grade fever.[23,27,35] Patients with spinal disease may complain of pain and limitation of motion, and occasionally diminished neural function.[23,36] Patients with early osteomyelitis may show no changes on routine radiographs and, in many cases, bones and soft tissues appear normal. The bone and gallium scans are almost always positive, even with early disease;[22,37,38] the computed tomography (CT) and magnetic resonance imaging (MRI) will usually show soft-tissue swelling and sites of edema within the bone[22,23,26,39,40] (Figure 3). With advancing disease, the pain becomes more severe and when the disease is metaphyseal, the joint often becomes limited in function.[22,23,34] Fever and symptoms of progressive systemic illness increase.[22,34] Radiographs may now show destructive changes in the cortex and soft-tissue enlargement at the site of the involucrum (Figure 4). Sequestrae are dense, while the remainder of the bone may be osteopenic.[22] CT and MRI scans are at this point diagnostic, with destructive damage to the bone, cloacae, involucrum, and sequestrae very evident on the imaging studies[22,23,26,39,40] (Figure 5). The bone may break at some point, and then the pain increases and the disability becomes extreme.[22]

As the amount of purulent fluid increases, it may ultimately break through the skin. With such an event, the pain often diminishes and the patient's temperature is reduced. The defect in the skin may be small or large and can be in multiple sites, all of which discharge at times copious amounts of purulent and sometimes foul-smelling material.[22,23,30,31,33,41-43]

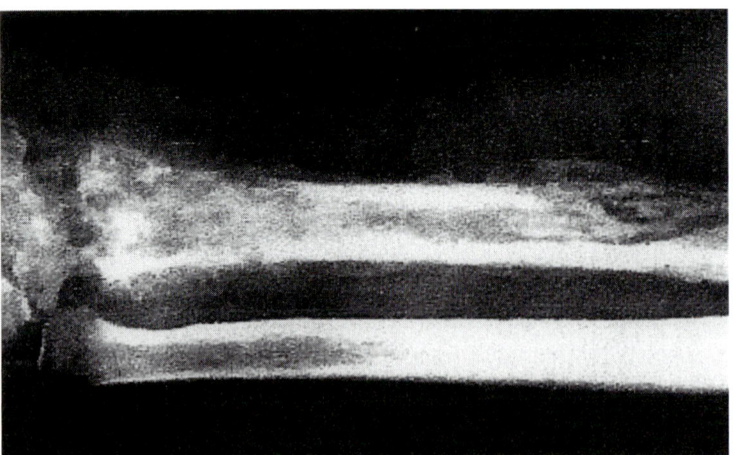

Figure 5
Chronic osteomyelitis shows excessive bone destruction with foci of osteonecrosis and marked involucrum formation.

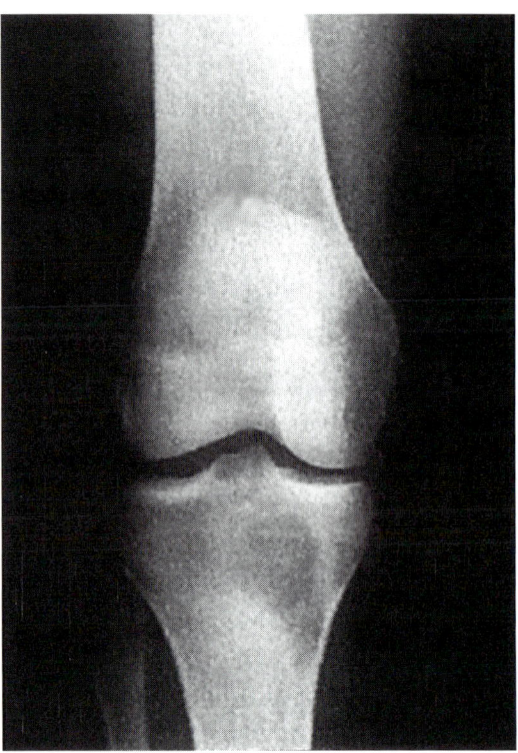

Figure 6
Brodie's abscess is a collection of low-grade osteomyelitis in a thin-walled bony shell, seen here in the proximal tibia.

Pathologic Organisms Associated with Hematogenous Osteomyelitis

The organism most frequently responsible for hematogenous osteomyelitis remains *S aureus* for all patients, but especially for infants and young children.[22-24,44-46] *Streptococcus pyogenes, S agalactiae, Escherichia coli,* and *Haemophilus influenzae* are also frequently seen in children. Other organisms include salmonella or *S pneumoniae,* both of which are common in patients with sickle cell anemia, and *Bartonella, Candida,* or *Mycobacterium avium,* which are occasionally noted in patients with HIV infection.[22-24,45-49]

Special Forms of Osteomyelitis

The form of the disease described above is the standard hematogenous osteomyelitic process, but a number of other forms exist, with some unusual features.

- *Thin-walled abscess of Brodie.*[8] These lesions have less excessive surrounding bone, and principally consist of a collection of purulent material inside the bone. The disease is believed to be milder than the standard form (Figure 6).
- *Sclerosing osteomyelitis of Garre.*[12] The bone surrounding a relatively small abscess is dense and usually does not demonstrate cloacae or sequestrae. The entire lesion is sometimes small in size and resembles an osteoid osteoma (Figure 7).

- *Vertebral disease.* Uncommon in adults, vertebral disease may present with bony collapse and localized collections of purulent material in the disk space and canal. The patient may develop neurologic problems, including Charcot's arthropathy of the feet.[22,34,49]
- *Gram-negative osteomyelitis in patients with sickle cell anemia.*[47] The infecting organism for patients with sickle cell anemia is usually salmonella. The disease may occur in multiple sites, including digits of hands and feet.[22,46,47]
- *Diskitis in children.* Ordinarily, vertebral osteomyelitis is rare and usually affects one segment. In children, the disk space may be involved and the two adjacent vertebrae show bony changes. The disease is relatively limited in severity and sometimes disappears spontaneously.[28,34,46]
- *Diaphyseal osteomyelitis.* Most of the bacterial hematogenous osteomyelitis affects the metaphyseal sites in the femur, tibia, etc, but these lesions are located in the diaphyseal regions of the bone and expand the cortex without

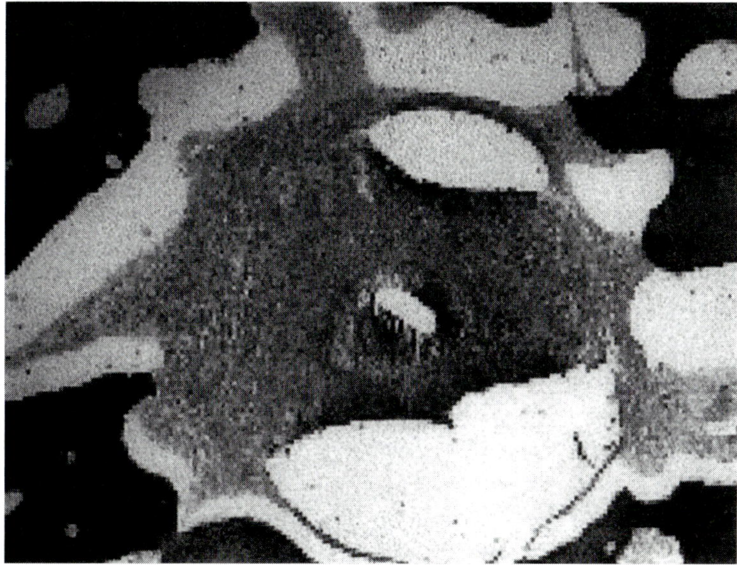

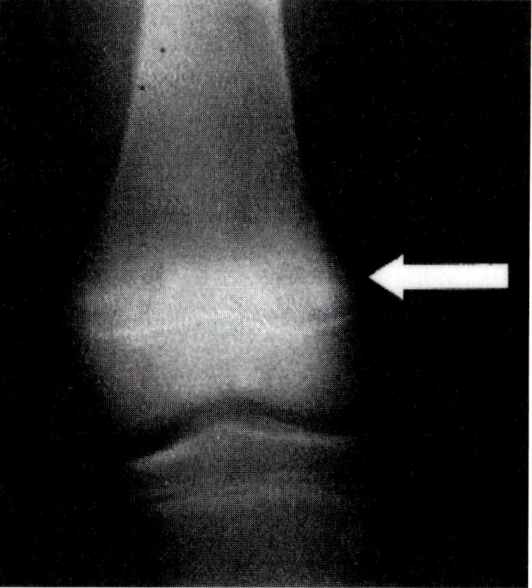

Figure 7
The characteristic histologic findings for a sclerosing osteomyelitis of Garre. Shown here are the collection of cells (bacteria is present within them), surrounded by areas of dense osteonecrotic bone. Hematoxylin and eosin × 40.

Figure 8
A relatively new entity is multicentric metaphyseal osteomyelitis in teenaged children. This often responds well to antibiotics, but may be present in several sites.

major destructive elements or necrotic segments.[22]

- *Multicentric metaphyseal osteomyelitis.* Lesions are more common in young children and frequently affect multiple metaphyseal sites adjacent to the calcified zone of the epiphyseal plates[22,34,39] (Figure 8).

The information above relates only to hematogenous osteomyelitis and does not apply to osteomyelitis occurring in relation to fractures, surgical procedures, insertion of allografts, major skin loss, burns, etc. The infecting organisms for these latter types are highly variable (although staphylococcus is still the most frequent), and the anatomic site, biology, and histologic structure may have little resemblance to that described above.

Treatment of Osteomyelitis

Many protocols have been proposed for the treatment of hematogenous and indeed other forms of osteomyelitis. The techniques include surgical and antibiotic treatments.

Treatment for Early or Mild Disease

The principal protocol is open biopsy to obtain culture material; abscess drainage; and, if necessary, simple débridement. For acute lesions, particularly in children, this is an effective approach and in fact may not be necessary if antibiotic solutions are effective in altering the changes. For Brodie's abscesses, simple drainage may be all that is necessary; if surgery is necessary for sclerosing lesions of Garre, simple excision of the small lesion may be effective.[22-24,29,34,35,39,50] Metaphyseal lesions at multiple sites in young people should probably be treated with antibiotics, as should the multiple sites seen in patients with sickle cell disease. For all the mild lesions, antibiotics are essential. Most effective for gram-positive staphylococci and streptococci are penicillin G, nafcillin, rifampin, ciprofloxacin, levofloxacin, gatifloxacin, clindamycin, linezolid, cotrimoxazole, and vancomycin. For gram-negative organisms, tobramycin, ampicillin, cefazolin, vancomycin, and gentamycin are often effective.[22-25,35,39,45-48] Most often these can be given intravenously initially, and then orally.

Treatment of Late or Extensive Osteomyelitis

Most of these patients will need surgery, and the procedures are principally those of débridement, extensive washing with antibiotic solutions, removal of dead tissue and damaged skin and soft tissue, insertion of antibiotic beads or polymethylmethacrylate with appropriate antibiotics, and prolonged immobilization, most often with drains including vacuum systems.[16,21,22,30,31,33,41-43,50-58] These patients usually require antibiotics for a prolonged period. Treatment of fractures or nonunions is often difficult and may require extensive multiple procedures, including insertion of hardware and even at times amputation.

Why are these lesions so difficult to treat with competent antibacterial regimens?[19] With mild disease, it is possible that the organisms gain an intracellular status and cannot be reached by the antibiotic agents.[44] Advanced disease has the ability to close off parts of the vascular system and maintain a large segment of the diseased bone in an avascular state.[22] Thus systemic antibiotics cannot penetrate the avascular bony blockade, and the bacteria (although isolated) continue to thrive. As noted above, a number of new approaches to these problems have been developed that involve special techniques for implantation of antibiotics.[16,31,33,42,43,45,46,48,50-56,58] Despite these advances, however, the credo "once an osteo, always an osteo" seems to maintain a remarkable credibility.

Summary

Hematogenous osteomyelitis was at one time a mysterious entity that caused severe problems for children and even adults. The treatment initially was ineffective, and sometimes caused great disability for the patient. Thanks to the development of antibiotics, as well as advancement in bacteriologic and imaging techniques, the hematogenous variant has become less of a problem. Many of the children who had severe problems now need no surgery and require only a short course of antibiotics. Although adults develop disease less frequently, it is often much more difficult to treat. In addition, the appearance of the adult lesion on imaging studies is sometimes difficult to distinguish from bone tumors, including Ewing's sarcoma, myeloma, or lymphoma. A much greater problem today is the often extensive bone infection that results from trauma, various forms of surgery, or in relation to disorders such as HIV, chronic pulmonary or renal disease, etc. These patients now far outnumber the hematogenous group and are in many ways much more difficult to treat.

References

1. Moodie RL: *Paleopathology: An Introduction to the Study of Ancient Evidences of Disease.* Urbana, IL, University of Illinois Press, 1923, pp 243-282.

2. Albucasis: *On Surgery and Instruments.* Translated by Spink MS, Lewis GL, Berkeley, CA, University of California Press, 1973, pp 347-348.

3. Celsus: *De Medicina.* Translated by Spencer WG, Cambridge, MA, Harvard University Press, 1953, pp 307-309.

4. Mackenzie A: A remarkable separation of part of the thigh bone. *Medical Observations and Inquiries* 1762;2:299-303.

5. Peltier LF: *Orthopedics: A History and Iconography.* San Francisco, CA, Norman Publishing Company, 1993, pp 101-120.

6. Bromfield W: *Chirurgical Observations and Cases.* London, England, T Cadell, 1773, pp 20-24.

7. Smith N: *Medical and Surgical Memoirs.* Baltimore, MD, William A. Francis, 1831, pp 98-100.

8. Brodie BC: An account of some cases of chronic abscesses of the tibia. *Med-Chir Trans* 1832;17:239-249.

9. Nelaton A: Elements de pathologie chirugicale. *Germer Bailliere* 1844;586:595-597.

10. Chassaignac E: De l'osteo-myelite. *Bull Mem Soc Chir Paris* 1852;3:431-436.

11. Becker J: Ein neuer microorganism. *Wien Mede Wschr* 1883;6:1410-1412.

12. Garre C: Ueber besondere formen und folge-zustande der acute infektiosen osteomyelitis. *Brun Beitr Klin Chir* 1893;10:241-298.

13. Starr CL: Acute hematogenous osteomyelitis. *Arch Surg* 1922;4:567-587.

14. Wilensky AO: *Osteomyelitis: Its Pathogenesis, Symptomatology and Treatment.* New York, NY, The Macmillan Company, 1934.

15. Armstrong B, Jarman TF: A method of dealing with chronic osteomyelitis by saucerization and skin grafting. *J Bone Joint Surg* 1936;18:387-398.

16. Bickel WH, Bateman JG, Johnson WE: Treatment of chronic hematogenous osteomyelitis by means of saucerization and bone grafting. *Surg Gynecol Obstet* 1953;96:265-274.

17. Orr HW: The treatment of osteomyelitis and other infected wounds by drainage and rest. *Surg Gynecol Obstet* 1927;45:446-464.

18. Altemeier WA: Penicillin therapy in acute osteomyelitis. *Surg Gynecol Obstet* 1945;81:138-157.

19. Chain E, Fleming A: Penicillin as a therapeutic agent. *Lancet* 1940;2:226-228.

20. Ciampolini J, Harding KG: Pathophysiology of chronic bacterial osteomyelitis: Why do antibiotics fail so often? *Postgrad Med J* 2000;76:479-483.

21. Cierny G III: Chronic osteomyelitis: Results of treatment. *Instr Course Lect* 1990;39:495-508.

22. Lazzarini L, Mader JT, Calhoun JH: Osteomyelitis in long bones. *J Bone Joint Surg Am* 2004;86:2305-2318.

23. Lew DP, Waldvogel FA: Osteomyelitis. *Lancet* 2004;364:369-379.

24. Song KM, Sloboda JF: Acute hematogenous osteomyelitis in children. *J Am Acad Orthop Surg* 2001;9:166-175.

25. Waldvogel FA, Medoff G, Swartz MN: Osteomyelitis: A review of clinical features, therapeutic considerations and unusual aspects. *N Engl J Med* 1970;282:260-266.

26. Kuhn JP, Berger PE: Computed tomographic diagnosis of osteomyelitis. *Radiology* 1979;130:503-506.

27. Cierny G III, Mader JT, Penninck JJ: A clinical staging for adult osteomyelitis. *Clin Orthop Rel Res* 2003;414:7-24.

28. Blyth MJ, Kincaid R, Craigen MA, Bennet GC: The changing epidemiology of acute and subacute haematogenous osteomyelitis in children. *J Bone Joint Surg Br* 2001;83:99-102.

29. Reinehr T, Burk G, Michel E, Andler W: Chronic osteomyelitis in childhood: Is surgery always indicated? *Infection* 2000;28:282-286.

30. Beals RK, Bryant RE: The treatment of chronic open osteomyelitis of the tibia in adults. *Clin Orthop Relat Res* 2005;433:212-217.

31. May JW Jr, Jupiter JB, Gallico GG III, Rothkopf DM, Zingarelli P: Treatment of chronic traumatic bone wounds: Microvascular free tissue transfer. A 13-year experience with 96 patients. *Ann Surg* 1991;214:241-252.

32. Tomford WW, Thornaphasuk J, Mankin HJ, Ferraro MJ: Frozen musculoskeletal allografts: A study of the clinical incidence and causes of infection associated with their use. *J Bone Joint Surg Am* 1990;72:1137-1143.

33. Zalavras CG, Patzakis MJ, Holtom P: Local antibiotic therapy in the treatment of open fractures and osteomyelitis. *Clin Orthop Relat Res* 2004;427:86-93.

34. Auh JS, Binns HJ, Katz BZ: Retrospective assessment of subacute or chronic osteomyelitis in children and young adults. *Clin Pediatr (Phila)* 2004;43:549-555.

35. Shih HN, Shih LY, Wong YC: Diagnosis and treatment of subacute osteomyelitis. *J Trauma* 2005;58:83-87.

36. Unkila-Kallio L, Kallio MJ, Eskola J, Peltola H: Serum C-reactive protein, erythrocyte sedimentation rate, and white blood cell count in acute hematogenous osteomyelitis of children. *Pediatrics* 1994;93:59-62.

37. Connolly LP, Connolly SA, Drubach LA, Jaramillo D, Treves ST: Acute hematogenous osteomyelitis of children: Assessment of skeletal scintigraphy-based diagnosis in the era of MRI. *J Nucl Med* 2002;43:1310-1316.

38. Losbona R, Rosenthall L: Observations of the sequential use of 99mTc-phosphate complex and 67 Ga imaging in osteomyelitis, cellulitis, and septic arthritis. *Radiology* 1977;123:123-129.

39. Hempfing A, Placzek R, Gottsche T, Meiss AL: Primary subacute epiphyseal and metaphyseal osteomyelitis in children: Diagnosis and treatment guided by MRI. *J Bone Joint Surg Br* 2003;65:559-564.

40. Ma LD, Frassica FJ, Bluemke DA, Fishman EK: CT and MRI evaluation of musculoskelelal infection. *Crit Rev Diagn Imaging* 1997;38:535-568.

41. Cierny G III, Mader J: The surgical treatment of adult osteomyelitis, in Evarts CM (ed): *Surgery of the Musculoskeletal System*. New York, NY, Churchill Livingstone, 1983, pp 15-35.

42. Mooney JF, Argenta LC, Marks MW, et al: Treatment of soft tissue defects in pediatric patients using the VAC system. *Clin Orthop Relat Res* 2000;376:26-31.

43. Parsons B, Strauss E: Surgical management of chronic osteomyelitis. *Am J Surg* 2004;188(suppl 1A):57-66.

44. Ellington JK, Harris M, Webb L, et al: Intracellular Staphyloccus aureus: A mechanism for the indolence of osteomyelitis. *J Bone Joint Surg Br* 2003;85:918-921.

45. Lazzarini L, Lipsky BA, Mader JT: Antibiotic treatment of osteomyelitis: What have we learned from 36 years of clinical trials? *Int J Infect Dis* 2005;9:127-138.

46. Mader JT, Calhoun J: Antimicrobial treatment of musculoskeletal disorders, in Evarts CM (ed): *Surgery of the Musculoskeletal System*, ed 2. New York, NY, Churchill Livingstone, 1990, vol 5, pp 4323-4336.

47. Epps CH Jr, Bryant DD III, Coles MJ, Castro O: Osteomyelitis in patients who have sickle cell disease: Diagnosis and management. *J Bone Joint Surg Am* 1991;73:1281-1294.

48. Mader JT, Shirtliff ME, Bergquist SC, Calhoun J: Antimicrobial treatment of chronic osteomyelitis. *Clin Orthop Relat Res* 1999;360:47-65.

49. Weinstein MA, Eismont FJ: Infections of the spine in patients with human immunodeficiency disease. *J Bone Joint Surg Am* 2005;87:604-609.

50. Perry CR, Pearson RL: Local antibiotic delivery in the treatment of bone and joint infections. *Clin Orthop Relat Res* 1991;263:215-226.

51. Adams K, Couch L, Cierny G, et al: In vitro and in vivo evaluation of antibiotic diffusion from antibiotic-impregnated polymethylmethacrylate beads. *Clin Orthop Relat Res* 1992;278:244-252.

52. Hashmi MA, Norman P, Saleh M: The management of chronic osteomyelitis using the Lautenbach method. *J Bone Joint Surg Br* 2004;86:269-275.

53. Liu SJ, Wen-Neng Ueng S, Lin SS, Chan EC: In vivo release of vancomycin from biodegradable beads. *J Biomed Mater Res* 2002;63:807-813.

54. McLaren AC: Alternative materials to acrylic bone cement for delivery of dept antibiotics in orthopaedic infections. *Clin Orthop Relat Res* 2004;427:101-106.

55. Minami A, Kaneda K, Itoga H: Treatment of infected segmental defect of a long bone with vascularized bone transfer. *J Reconstr Microsurg* 1992;8:75-82.

56. Rutledge B, Huyette D, Day D, Anglen J: Treatment of osteomyelitis with local antibiotics delivered via bioabsorbable polymer. *Clin Orthop Relat Res* 2003;411:280-287.

57. Simpson AH, Deakin M, Latham JM: Chronic osteomyelitis: The effect of the extent of the surgical resection on infection-free survival. *J Bone Joint Surg Br* 2001;83:403-407.

58. Scott DM, Rotschafer JC, Behrens F: Use of vancomycin and tobramycin polymethylmethacrylate impregnated beads in the management of chronic osteomyelitis. *Drug Intell Clin Pharm* 1988;22:480-483.

Chapter 6

Articular Cartilage Healing and Osteoarthritis

Articular cartilage is a wonderfully unique tissue in many respects. Covering the bones of the joints, the cartilage provides a system with a remarkable capacity for frictionless and pain-free joint movement (Figure 1). The tissue has no blood, lymphatic, or nerve supply and hence lives in a world of "splendid isolation" from the rest of the body. There is no reason to believe that the other body systems have any recognition of the existence, chemical composition, or activities of the cartilage. The cells derive their nutrition by a double diffusion system: first from the blood stream to the synovium, and from there to the synovial fluid; and second, by transport across the cartilage external membrane, which limits material by both size and chemical structure. In fact, the cartilage chemical construct prevents the ingress of unwanted materials and the egress of important agents required by the cartilage for normal function. The matrix of cartilage consists of some unique components, namely special collagens and large molecules known as aggrecan, which consist principally of glycosaminoglycans on a protein string. A large number of aggrecan molecules are attached to a filament of hyaluronic acid; multiple segments provide a major component of the cartilage structure, its relation to water content, and its resiliency. Unfortunately, cartilage in adults has a very limited capacity for repair. With acute or chronic injury, the cartilage can be damaged and over time develop osteoarthritis.

Cartilage Structure and Composition

Articular cartilage has five distinct zones[1-6] (Figure 2). On the surface of the cartilage is a fine acellular filamentous zone called the lamina splendens. Beneath that is a zone occupying less than one fourth of the cartilage structure. This area, rich in collagen, is called the gliding zone. Beneath the gliding zone is the transitional zone, in which the cells are randomly arranged and the chemi-

cal components dominate the composition. Below that component, which occupies well over two thirds of the structure, is the radial zone, in which the cells are arranged in short columns at right angles to the surface. Beneath the radial zone is the calcified zone, which lies adjacent to the bony end plate of the subjacent osseous segment. The radial zone is separated from the calcified zone by the tidemark, a linear slightly, wavy bluish line seen best on hematoxylin- and eosin-stained sections.[1-5]

Articular cartilage consists of three major components—cells, matrix, and water—that all have a role and relationship to one

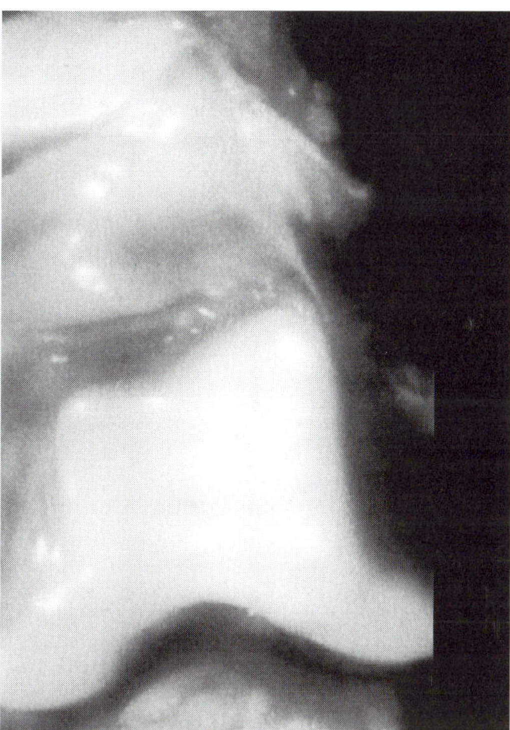

Figure 1

Normal cartilage in a knee joint. The coefficient of friction of the patella riding on the distal femur is approximately one fifth that of ice on ice. Despite the fact that the cartilage structure contains 70% water, the cartilage looks firm and clearly resistant to impact.

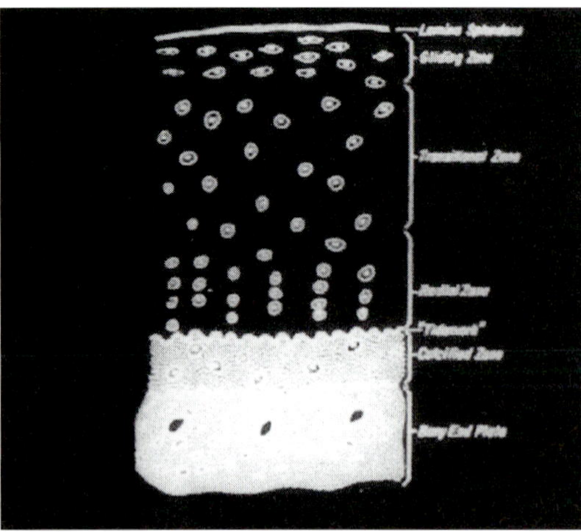

Figure 2
Cartilage organization includes the lamina splendens on the surface; the gliding zone, where the cells are longitudinally ordered and make collagen fibers that provide a "skin" to the structure; the transitional zone; the radial zone, where the cells are lined perpendicular to the surface; the tidemark, which separates the radial zone from the calcified zone; the calcified zone, in which the cells may not be alive or functional; and the bony end plate consisting of mature, quite dense bone.

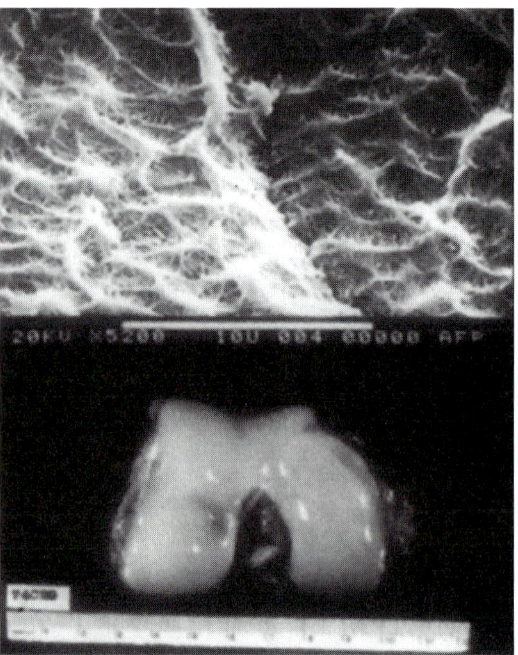

Figure 3
Although the surface of cartilage seems smooth, electron microscopy suggests that it is quite irregular in structure. Water discharged from the cartilage during pressure lies on the surface attached to the lamina splendens and represents the system for smooth functional movement with weight bearing.

another.[1-3] The number of cells is sparse by comparison with most other body tissues; the cells are separated from one another and seem to have no direct contact or relationship.[1,2,4,7-11] The cells vary somewhat in size and shape. The cells of the surface layer are elongated, resembling fibroblasts, and actually synthesize a large number of linearly placed collagen fibers in the surface layer (called by some the "skin" of the cartilage).[2,3,7,12-15] The cells of the intermediate zone of the cartilage are randomly arranged and moderate in size; they have components suggestive of active synthetic activities, as well as lysosomal bodies that contain enzymes.[1,2,4,7,14] The cells of the radial zone are smaller and less active in appearance; the cells of the calcified layer seem to be dead or at least dormant.[1,4,7,16] Beneath this region is the subchondral bone, which in adults does not provide nutrients to the cartilage but may affect the distribution and structure of the cartilage.[5,6,17]

Cartilage is heavily hydrated; approximately 70% of the material in cartilage is water, most of which is in the form of a gel.[3,4,18,19] With pressure on the cartilage surface, such as occurs with standing or especially compressive movement, the water passes off to the surface to attach to a part of the lamina splendens and forms the lubrication system.[4,15,19] Thus normal cartilage never touches cartilage in compressive movement; rather, the water abuts on the water in the surface system[4,15,19] (Figure 3).

The remaining materials consist of collagen, proteoglycan, and noncollagenous proteins. The collagens account for approximately 60% of the dry weight of the cartilage and include principally type II, but also smaller concentrations of types VI, IX, X, and XI, all of which play some role in the structure of the cartilage and to a limited extent the relationship of the cells to one another.[2-4,12,13,20] The proteoglycans consist of a core protein and negatively charged repeating disaccharides, which not only remain stiffly extended in space but also attract cations.[1-4,21] The glycosaminoglycans include chondroitin-4 sulfate, chondroitin-6 sulfate, and keratan sulfate.[3,4,21] These materials are fixed to protein cores with the aid of link proteins, and the entire structure—which is quite sizable—is now termed aggrecan molecules.[2,22-24] The aggrecan molecules in turn attach to a long filament of hyaluronic acid; these macromolecules, known as proteoglycan aggregates, are enormous in size and fill the intrafibrillar space.[1-4,22] Considerable alteration occurs in the aggrecan components with advancing age, with a fairly marked reduction in size and change in structure.[1,2,25,26]

Three other forms of proteoglycans are present in small concentrations—decorin, biglycan, and fibromodulin; all of them bind to type II collagen and are also involved in preventing the healing of cartilage defects, partly by interfering with transforming growth factor beta (TGF-β).[1,27-29] Other proteinaceous materials are present in low concentrations; these include anchorin CII, cartilage oligomeric protein, fibronectin, thrombospondin, and tenascin, all of which have roles in binding cells to collagen or maintaining the organization of the matrix.[2,5,30-39]

Chondrocyte Function

Despite the absence of blood supply, the low oxygen tension of articular cartilage (approximately 8%), and the low temperature of many joints (knee joint, approximately 34°C; ankle joint, 27°C), chondrocytes are active cells in terms of production of materials and, in children, cell replication.[2-4,16,40-43]

Chondrocytes synthesize proteoglycans, the link proteins, and other proteinaceous materials, sometimes at a fairly rapid rate.[1-4,21-24,44-46] They not only synthesize collagen, but once the material is produced and is outside the cell, the chondrocyte acts to cleave the molecules and set up crosslinks to increase the quality and organization of the structure.[3,4,11,13,20,41,47] Chondrocytes are also responsible for developing the degradative cascade, which includes interleukins, matrix metalloproteases (MMPs), collagenase, and aggrecanase.[1-4,44,48,49] In addition, however, the cells are responsible for producing other materials such as TGF-β, tissue inhibitors of metalloproteases, insulin-like growth factors, and plasminogen activator inhibitors, all of which diminish or prevent the action of the degradative materials.[3,4,36,37,49,50] Of considerable interest is how these activities are regulated in normal cartilage; it seems logical that weight-bearing movement and appropriate exercise activity are the logical activators of the materials that inhibit degradation.[3,4,15,51] This is one explanation for the role of controlled exercise in the prevention and treatment of cartilage injuries, even in elderly persons.[26,51-54]

Cartilage Synthesis and Response to Injury

Chondrocytes in immature individuals have the capacity to divide and enlarge the cartilaginous structure.[1-4,16,25] Not only is there evidence for DNA synthesis, but the rates of synthesis of collagen, proteoglycans, and other proteins are greater than those of adult cartilaginous tissues. With cessation of length growth, chondrocytes in normal cartilage no longer have the capacity to divide.[3,4,26,42] In three circumstances, however, the chondrocytes can regain this ability and actively synthesize new cells in support of the cartilage structure: cartilage injury that does not enter the underlying bone; cartilage injury in which the underlying bone is damaged; and osteoarthritis.

The response of connective and other tissues injuries includes four phases. The first of these is avascular, and consists of necrosis of tissue in response to the injury. The second is vascular and consists of inflammation, vascular dilatation, transudation, exudation, and organization of the fibrin clot into a vascular granulation tissue. The third phase is also vascular, and consists of fibrous (or osseous for bone injuries) repair, organization and fibrogenesis (osteogenesis for bone) of the granulation tissue, and scar (bone) formation. The final phase is one of scar (bone) remodeling.[1,4,44,54]

Cartilage injuries that do not penetrate the calcified layer usually respond in a classic fashion—death of cells at the sites of the injury and a modest biologic response related principally to the synovial inflammation. Because there is no blood supply, phase 2 is basically absent. Despite the absent blood supply, however, a modest DNA synthetic activity can often been seen in the cartilage; this rarely lasts longer than 2 weeks.[1,3,4,44,54] No remodeling can occur, and in fact the extent of the injury present initially remains the same regardless of the duration of follow-up.[1,3,4,44,52,54,55]

Those cartilage injuries that penetrate into the underlying bone cause a major response in the osseous tissues, which follows the pattern described above for response to injury. Death of tissue occurs in phase 1, followed by a marked vascular response in phase 2 with development of vascular granulation tissue. Although phase 3 should consist of bone formation, quite strikingly the response is one of production of cartilage, which augurs a good result. Regrettably, most of the time the material synthesized by the new chondrocytes seems to have too much type I collagen and other bone materials; in a relatively short period, it breaks down and becomes locally osteoarthritic.[1,3,4,44,52,54,55] Even if the response is partially competent, the amalgamation of the new material into the adjacent cartilage sites is poor and the fibrous "skin" is not ordinarily restored.[4,44,52]

Osteoarthritis

Osteoarthritis is a common progressive disorder of unknown cause, usually occurring late in life and principally affecting the hands and weight-bearing joints. The syndrome is characterized clinically by pain, deformity, and limitation of motion and pathologically by focal erosive lesions, cartilage destruction, subchondral bony sclerosis, cyst formation, and marginal osteophytes.[1,3,4,44,56]

Many etiologic factors have been postulated for osteoarthritis.[1,3,4,44] Although these include aging, this is not in itself accurate because the chemical changes that occur in cartilage with age are not those of osteoarthritis.[4,13,25,26,44] It seems more likely that the changes that occur with age are a prerequi-

site to the development of osteoarthritis. Genetic causes have been studied over the years, and although some genetic disorders include osteoarthritis as a characteristic, this is usually not a factor in most patients.[4,51] Nevertheless, study of family history may be helpful, particularly for hand and foot deformities. Hormonal changes have not been a noticeable cause, nor has biochemical alterations (with the exception of entities such as alkaptonuric ochronosis, hyperparathyroidism, renal osteodystrophy, or other diseases that cause calcification in joints). Paget's disease, in which the components of the joints are different sizes, may be a factor, as might unusual disorders such as Jaffe-Campanacci disease or Erdheim-Chester disease.[3,4,51]

Inflammatory disease may be a major issue in that the principal initiator of the degradative cascade in articular cartilage is probably synovial interleukin-1, which turns on the cartilage MMPs, leading to production of collagenase and aggrecanase.[1,3,4,10,20,35,44,48,49] Another possible explanation is related to damage to cartilage, which releases material that the body and, more specifically, the synovium does not recognize.[3,4] This leads to synovial inflammation and release of interleukins that begin the degradative cascade.[4,35] There can be little doubt, however, that most of the osteoarthritic changes seen in patients result from some form of mechanical injury, even slight or mild repetitive ones.[1,3,4,33,51-54,56] Increased body weight may be a problem as well. Regardless of cause, osteoarthritis is clearly the most common arthritic orthopaedic disorder and is certainly a major cause of disability.[3,4]

Histologic, Biochemical, and Clinical Characteristics of Osteoarthritis

Sequential histologic alterations in osteoarthritic cartilage show initial diminished staining of the tissue, irregularity of the surface of the cartilage, and clefts that descend deeper and deeper into the cartilaginous tissue.[1,3,4,17,44,57] The tidemark is violated by blood vessels, and the most striking feature is the presence of increased numbers of cells, often in clones, which appear to be attempting a restoration of the structure of the tissue[3-5,54,57] (Figure 4). The disease worsens, the clefts get deeper, and eventually the sur-

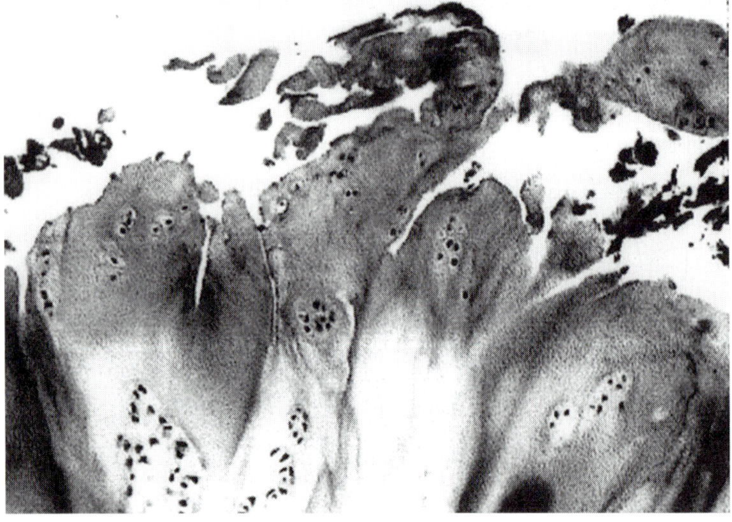

Figure 4

A histologic picture of osteoarthritic cartilage shows fragmentation of the surface, clefts, and cellular proliferation in clones. Hematoxylin and eosin × 40.

face is left with no cartilage at all, only the underlying dense and sometimes cyst-containing and osteonecrotic bone[4,57] (Figure 5). At the same time, cartilage and bone structures appear at the margins of the diseased joint; these are known as osteophytes.[3,4,6,17,50,57] The cartilage in this tissue is newly formed, as is the bone, and seems to represent an attempt at repair. Cysts may be very large and can occur on both sides of the joints[3,4,57] (Figure 5, *B*).

Biologically, the cartilage undergoes some major changes. There is an often marked increase in water content, and cartilage swelling occurs.[3,4,9,18,19,44] The proteoglycans are markedly diminished in concentration as are the collagens, but usually there is no change in the principal collagen type, which remains type II.[1,3,4,12,13,20,22,23,41,44,45,58] Materials of the degradative cascade are markedly increased in concentration and actively destructive of the cartilage. These materials include MMP-protease activator, an array of MMPs, synovial and cartilage interleukin-1, prostromelysin, procollagenase, proaggrecanase, plasminogen activator, and prostaglandins, all of which serve to produce collagenase, aggrecanase, and other materials that destroy the matrix of the cartilage.[1,3,4,10,35,43,48] The inhibitors of these materials include TGF-β, tissue inhibitors of matrix proteases, and plasminogen activator inhibitor, all of which attempt to reverse the action of the degradative agents but over time are unsuccessful and the cartilage disappears.[3,4,40,55]

Clinically, the joints become enlarged with fluid, can become profoundly limited in motion, display a creaking noise, and sometimes cause major disability. Imaging studies show the classic changes of narrow joints, dense subchondral bone sites, cysts, osteophytes, and sometimes fractured segments within the joints.[14,44,57] Computed tomography, magnetic resonance imaging (MRI), and high-resolution spectroscopy are useful in defining the extent of the disease and the possibility of surgical correction without total joint replacement.[59-61] A recent approach to defining the extent of the disease and, theoretically, the effect of treatment is the use of special stains using MRI. Gadolinium (DPTA)-2 is a special stain for glycosaminoglycan that can show the extent of cartilage damage more effectively than proton density or gadolinium alone.[59,60]

Treatment of Osteoarthritis

Numerous methods have been introduced over the years for the treatment of osteoarthritis.

- Anti-inflammatory drug treatment. Aspirin, acetaminophen, nonsteroidal anti-inflammatory drugs (Cox-1 inhibitors), Cox-2 inhibitors, and corticosteroids have all been used with some success. The approaches depend principally on reducing the inflammatory response in the synovium and possibly in the underlying bone and the adjacent cystic structures.[3,44,62,63]

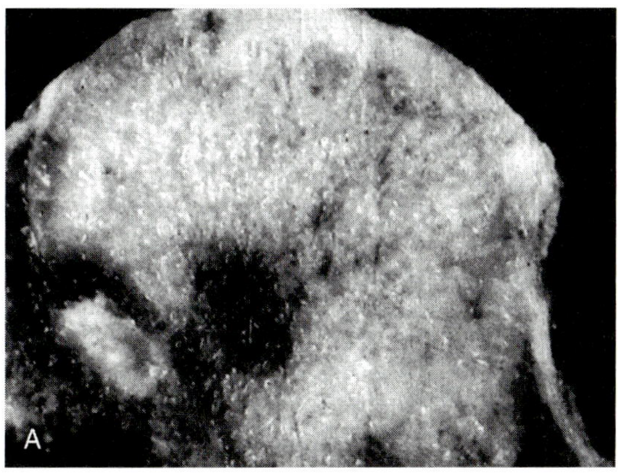
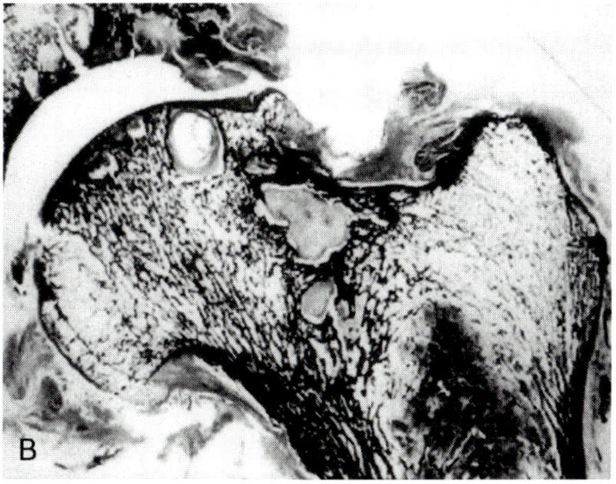

Figure 5
A, Cut section of the proximal femur showing the changes that occur with osteoarthritis. Note the osteophytes, the loss of surface cartilage, the small cysts, and the subchondral bone sclerosis. **B,** Radiographic image of a thin section of the same tissue, showing the cysts, osteophytes, and cartilage changes.

- Radiation treatment has been tried using approximately 60 Gy given over a prolonged period of time, but seems to be of limited value.[64]
- Injections of corticosteroids and hyaluronic analogs have resulted in mild to moderate improvement in patient complaints.[4,14,44,62,65]
- Recently, the introduction of chondroitin sulfate and glucosamine seems to provide some improvement for patients with osteoarthritis.[3,4,62]
- Physiotherapy designed to strengthen muscles about the damaged joint has a limited success rate, but is certainly an important addition to the treatment program.[4,44,53,62]
- Arthroscopic "washout" may be temporarily successful.[62,66-68]
- Deep cartilage defects can be treated by chondroplastic procedures producing tiny defects in the underlying bone, with autologous cartilage transplants, with cryopreserved allogeneic periosteum, or even with cartilage incubated with TGF-β.[1,40,44,55,69-73] Stem cells have also been introduced in scaffolds, but thus far have shown only limited success.[62,70,74]
- Another system recently introduced uses small segments of cartilage obtained from a condylar site in the joint, a technique known as mosaicplasty.[69,75]
- Allograft transplantation has achieved some success for condylar defects, particularly in the distal femur or proximal tibia.[1,4]
- Major surgical efforts such as osteotomy have a long history with limited success unless a specific error is to be corrected.[69,76] In the past, arthrodesis

has been advocated for certain types of osteoarthritic lesions such as those affecting the feet or hand bones[62,69]
- Total joint replacement surgery for hip, knee, or shoulder is usually successful, particularly for older patients.[48,62,77]

Current Status of Prevention, Assessment, and Treatment of Osteoarthritis

Although we now know a great deal more about the causes of osteoarthritis, it is clear that the extended life spans achieved over the past 40 or so years has enormously increased the number of patients with clinical osteoarthritis to the extent that it is now the most prevalent disease of the aged population. Some types of exercise, injury, and excessive weight clearly take a toll on the joints as do genetic factors and sometimes medication. We can make the diagnosis more readily on physical examination; clearly define the extent of the disease using imaging studies; and have an array of treatment protocols, some of which are modestly successful in reducing the patient's disability and restriction of activity but none that really "cure" the disease. The hope for the future is that agents can be identified that are the cause of cartilage degradation and methods of interfering with their actions can be sought by genetic means. Likewise it would be of great value if we could discover the agents that enhance cartilage repair, and introduce some genetic systems for activating them. Using these types of approaches, it is possible that the diagnosis could be made early in the course of the disease and that cartilage repair can take place prior to the end-stage disease that is now frequently seen in patients with osteoarthritis.

References

1. Buckwalter JA, Mankin HJ: Articular cartilage: Degeneration and osteoarthritis, repair, regeneration, and transplantation. *Instr Course Lect* 1998;47:487-504.

2. Buckwalter JA, Mankin HJ: Articular cartilage: Tissue design and chondrocyte-matrix interactions. *Instr Course Lect* 1998;47:477-486.

3. Buckwalter JA, Mankin HJ, Grodzinsky AJ: Articular cartilage and osteoarthritis. *Instr Course Lect* 2005;54:460-480.

4. Mankin HJ, Mow VC, Buckwalter JA, et al: Articular cartilage structure, composition and function, in Buckwalter JA, Einhorn TA, Simon SR (eds): *Orthopaedic Basic Science*, ed 2. Rosemont, IL, American Academy of Orthopaedic Surgeons, 2000, pp 443-470.

5. Redler I, Mow VC, Zimny ML, Mansell J: The ultrastructure and biomechanical significance of the tidemark of articular cartilage. *Clin Orthop Relat Res* 1975;112:357-362.

6. Reimann I, Mankin HJ, Trahan C: Quantitative histologic analyses of articular cartilage and subchondral bone from osteoarthritic and normal human hips. *Acta Orthop Scand* 1977;48:63-73.

7. Aydelotte MB, Schumacher BL, Kuettner KE: Heterogeneity of articular chondrocytes, in Kuettner KE, Schleyerbach R, Peyron JG, Hascall VC (eds): *Articular Cartilage and Osteoarthritis*. New York, NY, Raven Press, 1992, pp 237-249.

8. Buckwalter JA, Rosenberg LC: Electron microscopic studies of cartilage proteoglycans: Direct evidence for the variable length of the chondroitin sulfate-

rich region of the proteoglycan subunit core protein. *J Biol Chem* 1982;257:9830-9839.

9. Mankin HJ, Lippiello L: Biochemical and metabolic abnormalities in articular cartilage from osteoarthritic human hips. *J Bone Joint Surg Am* 1970;52:424-434.

10. Mankin HJ, Dorfman H, Lippiello L, Zarins A: Biochemical and metabolic abnormalities in articular cartilage from osteo-arthritic human hips: II. Correlation of morphology with biochemical and metabolic data. *J Bone Joint Surg Am* 1971;53:523-537.

11. Marcelino J, McDevitt CA: Attachment of articular cartilage chondrocytes to the tissue form of type VI collagen. *Biochim Biophys Acta* 1995;1249:180-188.

12. Eyre DR, Wu JJ, Woods P: Cartilage-specific collagens: Structural studies, in Kuettner KE, Schleyerbach R, Peyron JG, Hascall VC (eds): *Articular Cartilage and Osteoarthritis.* New York, NY, Raven Press, 1992, pp 119-131.

13. Eyre DR: Collagen structure and function in articular cartilage: Metabolic changes in the development of osteoarthritis, in Kuettner KE, Goldberg VM (eds): *Osteoarthritic Disorders.* Rosemont, IL, American Academy of Orthopaedic Surgeons, 1995, pp 219-227.

14. Kuettner KE, Schleyerbach R, Peyron JG, Hascall VC (eds): *Articular Cartilage and Osteoarthritis.* New York, NY, Raven Press, 1992.

15. Setton LA, Zhu W, Mow VC: The biphasic poroviscoelastic behavior of articular cartilage: Role of the surface zone in governing the compressive behavior. *J Biomech* 1993;26:581-592.

16. Hoffman LM, Weston AD, Underhill TM: Molecular mechanisms regulating chondroblast differentiation. *J Bone Joint Surg Am* 2003;85(suppl 2):124-132.

17. Oegema TR, Thompson RC: Histopathology and pathobiochemistry of the cartilage-bone interface in osteoarthritis, in Kuettner KE, Goldberg VM (eds): *Osteoarthritic Disorders.* Rosemont, IL, American Academy of Orthopaedic Surgeons, 1995, pp 205-217.

18. Mankin HJ: The water of articular cartilage, in Simon WH (ed): *The Human Joint in Health and Disease.* Philadelphia, PA, University of Pennsylvania Press, 1978, pp 37-42.

19. Maroudas A, Schneiderman R: "Free" and "exchangeable" or "trapped" and "nonexchangeable" water in cartilage. *J Orthop Res* 1987;5:133-138.

20. Sandell LJ: Molecular biology of collagens in normal and osteoarthritic cartilage, in Kuettner KE, Goldberg VM (eds): *Osteoarthritic Disorders.* Rosemont, IL, American Academy of Orthopaedic Surgeons, 1995, pp 131-146.

21. Roughley PJ, Lee ER: Cartilage proteoglycans: Structure and potential functions. *Microsc Res Tech* 1994;28:385-397.

22. Hardingham TE, Fosang AJ, Dudhia J: Aggrecan, the chondroitin/keratan sulfate proteoglycan from cartilage, in Kuettner KE, Schleyerbach R, Peyron JG, Hascall VC (eds): *Articular Cartilage and Osteoarthritis.* New York, NY, Raven Press, 1992, pp 5-20.

23. Sandell LJ, Chansky H, Zamparo O, Hering TM: Molecular biology of cartilage proteoglycans and link protein, in Kuettner KE, Goldberg VM (eds): *Osteoarthritic Disorders.* Rosemont, IL, American Academy of Orthopaedic Surgeons, 1995, pp 117-130.

24. Tang LH, Buckwalter JA, Rosenberg LC: The effect of link protein concentration on articular cartilage proteoglycan aggregation. *J Orthop Res* 1996;14:334-339.

25. Buckwalter JA, Roughley PJ, Rosenberg LC: Age-related changes in cartilage proteoglycans: Quantitative electron microscopic studies. *Microsc Res Tech* 1994;28:398-408.

26. Martin JA, Buckwalter JA: The role of chondrocyte senescence in the pathogenesis of osteoarthritis and in limiting cartilage repair. *J Bone Joint Surg Am* 2003;85(suppl 2):106-110.

27. Hedlund H, Mengarelli-Widholm S, Heinegard D, Reinhot FP, Svensson O: Fibromodulin distribution and association with collagen. *Matrix Biol* 1994;14:227-232.

28. Hildebrand A, Romaris M, Rasmussen LM, et al: Interaction of the small interstitial proteoglycans biglycan, decorin and fibromodulin with transforming growth factor beta. *Biochem J* 1994;302:527-534.

29. Poole AR, Rosenberg LC, Reiner A, Ionescu M, Bogoch E, Roughley PJ: Contents and distributions of the proteoglycans decorin and biglycan in normal and osteoarthritic human articular cartilage. *J Orthop Res* 1996;14:681-689.

30. Chevalier X, Groult N, Larget-Piet B, Zardi L, Hornebeck W: Tenascin distribution in articular cartilage from normal subjects and from patients with osteoarthritis and rheumatoid arthritis. *Arthritis Rheum* 1994;37:1013-1022.

31. Chevalier X: Fibronectin, cartilage, and osteoarthritis. *Semin Arthritis Rheum* 1993;22:307-318.

32. DiCesare PE, Morgelin M, Mann K, Paulsson M: Cartilage oligomeric protein and thrombospondin 1: Purification from articular cartilage, electron microscopic structure, and chondrocyte binding. *Eur J Biochem* 1994;223:927-937.

33. Farquhar T, Xia Y, Mann K, et al: Swelling and fibronectin accumulation in articular cartilage explants after cyclical impact. *J Orthop Res* 1996;14:417-423.

34. Hayashi T, Abe E, Jasin HE: Fibronectin synthesis in superficial and deep layers of normal articular cartilage. *Arthritis Rheum* 1996;39:567-573.

35. Lohmander LS, Saxne T, Heinegard DK: Release of cartilage oligomeric protein (COMP) into joint fluid after knee injury and in osteoarthritis. *Ann Rheum Dis* 1994;53:8-13.

36. Martin JA, Miller BA, Scherb MB, Lembke LA, Buckwalter JA: Co-localization of insulin-like growth factor binding protein 3 and fibronectin in human articular cartilage. *Osteoarthritis Cartilage* 2002;10:556-563.

37. Martin JA, Buckwalter JA: Human chondrocyte senescence and osteoarthritis. *Biorheology* 2002;39:145-152.

38. Nishida K, Inoue H, Murakami T: Immunohistochemical demonstration of fibronectin in the most superfical layer of normal rabbit articular cartilage. *Ann Rheum Dis* 1995;54:995-998.

39. Pfaffle M, Borchert M, Deutzmann R, et al: Anchorin CII, a collagen-binding chondrocyte surface protein of the calpactin family. *Prog Clin Biol Res* 1990;349:147-157.

40. Frenkel SR, Saadeh PB, Mehrara BJ, et al: Transforming growth factor beta superfamily members: Role in cartilage modeling. *Plast Reconstr Surg* 2000;105:980-990.

41. Lippiello L, Hall D, Mankin HJ: Collagen synthesis

in normal and osteoarthritic human cartilage. *J Clin Invest* 1977;59:593-600.

42. Martin JA, Buckwalter JA: The role of chondrocyte-matrix interactions in maintaining and repairing articular cartilage. *Biorheology* 2000;37:129-140.

43. Trippel SB: Growth factor actions on articular cartilage. *J Rheumatol Suppl* 1995;43:129-132.

44. Buckwalter JA, Mankin HJ: Articular cartilage: Degeneration and osteoarthritis, repair, regeneration, and transplantation. *Instr Course Lect* 1998;47:487-504.

45. Cs-Szabo G, Roughley PJ, Plaas AH, Glant TT: Large and small proteoglycans of osteoarthritic and rheumatoid articular cartilage. *Arthritis Rheum* 1995;38:660-668.

46. Heinegard D, Lorenzo P, Sommarin Y: Articular cartilage matrix proteins, in Kuettner KE, Goldberg VM (eds): *Osteoarthritic Disorders*. Rosemont, IL, American Academy of Orthopaedic Surgeons, 1995, pp 229-237.

47. Hedbom E, Heinegard D: Interaction of a 59-kDa connective tissue matrix protein with collagen I and collagen II. *J Biol Chem* 1989;264:6898-6905.

48. Ehrlich MG, Armstrong AL, Treadwell BV, Mankin HJ: The role of proteases in the pathogenesis of osteoarthritis. *J Rheumatol* 1987;14:30-32.

49. Testa V, Capasso G, Maffulli M, Sgambato A, Ames PR: Proteases and antiproteases in cartilage homeostasis: A brief review. *Clin Orthop Relat Res* 1994;308:79-84.

50. van-Beuningen HM, Kraan PM, Arntz OJ, Berg WB: Transforming growth factor-beta 1 stimulates articular chondrocyte proteoglycan synthesis and induces osteophyte formation in the murine knee joint. *Lab Invest* 1994;71:279-290.

51. Felson DT: The epidemiology of osteoarthritis: Prevalence and risk factors, in Kuettner KE, Goldberg VM (eds): *Osteoarthritic Disorders*. Rosemont, IL, American Academy of Orthopaedic Surgeons, 1995, pp 13-24.

52. Buckwalter JA: Articular cartilage injuries. *Clin Orthop Relat Res* 2002;402:21-37.

53. Buckwalter JA: Sports, joint injury, and posttraumatic osteoarthritis. *J Orthop Sports Phys Ther* 2003;33:578-588.

54. Fukui N, Purple CR, Sandell LJ: Cell biology of osteoarthritis: The chondrocyte's response to injury. *Curr Rheumatol Rep* 2001;3:496-505.

55. Hunziker EB: Articular cartilage repair: Basic science and clinical progress. A review of the current status and prospects. *Osteoarthritis Cartilage* 2002;10:432-463.

56. Dieppe P: The classification and diagnosis of osteoarthritis, in Kuettner KE, Goldberg VM (eds): *Osteoarthritic Disorders*. Rosemont, IL, American Academy of Orthopaedic Surgeons, 1995, pp 5-12.

57. Schiller AL: Pathology of osteoarthritis, in Kuettner KE, Goldberg VM (eds): *Osteoarthritic Disorders*. Rosemont, IL, American Academy of Orthopaedic Surgeons, 1995, pp 95-101.

58. Mankin HJ, Johnson ME, Lippiello L: Biochemical and metabolic abnormalities in articular cartilage from osteoarthritic human hips: III. Distribution and metabolism of amino sugar-containing macromolecules. *J Bone Joint Surg Am* 1981;63:131-139.

59. Burgkart R, Glaser C, Hyhlik-Durr A, Englmeier KH, Reiser M, Eckstein F: Magnetic resonance imaging-based assessment of cartilage loss in severe osteoarthritis: Accuracy, precision and diagnostic value. *Arthritis Rheum* 2001;44:2072-2077.

60. Burstein D, Gray M: New MRI techniques for imaging cartilage. *J Bone Joint Surg Am* 2003;85(suppl 2):70-77.

61. Seog J, Dean D, Plaas AHK, et al: Direct measurement of glycosaminoglycan intermolecular interactions via high resolution force spectroscopy. *Macromolecules* 2002;35:5601-5615.

62. Lyman S, Sherman S, Dunn WR, Marx RG: Advancements in the surgical and alternative treatment of arthritis. *Curr Opin Rheumatol* 2005;17:129-133.

63. Weaver AL: Rofecoxib: Clinical pharmacology and clinical experience. *Clin Ther* 2001;23:1323-1338.

64. Seegenschmiedt MH, Katalinic A, Makoski H, Haase W, Gademann G, Hassenstein E: Radiation therapy for benign diseases: Patterns of care study in Germany. *Int J Radiat Oncol Biol Phys* 2000;47:195-202.

65. Evanich JD, Evanich CJ, Wright MB, Rydlewicz JA: Efficacy of intra-articular hyaluronic acid injections in knee osteoarthritis. *Clin Orthop Relat Res* 2001;390:173-181.

66. Calvert GT, Wright RW: The use of arthroscopy in the athlete with knee osteoarthritis. *Clin Sports Med* 2005;24:133-152.

67. Livesley PJ, Doherty M, Needhoff M, Moutlon A: Arthroscopic lavage of osteoarthritic knees. *J Bone Joint Surg Br* 1991;73:922-926.

68. Wray NP, Moseley JB, O'Malley K: Arthroscopic treatment of osteoarthritis of the knee. *J Bone Joint Surg Am* 2003;85:381.

69. Buckwalter JA, Lohmander S: Operative treatment of osteoarthrosis: Current practice and future development. *J Bone Joint Surg Am* 1994;76:1405-1418.

70. Hidaka C, Goodrich LR, Chen CT, Warren RF, Crystal RG, Nixon AJ: Acceleration of cartilage repair by genetically modified chondrocytes over expressing bone morphogenetic protein-7. *J Orthop Res* 2003;21:573-583.

71. Peterson L, Minas T, Brittberg M, Lindahl A: The treatment of osteochondritis dissecans of the knee with autologous chondrocyte transplantation: Results at two to ten years. *J Bone Joint Surg Am* 2003;85(suppl 2):17-24.

72. Richardson JB, Caterson B, Evans EH, Ashton BA, Roberts S: Repair of human articular cartilage after implantation of autologous chondrocytes. *J Bone Joint Surg Br* 1999;81:1064-1068.

73. Trippel SB, Ghivizzani SC, Nixon AJ: Gene-based approaches for the repair of articular cartilage. *Gene Ther* 2004;11:351-359.

74. Grande DA, Mason J, Light E, Dines D: Stem cells as platforms for delivery of genes to enhance cartilage repair. *J Bone Joint Surg Am* 2003;85(suppl 2):111-116.

75. Hangody L, Fules P: Autologous osteochondral mosaicplasty for the treatment of full-thickness defects of weight-bearing joints: Ten years of experimental and clinical experience. *J Bone Joint Surg Am* 2003;85(suppl 2):25-32.

76. Weisl H: Intertrochanteric osteotomy for osteoarthritis: A long-term follow-up. *J Bone Joint Surg Br* 1980;62:37-42.

77. Ethgen O, Bruyere O, Richy F, Dardennes C, Reginster JY: Health-related quality of life in total hip and knee arthroplasty: A qualitative and systematic review of the literature. *J Bone Joint Surg Am* 2004;86:963-974.

Chapter 7

Pigmented Villonodular Synovitis of Joints, Bursae, and Tendon Sheaths

Pigmented villonodular synovitis (PVNS) is a proliferative disorder arising principally from synovium but occasionally from bursae or tendon sheaths. The disease is characterized by a unique gross and histologic structure consisting of brownish villous and nodular masses arising on the surface of synovial tissue that consist of fibrous elements, hemosiderin-containing macrophages, lipid cells, multinucleated giant cells, and some inflammatory cells. The lesions may be aggressive and destroy the adjacent bone or relatively benign, assuming a solitary nodular pattern. Although the early literature suggested that the tumors were sometimes malignant, it is now evident that the lesions are for the most part locally aggressive, but only very rarely metastasize and even less commonly cause patient death. The entities are now known as giant cell tumors of synovium rather than PVNS, but the latter name still persists in most literary reviews and orthopaedic and pathologic programs.

Nomenclature and History

Over the years, various names have been applied to PVNS based in part on the tissue within the structures. Early studies showed that some lesions had a high number of cells containing fat, thus they were called a xanthoma, fibroxanthoma, or xanthogranuloma.[1-5] Because of the extensive hemosiderin deposits, the lesions were once described as hemosiderosis or hemochromatosis.[6,7] The presence of giant cells led to the term giant cell tumor of synovial membrane or tendon sheath or giant cell synovioma; these terms are currently considered more accurate than the descriptive term PVNS.[1,8-11] Unfortunately, the terminology incorporating synovioma suggests a relationship to synovial sarcoma or malignant synovioma of soft tissues, which provides an inappropriate sug-

gestion of malignancy.[5,12,13] According to Jaffe,[7] the confusion with malignant disease has allowed terms such as fibrohemosideric sarcoma or malignant polymorphocellular tumor to be introduced. Although the lesions may be locally destructive, only a few reported cases support the possibility of malignancy.[14-18]

In 1941, Jaffe, Lichtenstein, and Sutro[19] introduced the term PVNS; until recently, this has remained the label of choice. Further nomenclature confusion currently exists because the disorder is not confined to joints but also occurs in tendon sheaths (giant cell tumor of tendon sheath)[4,9,11,13,20,21] and adjacent to joints but extra-articular (pigmented villonodular bursitis).[1,5,7,13]

Historically, the first account of a disorder that could later be defined as PVNS was that of Chassaignac,[22] who in 1852 described nodular tumors of the hand. In 1865, Simon[23] described a nodular mass in the knee, and in 1928 Mandl[24] defined the disease as arising from a hematologic tumor. These and other reports strongly suggested that the lesion had characteristics of a malignant tumor of soft tissue.[5,25] It was not until 1912 that Dowd defined the benign nature of the process.[8] DeSanto and Wilson[2] proposed in 1939 that the lesion was associated with high blood cholesterol, but this was never substantiated. The clear definition of the disease and the introduction of the name pigmented villonodular synovitis was the result of the seminal article by Jaffe, Lichtenstein, and Sutro[19] in the *Archives of Pathology* in 1941. Young and Hudacek[26] produced changes similar to PVNS by repeated injections of blood into dog knees. Geschickter and Copeland[17] conducted additional studies in an attempt to define the cause of PVNS, including a relationship to blood in the joint, but they could not arrive at a satisfactory conclusion. Breimer and Freiberger[27] first described the

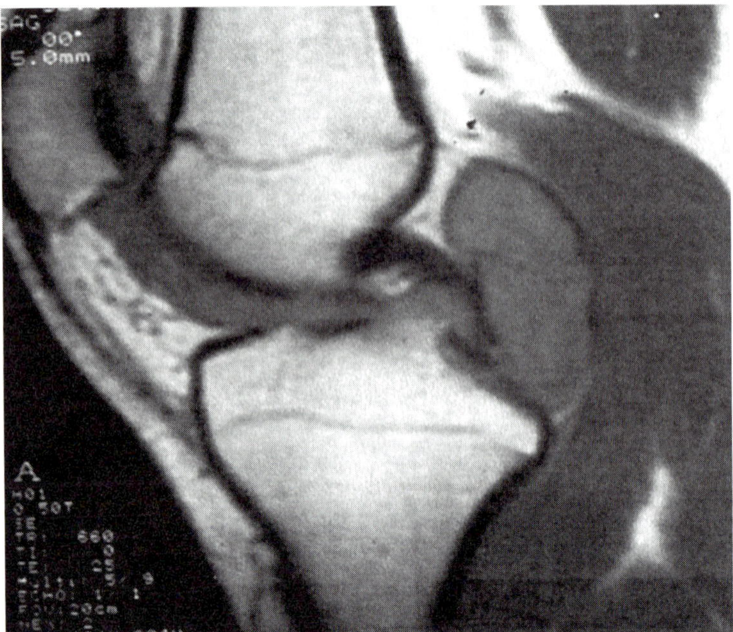

Figure 1

Magnetic resonance imaging study of pigmented villonodular synovitis of the knee joint. Note the dark images on T1 both anteriorly and posteriorly in the joint.

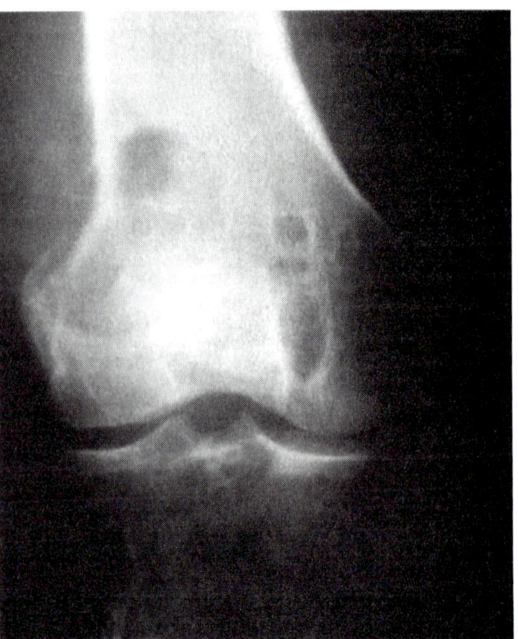

Figure 2

Radiograph of the knee joint in a patient with pigmented villonodular synovitis. Note the destructive areas in the distal femur and the soft-tissue mass surrounding the bony parts, reflecting the marked degree of synovial enlargement.

periarticular destructive bone lesions associated with the disease in 1958; this finding was supported by McMaster[28] in his 1960 article. Additional early references included the description of extra-articular lesions of the knee by Peterson and associates[29] in 1958, the description of lesions in the hand by Phalen and colleagues[10] in 1959, and a review of radiologic characteristics by Smith and Pugh[30] in 1962. Localized forms of the disease within the joint, which were thought to have a better prognosis, were identified by Lichtenstein[31] in 1955, by Phalen and associates[10] in 1959, and by Granowitz and Mankin[32] in 1967. These relatively small nodular lesions became known as pigmented nodular synovitis.[1,5,32]

Biology of PVNS

Several studies have identified clonal abnormalities in the diffuse form of PVNS within a joint that strongly suggest a neoplastic origin. Dal Cin and associates[33] found clonal abnormalities within the tissue in t(1;2) (p11;q35-36) or t(1;5(p11;q22) and t(2;16) (q33;q24); rearrangements of 1p11-13 were most common. The number of variations observed, however, suggests that the lesions have a multiplicity of causes or that as part of the disease process, the disorder itself in-

duces a large number of nuclear abnormalities. A recent study by Ijiri and associates[34] suggests that humanin peptide, a material that interferes with apoptotic activity, is present in the diffuse form of the disease but is less common in the nodular form. Berger and associates[35,36] have suggested that the expression of bc-2 and Ki-57 and p53 may also interfere with apoptotic activity, thus increasing the survival rate for the tissue and leading to the slow but permanent progression of the lesions.

As noted in the discussion of the history of the disease, a malignant form of the disorder, particularly one growing outside the joints (tendon sheath or bursa), has been described.[14,16,18] The lesion is rare and seems to bear some resemblance to clear cell sarcoma of soft tissues, epithelioid sarcoma, fibrosarcoma, and malignant fibrous histiocytoma.[13,14] Metastases can occur from such lesions, and deaths have been reported.[14-18] The relationship to the benign form of the disease is not clear; despite several case reports by Bertoni and associates[14] and Schajowicz,[13] PVNS confined within a joint rarely, if ever, undergoes malignant degeneration.

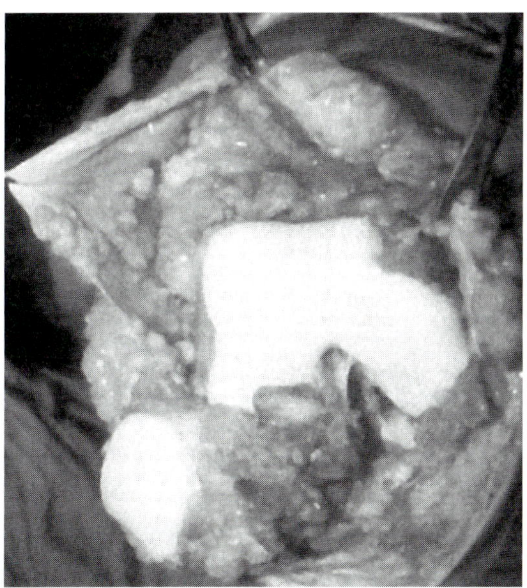

Figure 3

Gross picture of pigmented villonodular synovitis of the knee joint showing the nodular masses, many colored with hemosiderin, and the effect on the cartilage margins.

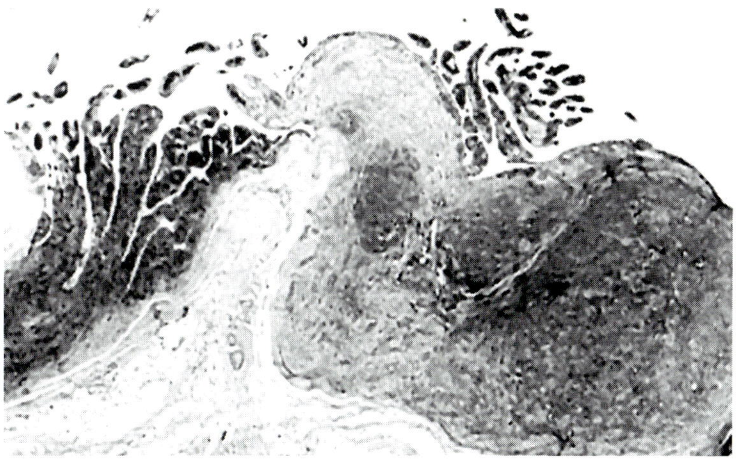

Figure 4

Histologic picture of pigmented villonodular synovitis showing the villous component (on the left side and on top) and the nodular component that illustrates monocytic infiltrate with frequent giant cells. Hematoxylin and eosin × 75.

Imaging and Histology

PVNS or tendinitis or bursitis is a soft-tissue disorder initially studied by standard radiography,[37] but best seen with magnetic resonance imaging.[20,38-43] Magnetic resonance imaging shows a low intensity on both T1 and T2, presumably related to the presence of hemosiderin in the tissue[39,42] (Figure 1). The exception to this rule is when the lesion invades and partially destroys the adjacent bone, an event that occurs with high frequency in hip disease and to a lesser degree (but still greater than 50%) in knee disease.[27,28,44-49] Under these circumstances, the masses may be seen on standard radiographs and in computed tomography studies, and can be readily detected by bone scan[7,27,28,30,37,44,49] (Figure 2). A recent report by Mackie[21] suggests that the lesions are positive on positron emission tomography scanning.

The gross pathology for all lesions, whether they are within the joint or bursa or tendon sheath, shows variable amounts of brownish fluid surrounding the lesion.[1,5,7,13,19,25,31,50,51] The lesion itself is usually irregular in structure, has some villous structures on the surface, and is often brown in color (Figure 3). The histologic picture is not uniform; different parts of the lesion may show variable cellular and extracellular tissue. The pattern includes fibroblastic cells, multiple capillaries, villi and clefts lined with synovial cells, macrophages containing hemosiderin, lipocytes, and a variable number of multinucleated giant cells, along with some inflammatory cells and macrophages[1,5,7,11,13,15,17,19,25,31,52-57] (Figure 4). Granular hemosiderin may be striking in concentration in the villous or nodular synovitis contained within the joint, while giant cells may dominate the picture in the extracellular lesions.[4-7,9,13,32,53,55,56,58-61]

Treatment of PVNS

Surgical resection of the lesional tissue remains the treatment of choice for PVNS.[1,10,15,25,46,47,53,58,59,62,63] The procedure should probably be done as an open procedure, and if necessary in the knee, both from the front and separately from the posterior aspect of the knee.[1,52,53,61,62] Hip surgery is best performed from an anterior or a lateral approach, but has a high rate of failure in terms of restoration of normal function.[45-47,64] Ankle and foot surgery is done principally from the dorsum and is usually successful;[59,65] hand surgery is less common, but also often successful.[10,48] Resection of tendinous or bursal lesions is direct, with the incision over the site of the disease; this procedure is for the most part successful unless tendons or nerves or vessels are too close to the lesion.[53,66]

Several problems are associated with surgery. Is it possible to do the procedure arthroscopically? The results of trials indicate that for nodular disease of the knee this is a reasonable approach, but for more extensive disease the recurrence rate is high.[67,68] A second question regards the value of dysprosium or yttrium injected into the knee instead of (or after) surgery; both appear to have some effect on rheumatoid synovitis.[62,69] However, the effect on the disease does not appear to be sufficient, and the recurrence rate is high.[62] Should radiation be added? There is little doubt that radiation may be effective for small lesions in the foot,[70] but less success has been achieved in restoring function for patients with knee or especially hip disease.[71] Are any chemotherapeutic agents available to slow the process of the disease? Some have been tried, but ultimately surgery is required. Finally, what if the disease has caused damage to the bone around the affected joint? Total hip replacement is the only solution for hip disease, and most of these patients require such a procedure because the destruction of bone is frequent.[1,44-47,53,64] Half or less of the knee disease patients require total knee replacement, but certainly it is a reasonable solution when enough bone has been damaged.[1,49,53,62] Metatarsal or metacarpal or phalangeal lesions may require resection of the damaged site, and either replacement with autograft or allograft chips or sometimes partial amputation.[10,65]

Summary

Pigmented villonodular synovitis and its clinical counterparts—giant cell tumors of tendon sheath, giant cell synovioma, nodular synovitis, and bursitis—remain mysterious entities. The genesis is unknown. There is no evidence for familial or genetic origin. The lesions do not seem to be typically neoplastic, although clonal abnormalities and the presence of some materials such as p53 strongly support this contention. The literature suggests that a malignant form exists, but there is no evidence to support the claim that it arises from or is the same as the benign disorder. The lesions are uncommon and appear to be relatively easily diagnosed, particularly if magnetic resonance imaging studies are conducted. Treatment seems to be principally surgical, but recurrences (particularly for diffuse knee disease) are frequent. Hip disease has a high failure rate partly because of peri-articular acetabular and femoral head destruction in the enclosed hip capsule, but also because surgical resection is difficult. The use of radiation is possibly helpful, particularly for recurrences, and there are as yet no known chemotherapeutic agents that are useful for control of the disorder. Fortunately, the diseases are rare; even more fortunately, they are often not very destructive to the joint, bone, or tendon.

References

1. Campanacci M: *Bone and Soft Tissue Tumors*, ed 2. New York, NY, Springer Verlag, 1999, pp 1289-1306.

2. DeSanto DA, Wilson PD: Xanthomatous tumors of joint. *J Bone Joint Surg* 1939;21:531-538.

3. Friedman M, Ginzler A: Xanthogranuloma of the knee joint: A report of two cases. *Bull Hosp Joint Dis* 1940;1:17-22.

4. Jones FE, Soule EH, Coventry MB: Fibrous xanthoma of synovium (giant-cell tumors of tendon sheath, pigmented nodular synovitis): A study of one hundred and eighteen cases. *J Bone Joint Surg Am* 1969;51:76-86.

5. Weiss SW, Goldblum JR: Benign tumors and tumor-like lesions of synovial tissue, in *Enzinger and Weiss's Soft Tissue Tumors*, ed 4. St. Louis, MO, Mosby, 2001, pp 1037-1062.

6. Collins DH: Haemosiderosis and haemochromatosis of synovial tissues. *J Bone Joint Surg Br* 1951;33:436-441.

7. Jaffe HL: *Tumors and Tumorous Conditions of the Bones and Joints*. Philadelphia, PA, Lea and Febiger, 1958, pp 532-557.

8. Dowd CN: Villous arthritis of the knee (sarcoma). *Ann Surg* 1912;56:363-366.

9. Fletcher AG Jr, Horn RC Jr: Giant cell tumors of tendon sheath origin. *Ann Surg* 1951;133:374-385.

10. Phalen GS, McCormack LJ, Gazale WJ: Giant-cell tumor of the tendon sheath (benign synovioma) in the hand: Evaluation of 56 cases. *Clin Orthop Relat Res* 1959;15:140-151.

11. Wright CJE: Benign giant cell synovioma: An investigation of 85 cases. *Br J Surg* 1951;38:257-281.

12. Jergesen HE, Mankin HJ, Schiller AL: Diffuse pigmented villonodular synovitis of the knee mimicking primary bone neoplasm: A report of two cases. *J Bone Joint Surg Am* 1978;60:825-829.

13. Schajowicz F: Tumors and tumor-like lesions of the synovial membrane, in *Tumors and Tumorlike Lesions of Bone and Joints*. New York, NY, Springer Verlag, 1981, pp 519-567.

14. Bertoni F, Unni KK, Beabout JW, Sim FH: Malignant giant cell tumor of the tendon sheaths and joints (malignant pigmented villonodular synovitis). *Am J Surg Pathol* 1997;21:153-163.

15. Campanacci M, Cerveletti C, Olmi R, Trentani C: Aspeti neoplastiformi della synovite villonodulare

pigmentosa. *Chir Organi Mov* 1972;60:463-474.

16. Guccion JG, Enzinger F: Malignant giant cell tumor of soft parts: An analysis of 32 cases. *Cancer* 1972;29:1518-1529.

17. Geschickter CF, Copeland MM: *Tumors of Bone,* ed 3. Philadelphia, PA, JB Lippincott, 1949, pp 357-363.

18. Kubak MW, Perlow S: Xanthomatous giant cell tumors arising in soft tissue: Report of an instance of malignant growth. *Arch Surg* 1949;59:909-916.

19. Jaffe HL, Lichtenstein L, Sutro CJ: Pigmented villonodular synovitis, bursitis and tenosynovitis. *Arch Pathol* 1941;31:731-765.

20. Jelinek JS, Kransdorf MJ, Shmookler BM, Aboulafia AA, Malawer MM: Giant cell tumor of the tendon sheath: MR findings in nine cases. *AJR Am J Roentgenol* 1994;162:919-922.

21. Mackie GC: Pigmented villonodular synovitis and giant cell tumor of tendon sheath: Scintigraphic findings in 10 cases. *Clin Nucl Med* 2003;28:881-885.

22. Chassaignac: Cancer de la gaine des tendons. *Gazette des hopitaux civils et miltaires* 1852:185-186.

23. Simon G: Extirpation einer sehr grossen mit dickem stiele augewachsenen knieglenken maus mit glucklichem erfolge. *Arch J Klin Chir* 1865;6:573-576.

24. Mandl F: Chronische arthritis villosa haemor-rhagica des Kniegelenkes. *Zentenlbl Chir* 1928;10:597-600.

25. Byers PD, Cotton RE, Deacon OW, et al: The diagnosis and treatment of pigmented villonodular synovitis. *J Bone Joint SurgBr* 1968;50:290-305.

26. Young JM, Hudacek AG: Experimental production of pigmented villonodular synovitis in dogs. *Am J Pathol* 1954;30:799-811.

27. Breimer CW, Freiberger RH: Bone lesions associated with villonodular synovitis. *Am J Roentgenol Radium Ther Nucl Med* 1958;79:618-629.

28. McMaster PE: Pigmented villonodular synovitis with invasion of bone: Report of six cases. *J Bone Joint Surg Am* 1960;42:1170-1183.

29. Peterson LFH, Johnson EW Jr, Woolner LB: Extra-articular pigmented villonodular synovitis of the knee. *Am J Clin Pathol* 1958;30:158-162.

30. Smith JH, Pugh DG: Roentgenographic aspects of articular pigmented villonodular synovitis. *Am J Roentgenol Radium Ther Nucl Med* 1962;87:1146-1156.

31. Lichtenstein L: Tumors of synovial joints, bursae and tendon sheaths. *Cancer* 1955;8:816-830.

32. Granowitz SP, Mankin HJ: Localized pigmented villonodular synovitis of the knee: Report of five cases. *J Bone Joint Surg Am* 1967;49:122-128.

33. Dal Cin P, Sciot R, Samson L, et al: Cytogenetic characterization of tenosynovial giant cell tumors (nodular tenosynovitis). *Cancer Res* 1994;54:3986-3987.

34. Ijiri K, Tsuruga H, Sakakima H, et al: Increased expression of humanin peptide in diffuse-type pigmented villonodular synovitis: Implication of its mitochondrial abnormality. *Ann Rheum Dis* 2005;64:816-823.

35. Berger I, Aulmann S, Ehemann V, Helmchen B, Weckauf H: Apoptosis resistance in pigmented villonodular synovitis. *Histol Histopathol* 2005;20:11-17.

36. Berger I, Rieker R, Ehemann V, Schmitz W, Autschbach F, Weckauf H: Analysis of chromosomal imbalances by comparative genomic hybridisation of pigmented villonodular synovitis. *Cancer Lett* 2005;220:231-236.

37. Lewis RW: Roentgen diagnosis of pigmented villonodular synovitis and synovial sarcoma of the knee joint: Preliminary report. *Radiology* 1947;49:26-38.

38. Bhimani MA, Wenz JF, Frassica FJ: Pigmented villonodular synovitis: Keys to early diagnosis. *Clin Orthop Relat Res* 2001;386:197-202.

39. Cheng XG, You YH, Liu W, Zhao T, Zu H: MRI features of pigmented villonodular synovitis (PVNS). *Clin Rheumatol* 2004;23:31-34.

40. Giannini C, Scheithauer BW, Wenger DE, Unni KK: Pigmented villonodular synovitis of the spine: A clinical, radiological and morphological study of 12 cases. *J Neurosurg* 1996;84:592-597.

41. Huang GS, Lee CH, Chan WP, Chen CY, Yu JS, Resnick D: Localized nodular synovitis of the knee: MR imaging and clinical correlates in 21 patients. *AJR Am J Roentgenol* 2003;181:539-543.

42. Hughes TH, Sartoris DJ, Schweitzer ME, Resnick DL: Pigmented villonodular synovitis: MRI characteristics. *Skeletal Radiol* 1995;24:7-12.

43. Weisz GM, Gal A, Kitchener PN: Magnetic resonance imaging in the diagnosis of aggressive villonodular synovitis. *Clin Orthop Relat Res* 1988;236:303-306.

44. Carr CR, Berley FV, Davis WC: Pigmented villonodular synovitis of the hip joint: A case report. *J Bone Joint Surg Am* 1954;36:1007-1013.

45. Chung SMK, Janes JM: Diffuse pigmented villonodular synovitis of the hip joint: Review of the literature and report of four cases. *J Bone Joint Surg Am* 1965;47:293-303.

46. Gitelis S, Heligman D, Morton T: The treatment of pigmented villonodular synovitis of the hip: A case report and literature review. *Clin Orthop Relat Res* 1989;239:154-160.

47. Gonzales Della Valle A, Piccaluga F, Potter HG, Salvati EA, Pusso R: Pigmented villonodular synovitis of the hip: 2- to 23- year followup study. *Clin Orthop Relat Res* 2001;388:187-199.

48. Schajowicz F, Blumenfeld I: Pigmented villonodular synovitis of the wrist with penetration into the bone. *J Bone Joint Surg Br* 1968;50:312-317.

49. Scott PM: Bone lesions in pigmented villonodular synovitis. *J Bone Joint Surg Br* 1968;50:306-311.

50. Gaubert J, Mazabraud A, Verdie JC, Cheneu J: Les synovites villonoulaires hemo-pigmentees des grosses articulations. *Rev Chir Orthop* 1974;60:265-298.

51. Greenfield M, Wallace KM: Pigmented villonodular synovitis. *Radiology* 1951;54:571-580.

52. Granowitz SP, D'Antonio J, Mankin HJ: The pathogenesis and long-term end results of pigmented villonodular synovitis. *Clin Orthop Relat Res* 1976;114:335-351.

53. Martin RC II, Osborne DL, Edwards MJ, Wrightson W, McMasters KM: Giant cell tumor of tendon sheath, tenosynovial giant cell tumor and pigmented villonodular synovitis: Defining the presentation, surgical therapy and recurrence. *Oncol Rep* 2000;7:413-419.

54. Shafer SJ, Larmon WA: Pigmented villonodular synovitis: A report of seven cases. *Surg Gynecol Obstet* 1951;92:574-580.

55. Nilsonne U, Moberger G: Pigmented villonodular synovitis of joints: Histological and clinical problems in diagnosis. *Acta Orthop Scand* 1969;40:448-460.

56. Oehler S, Fassbender HG, Neureiter D, Meyer-Scholten C, Kirchner T, Aigner T: Cell populations involved in pigmented villonodular synovitis of the knee. *J Rheumatol* 2000;27:463-470.

57. Shafer SJ, Larmon WA: Pigmented villonodular synovitis. *Surg Gyne Obstet* 1951;92:574-580.

58. Arthaud JB: Pigmented nodular synovitis: Report of 11 lesions in non-articular locations. *Am J Clin Pathol* 1972;58:511-517.

59. Brien EW, Sacoman DM, Mirra JM: Pigmented villonodular synovitis of the foot and ankle. *Foot Ankle Int* 2004;25:908-913.

60. Eisenstein R: Giant-cell tumor of tendon sheath: Its histogenesis as studied in the electron microscope. *J Bone Joint Surg Am* 1968;50:476-486.

61. Fraire AE, Fechner RE: Intra-articular localized nodular synovitis of the knee. *Arch Pathol* 1972;93:473-476.

62. Chin KR, Barr SJ, Winalski C, Zurakowski D, Brick GW: Treatment of advanced primary and recurrent diffuse pigmented villonodular synovitis of the knee. *J Bone Joint Surg Am* 2002;84:2192-2202.

63. Levin EJ, Gannon WS: Diffuse villonodular synovitis of the shoulder. *Am J Roentgenol Radium Ther Nucl Med* 1963;89:1302-1304.

64. Vastel L, Lambert P, De Pinieux G, Charrois O, Kerboull M, Courpied JP: Surgical treatment of pigmented villonodular synovitis of the hip. *J Bone Joint Surg Am* 2005;87A:1019-1024.

65. Saxena A, Perez H: Pigmented villonodular synovitis about the ankle: A review of the literature and presentation in 10 athletic patients. *Foot Ankle Int* 2004;25:819-826.

66. Sherry JB, Anderson W: The natural history of pigmented villonodular synovitis of tendon sheaths. *J Bone Joint Surg Am* 1955;37:1005-1011.

67. De Ponti A, Sansone V, Malchere M: Result of arthroscopic treatment of pigmented villonodular synovitis of the knee. *Arthroscopy* 2003;19:602-607.

68. Kim SJ, Shin SJ, Choi NH, Choo ET: Arthroscopic treatment for localized pigmented villonodular synovitis of the knee. *Clin Orthop Relat Res* 2000;379:224-230.

69. Shabat S, Kollender Y, Merimsky O, et al: The use of surgery and yttrium 90 in the management of extensive and diffuse pigmented villonodular synovitis of large joints. *Rheumatology (Oxford)* 2002;41:1113-1118.

70. Friedman M, Schwartz EE: Irradiation therapy of pigmented villodular synovitis. *Bull Hosp Joint Dis* 1957;18:19-32.

71. O'Sullivan B, Cummings B, Catton C, et al: Outcome following radiation treatment for high-risk pigmented villonodular synovitis. *Int J Radiat Oncol Biol Phys* 1995;15:777-786.

Chapter 8

Synovial Chondromatosis

Synovial chondromatosis is an intriguing entity; although the disease is rare, numerous reports have appeared in the literature. The disorder is characterized by chondral and chondro-osseous nodules in the synovium or free in a joint. The disorder is relatively easy to diagnose radiographically, based on the presence of calcification of the cartilaginous nodules when they are in the synovium, and even more evident when the nodules are free within the joint. Hundreds of small round nodular cartilaginous and bony structures can be present, most often contained within the joint capsule of the knee, shoulder, hip, elbow, and even the temporomandibular joint. The disorder can also exist extra-articularly in tendinous structures and bursae.

Nomenclature and History

Synovial chondromatosis is linguistically defined as a cartilage lesion arising from and located within synovial tissues, usually of the joint (most often the knee) but occasionally in relation to tendons, ligaments, and bursae. The difficulty with language is related to the fact that the cartilaginous bodies that arise within the synovium are similar in structure to epiphyseal cartilage, rather than articular cartilage, and hence undergo enlargement and ossification.[1-4] When they break free of the synovium, the blood supply is insufficient to support the bone; the segment dies, but the calcified dead bone is still retained within and surrounded by living and often heavily calcified cartilage.[3,4] This leads to a second name for the disease—synovial osteochondromatosis. In addition, because one of the early descriptions was rendered by Paul Friedrich Reichel[5] in 1900, the disease is also known as Reichel syndrome or Reichel-Jones-Henderson syndrome (to include two other early describers of the lesion).[6-8]

The first recorded description of an entity in which bony lesions were present within a joint was that of Cruveilhier in 1835.[9] The nature of these lesions was, however, unclear until Kolliker[10] identified the segments as containing cartilage as well as bone in his 1853 text. Reichel's findings,[5] both clinically and radiographically (a technology that became available in the late 1890s), supported the finding of bone inside of cartilage, but it was Lexer[11] who in 1907 defined a relationship of the small osteocartilaginous bodies to the synovium and showed that they actually arose within the synovial tissue in the joint. A decade later, Henderson[6] and Fisher[12] further implicated the synovium as the origin rather than the articular cartilage. Two major contributors to the understanding of the disorder were Henderson[7] and Jones,[8] who published descriptions of the pathologic production of the lesions by the synovial tissues in 1923 and 1924 and established without equivocation not only the synovial origin of the process but the relationship to the epiphyseal type of cartilage rather than articular. Rixford[13] further defined this relationship in 1930 and indicated a possible relation to sarcomas. In his 1958 book on bone and joint pathology, Henry Jaffe[3] provided descriptive histologic sections that showed the stages of the segments, ranging from cartilaginous to cartilaginous tissue that creates living bone and finally to free segments with living cartilaginous tissue enclosing calcified dead bone. The extent of the joint destruction that can occur was further defined by Wilmoth[14] in 1941, by Mussey and Henderson[15] in 1949, by Jeffreys[16] in 1967, and finally by Milgram[4] in his 1977 report on 30 cases. Of some concern were the early studies by Riemann and Kienbock[17] in 1931, Geschickter and Copeland[18] in 1949, Nixon and associates[19] in 1960, and Mullins and colleagues[20] in 1965—all of whom identified chondrosarcomas that appeared to have arisen from the synovial chondromatous cartilage lesions.

The Disease Process

Synovial chondromatosis is a generally benign process in which small round islands of cartilage arise in synovium—often of the knee; less commonly in the temporoman-

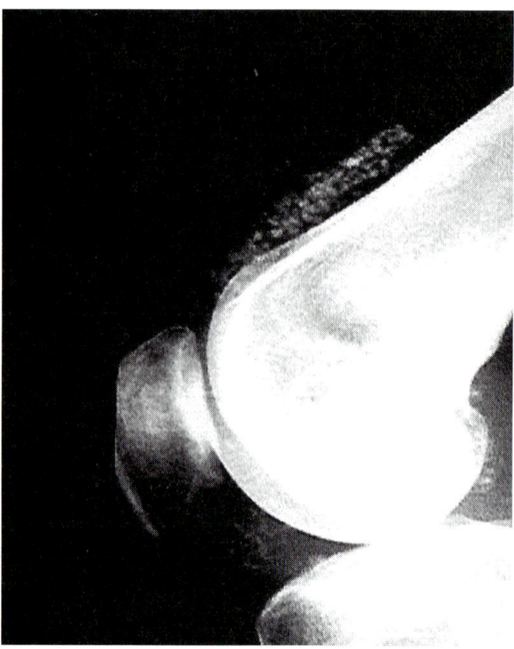

Figure 1
Earliest phase of synovial chondromatosis in a knee joint. There are faint calcifications posteriorly and anteriorly in the region of the cruciate ligaments. In the part of the joint superior to the patella, the nodules are small but clearly distinct.

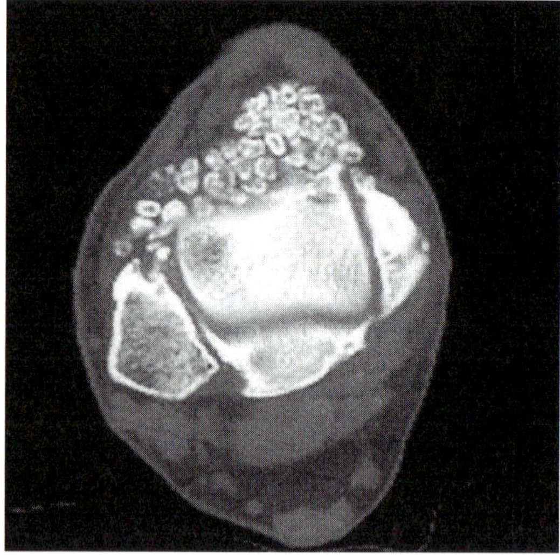

Figure 2
Later phases of synovial chondromatosis show multiple, distinct, round, heavily calcified nodules anteriorly.

dibular joint, hip, elbow, or shoulder; and even less frequently in other sites such as the hands or feet and structures such as tendon sheaths and bursae.[1-4,14,16,21-44] The disease appears to be more frequent in young adults and consistently more common in males than females.[1,3,37] Initially the joint becomes swollen and imaging studies often define synovial enlargement.[23] The disease process was defined by Milgram[45] in 1977 as occurring in three phases. Phase 1 shows cartilaginous nodules within the synovium. These sometimes become calcified, but in addition the nodules act as epiphyseal-type chondrocytic structures rather than hyaline cartilage and thus make bone by endochondral ossification. At this point the lesion is not calcified on imaging studies, but will result in a positive bone scan. Phase 2 shows both active intrasynovial proliferation of nodules leading to enlargement, but also breaking away from the surface of the synovium to become first loosely attached and then free within the joint. Because bone requires a vascular supply, the bone dies; however, the calcified cartilage, which is avascular, survives on the basis of synovial fluid nutrition for the cells.[2,3,37] Phase 3

shows a gradual enlargement of the segments that lie within the joint but no longer have any contact with the synovium. At times, however, there are large collections of fluid within the joint and some nonspecific synovitis.[2,3,21,28,29,31,46] In addition, the presence of the osteocartilaginous free bodies in the joint may lead to bone destruction and ultimately progress to cause osteoarthritis.[26,28,29,37,46] This is especially true for the hip joint and sometimes for the knee or elbow as well.

The origin of synovial chondromatosis is unclear. The occasional occurrence of malignancy in the joint in the form of a chondrosarcoma suggests that the disease is neoplastic, but attempts to study the tissue to further identify the cause have not been helpful. The cells fail to stain for C-erb-B2 or Ki-67, and are nonreactive for p53.[47] Some evidence suggests that fibroblast growth factor-3 may play a role in growth of the lesions, and a recent report on three cases has implicated abnormalities on chromosome 6 for two of them.[48,49] Increased levels of chondrocalcin and fibroblast growth factor-9 have been found in the synovial fluid, indicating that they may play a role in the disease progression.[50,51] A study using flow cytometry demonstrated that only one of 20 cases has a nondiploid pattern,[52] and only one of 14 patients in the series in the Massachusetts General Hospital Orthopaedic Oncology Database was found to have an aneuploid synovial chondromatosis.[53] That patient developed a chondrosarcoma of the shoulder site as well as pulmonary metastases. With the exception of the rare cases of chondrosarcoma arising in the lesions, the overall impression from these data is that the standard synovial chondromatosis lesion is probably nonneoplastic and may actually be metaplastic, evolving out of some as yet undiscovered synovial tissue metabolic or biochemical abnormality.[1,2]

Imaging and Histologic Characteristics

In Milgram phase 1 disease, the bone and joint radiographs may show only a diffuse swelling and perhaps faint calcification of the cartilaginous bodies still in the synovium[1,2,35] (Figure 1). With magnetic resonance imaging (MRI), the lesion will appear as a positive on T1 because of the vascularity, and occasionally on T2 as well.[29,35,54-56] With phase 2 disease, the lesions are visible on standard radiographs and show multiple sites of calcification and internal ossification of the nodules (Figure 2). They show up quite noticeably on computed tomography and MRI, and the bone scan is now positive.[54,56] The imaging for Milgram phase 3 reveals calcified nodules in the joint that are essentially free of the synovium, often causing a marked degree of capsular enlargement and joint distortion.[29,35,54-56] Osteophytes, bone and cartilage destruction, and subsequent osteoarthritic changes may become apparent at late stages of the disease[1,8,46] (Figure 3).

The histologic pattern is very striking. Initially the synovium shows small islands of cartilage surrounded by fibrous capsule and synovial tissue. The cartilage tissue is initially richly cellular, and shows some suggestion of cell replication[1-4,22,37] (Figure 4). Within a relatively short period of time the small cartilage foci calcify, leading to a moderately heavy incrustation on histologic study. Some of the nuclei in this system are quite plump and show evidence of active DNA synthesis in the form of double nuclei. The cartilaginous tissue then begins endochondral ossification and makes bone, which increases the amount of calcific material within the nodule[1-4,22,37] (Figure 5). When the nodules become larger, they lose their synovial support, become avascular,

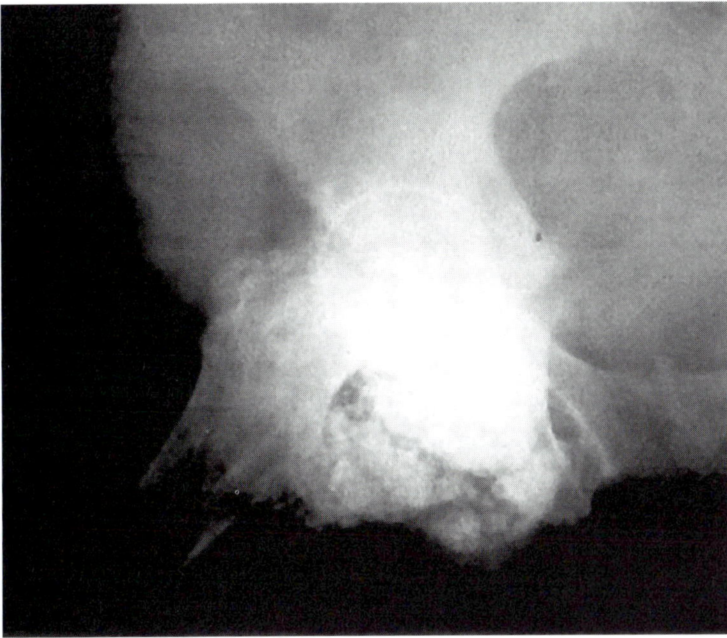

Figure 3
Severe changes of synovial chondromatosis have virtually destroyed this hip joint. The joint space is narrowed and the entire joint space is filled with nodular material.

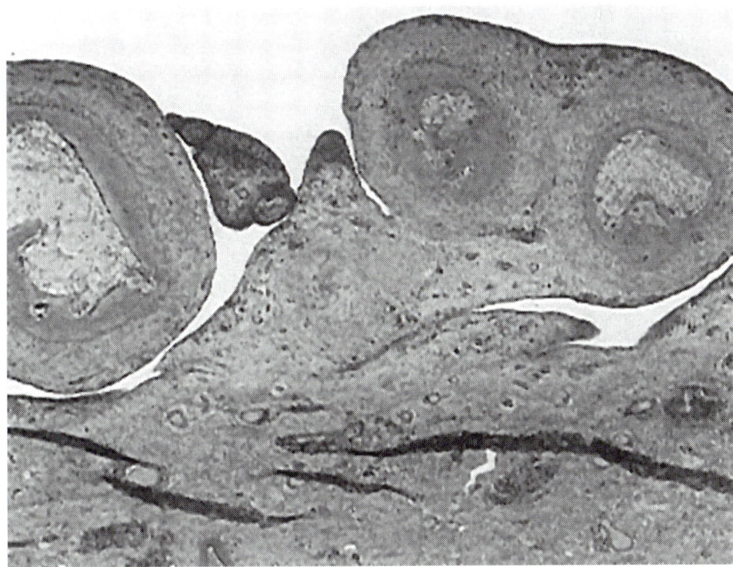

Figure 4
Histologic picture of the early phase of synovial chondromatosis, showing the nodular masses arising from the fibrotic synovial tissue. The central portion shows irregular cartilaginous tissue. Hematoxylin and eosin × 100.

and the bone dies. The nodules still maintain their heavy calcification; sometimes enormous numbers can be found throughout the joint and are clearly visible on imaging[1,2,37] (Figure 6).

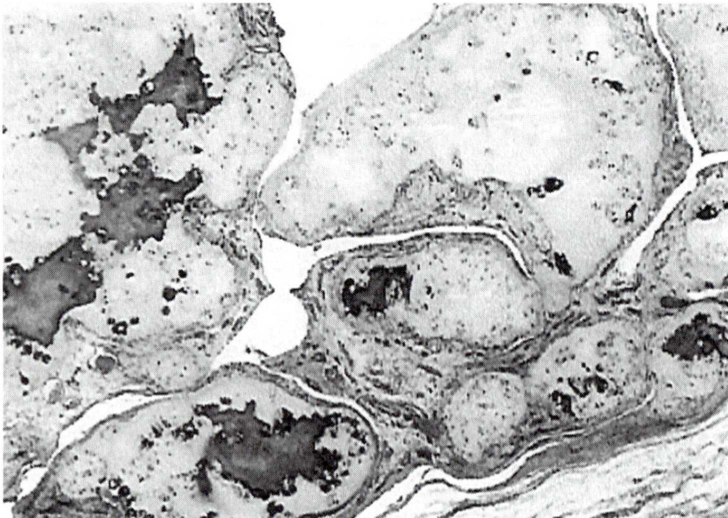

Figure 5

Histologic picture showing calcification in the cartilage and early bone formation occurring by endochondral ossification. Hematoxylin and eosin × 150.

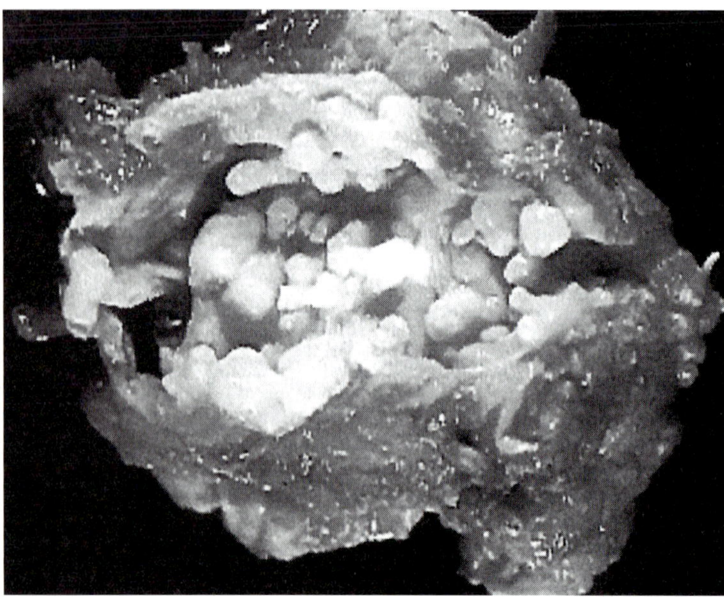

Figure 6

The joint structure in the synovium of a patient with extensive synovial chondromatosis. Note the calcified cartilaginous ossific bodies and the relationship to the markedly hypertrophic synovium.

Bursal and tenosynovial lesions are essentially identical but usually have fewer nodules, which are smaller in size and more irregular in outline. They remain quite evident on imaging.[25,30,32,34,38,39,41,43,44]

Malignant Degeneration

The synovial tissue of major joints does not usually undergo malignant degeneration, and nearly all synovial sarcomas and clear cell sarcomas occur outside the joint.[1,37,57] In 1991, Bertoni and associates[57] reported on chondrosarcomas arising from the synovium but declared it to be a rare phenomenon. Similarly, hyaline articular cartilage of the knee, hip, or other joints does not undergo malignant degeneration; although chondrosarcomas can arise in the rib cartilage or spinal segments, virtually none occur in relation to the hyaline cartilage from knee, hip, shoulder, or other sites.[1-3,37,57] Since the earliest identification of the syndrome, however, there have been reports of chondrosarcomas that seem to arise in relation to synovial chondromatosis in the knee, hip, shoulder, or even temporomandibular joint.[17-20,37,58-60] These may be quite malignant, and can metastasize and cause death. Fortunately such lesions are rarely encountered and most often occur after long periods of observation of a stable, benign synovial chondromatosis.

Treatment of Synovial Chondromatosis

Surgical resection of the lesions, and for most cases, the synovium as well is the principal method of treatment.[1,21,26,29,61,62] In some, the disease may develop quite slowly and, after Milgram phase 3, become stable.[38,63,64] Patients in this fortunate state may be monitored periodically with imaging studies and perhaps will only need surgical removal if symptoms supervene or the lesions appear larger on imaging studies.[63,64] Arthroscopic removal of the tissues including the nodules and the synovium is sometimes possible for synovial chondromatosis of the knee or shoulder, but may not be possible for the hip, elbow, or temporomandibular joint.[26,61,65] The key issue is one of recurrence, which frequently occurs no matter how the patient is treated. It is not the free bodies that are the problem; rather, it is the synovium that may begin another round of cartilage metaplasia. Bursal and tendinous lesions can be resected as necessary, but also may recur locally if the margins are not wide.[25,30,38,39,41,44]

Summary

Synovial chondromatosis or osteochondromatosis is an unusual entity, which probably represents a synovial metaplasia to form cartilaginous bodies that subsequently produce bone by endochondral ossification. Over time, the lesions result in many calcific cartilaginous and ossific nodules that are present throughout the joint. They cause symptoms such as swelling, tenderness, and limitation of movement. The lesions are best treated by resection of not only the nodular tissue, but by a synovectomy as well. Many patients recover nicely from this disorder, and development of a malignant form of the disease is fortunately very rare.

References

1. Campanacci M: *Bone and Soft Tissue Tumors*, ed 2. New York, NY, Springer Verlag 1999, pp 1289-1306.

2. Dorfman HD, Czerniak B: *Bone Tumors*. St. Louis, MO, Mosby, 1998, pp 1041-1061.

3. Jaffe HL: *Tumors and Tumorous Conditions of Bones and Joints*. Philadelphia, PA, Lea and Febiger, 1958, pp 558-576.

4. Milgram JW: Synovial chondromatosis: A histopathological study of thirty cases. *J Bone Joint Surg Am* 1977;59:792-801.

5. Reichel PF: Chondromatose der Kniegelenkskapsel. *Arch Klin Chir Berlin* 1900;61:717-724.

6. Henderson MS: Osteocartilaginous joint bodies. *Railway Surg J* 1918;25:49-53.

7. Henderson MS, Jones HT: Loose bodies in joints and bursae due to synovial osteochondromatosis. *J Bone Joint Surg* 1923;5:400-424.

8. Jones HT: Loose body formation in synovial osteochondromatosis with special reference to the etiology and pathology. *J Bone Joint Surg* 1924;6:407-458.

9. Cruveilhier J: Anatomie pathologique du corps humain. *Paris Bailliere* 1835:1829-1832.

10. Kolliker A: *Manual of Human Histology*. London, England, Sydenham Society, 1853, pp 326-329.

11. Lexer E: Gelenkchondrome. *Deutsche Zeitschrift F Chir* 1907;88:311-323.

12. Fisher AGT: A study of loose bodies composed of cartilage or of cartilage and bone occurring in joints, with special reference to their pathology and etiology. *Br J Surg* 1921;8:493-521.

13. Rixford E: Osteochondromatosis. *Ann Surg* 1930;92:673-680.

14. Wilmoth CL: Osteochondromatosis. *J Bone Joint Surg* 1941;23:367-374.

15. Mussey RD Jr, Henderson MS: Osteochondromatosis. *J Bone Joint Surg Am* 1949;31:619-627.

16. Jeffreys TE: Synovial chondromatosis. *J Bone Joint Surg Br* 1967;49:530-534.

17. Riemann H, Kienbock R: Über Gelenks-osteochondromatoses mie sarcombildung. *Röentgenpraxis* 1931;3:942-944.

18. Geschickter CF, Copeland MM: *Tumors of Bone*, ed 3. Philadelphia, PA, JB Lippincott Co, 1949, pp 697-701.

19. Nixon JE, Frank GR, Chambers G: Synovial osteochondromatosis with report of four cases, one showing malignant change. *US Armed Forces Med J* 1960;11:1434-1445.

20. Mullins F, Berard W, Eisenberg SH: Chondrosarcoma following synovial chondromatosis: A case study. *Cancer* 1965;18:1180-1188.

21. Bloom R, Pattinson JN: Osteochondromatosis of the hip joint. *J Bone Joint Surg Br* 1951;33:80-84.

22. Chillemi C, Marinelli M, deCupis V: Primary synovial chondromatosis of the shoulder: Clinical, arthroscopic and histopathologic aspects. *Knee Surg Sports Traumatol Arthrosc* 2005;13:483-488.

23. Crotty JM, Monu JU, Pope TL Jr: Synovial osteochondromatosis. *Radiol Clin North Am* 1996;34:327-342.

24. Edeiken J, Edeiken BS, Ayala AG, et al: Giant solitary synovial chondromatosis. *Skeletal Radiol* 1994;23:23-29.

25. Fetsch JF, Vinh TN, Remotti F, Walker EA, Murphey MD, Sweet DE: Tenosynovial (extraarticular) chondromatosis: An analysis of 37 cases of an underrecognized clinicopathologic entity with a strong predilection for the hands and feet and a high local recurrence rate. *Am J Surg Pathol* 2003;27:1260-1268.

26. Gilbert SR, Lachiewicz PF: Primary synovial osteochondromatosis of the hip: Report of two cases with long-term follow-up after synovectomy and a review of the literature. *Am J Orthop* 1997;26:555-560.

27. Jazrawi LM, Ong B, Jazrawi AJ, Rose D: Synovial chondromatosis of the elbow. *Am J Orthop* 2001;30:223-224.

28. McFarland EG, Neira CA: Synovial chondromatosis of the shoulder associated with osteoarthritis: Conservative treatment in two cases and review of the literature. *Am J Orthop* 2000;29:785-787.

29. McGrory JE, Rock MG: Synovial chondromatosis of the shoulder. *Am J Orthop* 2000;29:793-795.

30. Milgram JW, Hadesman WM: Synovial osteochondromatosis in the subacromial bursa. *Clin Orthop Relat Res* 1988;236:154-159.

31. Murphy FP, Dahlin DC, Sullivan CR: Articular synovial chondromatosis. *J Bone Joint Surg Am* 1962;44:77-86.

32. Robinson P, White LM, Kandel R, Bell RS, Wunder JS: Primary synovial osteochondromatosis of the hip: Extracapsular patterns of spread. *Skeletal Radiol* 2004;33:210-215.

33. Rosati LA, Stevens C: Synovial chondromatosis of the temporomandibular joint presenting as an intracranial mass. *Arch Otolaryngol Head Neck Surg* 1990;116:1334-1337.

34. Roulot E, Le Viet D: Primary synovial osteochondromatosis of hand and wrist: Report of a series of 21 cases and literature review. *Rev Rhum Engl Ed* 1999;66:256-266.

35. Ryan RS, Harris AC, O'Connell JX, Munk PL: Synovial osteochondromatosis: The spectrum of imaging findings. *Australas Radiol* 2005;49:95-100.

36. Sarmiento A, Elkins RW: Giant intra-articular osteochondroma of the knee. *J Bone Joint Surg Am* 1975;57:560-561.

37. Schajowicz F: Tumors and tumor-like lesions of the

synovial membrane, in *Tumors and Tumorlike Lesions of Bone and Joints*. New York, NY, Springer Verlag, 1981, pp 519-567.

38. Sim FH, Dahlin DC, Ivins JC: Extra-articular synovial chondromatosis. *J Bone Joint Surg Am* 1977;59:492-495.

39. Tibrewal SB, Iossifidis A: Extra-articular synovial chondromatosis of the ankle. *J Bone Joint Surg Br* 1995;77:659-660.

40. Trias A, Quintana O: Synovial chondrometaplasia: Review of world literature and study of 18 Canadian cases. *Can J Surg* 1976;19:151-158.

41. Van P, Wilusz PM, Ungar DS, Pupp GR: Synovial chondromatosis of the subtalar joint and tenosynovial chondromatosis of the posterior ankle. *J Am Podiatr Med Assoc* 2006;96:59-62.

42. von Lindern JJ, Theuerkauf I, Niederhagen B, Berge S, Appel T, Reich RH: Synovial chondromatosis of the temporomandibular joint: Clinical, diagnostic and histomorphologic findings. *Oral Surg Oral Med Oral Pathol Oral Radiol Endod* 2002;94:31-38.

43. Wagner S, Bennek J, Grafe G, et al: Chondromatosis of the ankle joint (Reichel syndrome). *Pediatr Surg Int* 1999;15:437-439.

44. Young-In Lee F, Hornicek FJ, Dick HM, Mankin HJ: Synovial chondromatosis of the foot. *Clin Orthop Relat Res* 2004;423:186-190.

45. Milgram JW: The classification of loose bodies in human joints. *Clin Orthop Relat Res* 1977;124:282-291.

46. Norman A, Steiner GC: Bone erosion in synovial chondromatosis. *Radiology* 1986;161:749-752.

47. Davis RI, Foster H, Biggart DJ: C-erb B-2 staining in primary synovial chondromatosis: A comparison with other cartilaginous tumours. *J Pathol* 1996;179:392-395.

48. Buddingh EP, Krallman P, Neff JR, et al: Chromosome 6 abnormalities are recurrent in synovial chondromatosis. *Cancer Genet Cytogenet* 2003;140:18-22.

49. Robinson D, Hasharoni A, Evron Z, Segal M, Nevo Z: Synovial chondromatosis: The possible role of FGF 9 and FGF receptor 3 in its pathology. *Int J Exp Pathol* 2000;81:183-189.

50. Fukuhara S, Kanazawa Y, Uchida S, Akahoshi S, Yoshioka T, Nakamura T: Increased levels of chondrocalcin in knee joint fluid in synovial chondromatosis: A case report. *Acta Orthop Scand* 2000;71:326-327.

51. Inoue K, Nakajima H, Ushiyama T, Hukuda S: Immunohistochemical identification of chondrocalcin in synovial chondromatosis. *Osteoarthritis Cartilage* 1996;4:287-288.

52. Coughlan B, Feliz A, Ishida T, Czerniak B, Dorfman HD: P53 expression and DNA ploidy of cartilage lesions. *Hum Pathol* 1995;26:620-624.

53. Mankin HJ: A computerized system for orthopaedic oncology. *Clin Orthop Relat Res* 2002;398:252-261.

54. De Beuckeleer LH, De Schepper AM, Ramon F, Somville J: Magnetic resonance imaging of cartilaginous tumors: A retrospective study of 79 patients. *Eur J Radiol* 1995;21:34-40.

55. Kim HG, Park KH, Huh JK, Song YB, Choi HS: Magnetic resonance imaging characteristics of synovial chondromatosis of the temporomandibular joint. *J Orofac Pain* 2002;16:148-153.

56. Shanley DJ, Evans EM, Buckner AB, Delaplain CB: Synovial osteochondromatosis demonstrated on bone scan: Correlation with CT and MRI. *Clin Nucl Med* 1992;17:338-339.

57. Bertoni F, Unni KK, Beabout JW, Sim FH: Chondrosarcomas of the synovium. *Cancer* 1991;67:155-162.

58. Hamilton A, Davis RI, Hayes D, Mollan RA: Chondrosarcoma developing in synovial chondromatosis: A case report. *J Bone Joint Surg Br* 1987;69:137-140.

59. Hermann G, Klein MJ, Abdelwahab IF, Kenan S: Synovial chondrosarcoma arising in synovial chondromatosis of the right hip. *Skeletal Radiol* 1997;26:366-369.

60. Perry BE, McQueen DA, Lin JJ: Synovial chondromatosis with malignant degeneration to chondrosarcoma: Report of a case. *J Bone Joint Surg Am* 1988;70:1259-1261.

61. Ogilvie-Harris DJ, Saleh K: Generalized synovial chondromatosis of the knee: A comparison of removal of the loose bodies alone with arthroscopic synovectomy. *Arthroscopy* 1994;10:166-170.

62. Shpitzer T, Ganel A, Engleberg S: Surgery for synovial chondromatosis: 26 cases followed up for 6 years. *Acta Orthop Scand* 1990;61:567-569.

63. Sviland L, Malcolm AJ: Synovial chondromatosis presenting as painless soft tissue mass: A report of 19 cases. *Histopathology* 1995;27:275-279.

64. Swan EF, Owens WF Jr: Synovial chondrometaplasia: A case report with spontaneous regression and a review of the literature. *South Med J* 1972;65:1496-1500.

65. Jeon IH, Ihn JC, Kyung HS: Recurrence of synovial chondromatosis of the glenohumeral joint after arthroscopic treatment. *Arthroscopy* 2004;20:524-527.

Chapter 9

Osteonecrosis

Osteonecrosis was originally called aseptic necrosis or avascular necrosis of bone, but both terms are somewhat misleading. The term "aseptic" was introduced before the development of antibiotics, when septic necrosis was a common disorder. The word "avascular" suggests (incorrectly) that the affected bone site is without a blood supply. The medical community has now chosen the word osteonecrosis to define the multiple entities that cause various forms of death of bone. Bone does indeed have a blood supply, which consists of two components.[1-8] The first component is the nutrient medullary blood supply, which arises in blood vessels from major vascular sources in the limb and enters the bone through small nutrient vascular channels regularly placed through the cortex. This system supplies blood to the medullary cavity and the internal half of the cortex. The second vascular system is a periosteal blood supply consisting of small blood vessels that provide a vascular supply to the external half of the cortex. The blood supply of bone is clearly a major factor in maintaining not only the viability of the cells in the marrow, but the vascularity of the cortices and the trabeculae. If this blood supply is interrupted or in any way impaired, the bone will undergo the disorder now known as osteonecrosis. The degree of bone death will depend on the nature, extent, and location of the vascular interruption or impairment.[1,2,7,9-12]

History of Osteonecrosis as a Disease Entity

The earliest writings related to the blood supply of bone were provided by Cooper[13] in the 19th century. In an 1822 treatise, he defined the effect of fractures on blood supply, particularly of the femoral neck and head. The blood supply was clearly challenged by such injuries; bone death appeared to be the major consequence and also represented the problem that interfered with healing.[3] It was the remarkable contribution by Johnson[6] in 1927 that clearly defined the vascular supply for the shaft of the bone. This was followed closely by Phemister's[14] presentation in 1930, which identified the disease now known as osteonecrosis and in fact defined some of the major causes of the problem. Phemister cited radiation as a possible cause, along with interference with circulation, infection, periosteal separation, and trauma; he also defined the nature of the histologic changes and the attempts at repair. Subsequent studies by Phemister and his colleagues Kahlstrom and Burton[15-17] showed that osteonecrosis could occur in patients who had not sustained trauma and who presented with defined disease. The causes of osteonecrosis for many of these patients are still somewhat shrouded in mystery. As Marcus Aurelius said, "Death, like birth, is a secret of nature."[18]

Over the next 50 years, numerous authors defined osteonecrosis both histologically and as a series of highly variable clinical syndromes. Further studies correlated causation of osteonecrosis with an array of illnesses and conditions, including obesity,[19,20] radiation,[21] bowel abnormalities,[22-24] acquired immunodeficiency syndrome (AIDS),[25-28] Gaucher disease,[29-32] renal failure,[33-35] alcoholism,[36-40] coagulopathies[20,41,42] genetic hematologic abnormalities,[43-48] pregnancy,[49,50] aging,[51] dysbarism,[52-54] and rheumatic afflictions.[55-59] In the past 30 years, it has become evident that the most common cause of nontraumatic bone death is the administration of corticosteroids and other agents that are used to reduce the immune response.[1,10,23,24,34,58-67]

Pathogenesis of Osteonecrosis

Bone has a rich blood supply that varies from site to site and provides both a medullary and cortical vascularity.[1-8] The medullary supply is almost entirely based on a set of nutrient channels arising from vessels lying longitudinally along the osseous structure that enter the medullary cavity at regular intervals. They supply not only the bone and cells of the medullary cavity, but in addition provide vasculature for the inner half of the cortices and the metaphysis as well as the

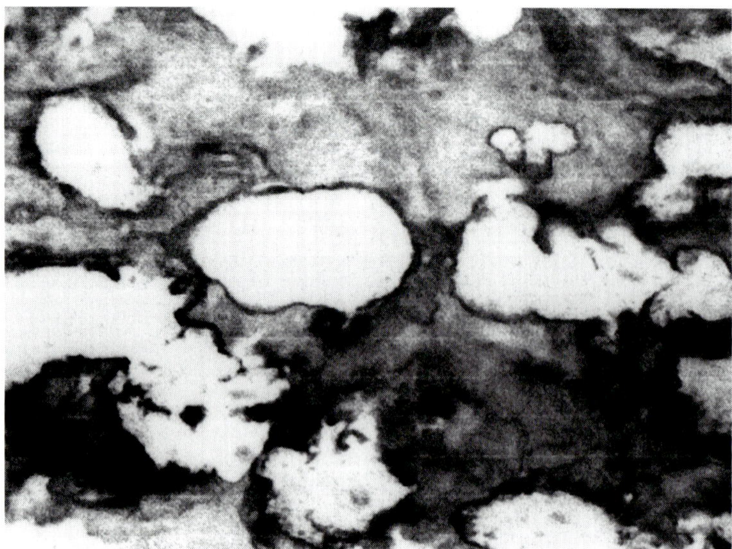

Figure 1
Histologic picture of a focus of medullary osteonecrosis. Fat cells have died, releasing free fatty acids that use calcium as counterions. The result is the irregular calcified material seen here. Hematoxylin and eosin × 20.

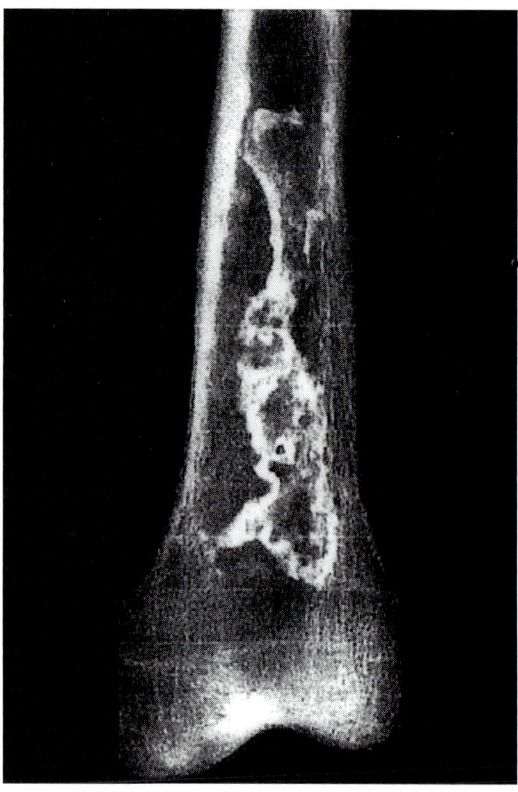

Figure 2
Radiographic appearance of a focus of medullary osteonecrosis, described as "smoke goes up the chimney".

ring of Ranvier. The other vascular systems are periosteal in origin with channels that are smaller in size. They provide the blood supply to the outer half of the cortices but are also major components of the metaphyseal region, which usually has a much better blood supply than the diaphyseal sites.[1-8]

Interruption of these channels, either as a result of trauma or in the course of surgery or because of an array of clinical disorders that affect the blood flow in the bones, leads to osteonecrosis.[1,2,7,9-12] There are two types of pathologic osteonecrotic disorders—medullary, and corticocancellous involving a joint. Medullary osteonecrosis is caused by interference in the blood supply to the medullary cavity, which results in not only trabecular bone death but in the death of the cells that inhabit the medullary cavity.[7,9,68-70] In young children, these represent marrow cells such as polymorphonucleocytes, lymphocytes, and monocytes, but in older individuals the majority of the cells are lipocytes. Because medullary osteonecrosis is most often a disease of mature individuals, most of the cells that die as a result of a medullary vascular injury are the lipocytes.[7,9] The damage to these cells releases free fatty acids in large quantities; they seek a counterion, and the major one available is obviously calcium. The result is the production of a calcium soap (calcium plus a free fatty acid), which is insoluble in body fluids.[7] This produces a mass of material that is seen histologically as fragments of acellular poorly stained material (Figure 1) and radiographically as an irregular densely calcified structure described as "smoke goes up the chimney"[7] (Figure 2). Most of these lesions are asymptomatic, with the possible exception of the "Gaucher crisis," a painful and markedly inflammatory process that occurs in patients with Gaucher disease in whom an enormous number of cells contain glucosyl ceramide, consisting of a glucose, sphingosine, and a free fatty acid.[29-32] Death of these cells can cause the release of agents that cause a major systemic inflammatory response.[29,30]

Corticocancellous osteonecrosis involving a joint is usually much more pernicious. The vascular compromise occurs in the proximal femur or proximal humerus, and less commonly the distal femur or proximal tibia, and is located in the metaphysis just subjacent to the joint.[9,71] The trabecular and often the subchondral bone die; the region calcifies to a lesser extent; and the cartilaginous surface loses its support, partly because of microfractures but also related to uncontrolled repair. The joint collapses and frequently the patients become profoundly symptomatic [7,9,68-70] (Figure 3).

The mechanisms by which blood supply can be interrupted in either of these pathologic disorders consist of four possible disorders.[7,72] The first of these is mechanical interruption of the blood supply. This may result from a fracture or dislocation of the hip or shoulder; both sites have tenuous blood supplies that can be easily completely or partially interrupted by an injury, even one as limited as a stress fracture or closed trauma.[1,10,11,62] The second is related to vascular thrombosis or embolism. Any process occluding the vessel that supports a segment of bone with poor collateral circulation can cause osteonecrosis. Blockages of this sort can result from thrombus or embolus, excessive circulating fat, air or nitrogen bubbles ("dysbarism") or abnormally shaped cells such as those occurring in sickle cell crisis.[19,20,43,45,48,52,53] The third form of disorder is injury or pressure to a vascular wall. Vascular walls can be temporarily or permanently damaged by radiation, inflammatory disorders, vasculitis, or excessive pressure by fat or marrow cells.[7,21,48,55,56,62,73] The fourth form of disorder that can lead to osteonecrosis is venous occlusion (Chandler's disease).[74,75] If the veins become occluded or compressed, venular pressure may exceed arteriolar pressure in a closed system; as a result, the arterial blood supply can be severely compromised. Even if the arteries are not occluded, the reduction in blood flow as a result of increased venular pressure can result in an arteriolar ischemia leading to cell death.[73] Venular pressure, particularly around the hip, can be increased as a result of large joint effusions or alterations in capsular structure and lead to cell death and pathologic osteonecrosis.[1,7,10]

Clinical Causes of Osteonecrosis

Although the four generic causes described above are the major explanations for the entity, an enormous number of clinical disorders have been described as being associated with osteonecrosis. The principal problem with this is that for many of the disorders listed, the nature of the effect on the bone blood supply is not really known

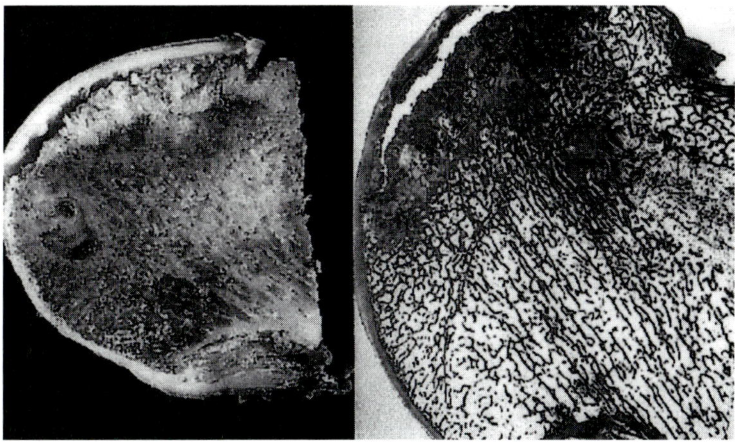

Figure 3
Subchondral osteonecrosis in the femoral head leading to collapse of the bone beneath the cartilage and ultimately an arthritic course, which can be quite severe and disabling. The photograph on the left is a gross photograph; the one on the right is a very low-power histologic study. Hematoxylin and eosin × 10.

or established. Some of the lists in the literature include as many as 100 entities that on occasion have been reported as being associated with osteonecrosis, but the 20 most frequent entities and their approximate causation are shown alphabetically in Table 1. Included in the table is an assessment of the likely causation according to the four principal mechanisms described above, with the addition of the all important fifth mechanism ("really not sure").

Most authorities now believe that the most frequent cause of osteonecrosis is corticosteroid treatment; the incidence ranges from 5% to 25% of patients who receive the medication.[1,10,23,24,34,58-67] In general, the drugs must be administered for more than 1 month and dosage must be greater than twice the normal adrenal output level. Patients at risk include those with allograft implants, connective tissue disorders, dermatologic problems, chronic pulmonary disease, inflammatory bowel disease, hematologic and ophthalmologic disorders, and many others. Corticosteroid-induced osteonecrosis may not occur for months or sometimes even years after treatment. Although the numbers are lower now than in the past, greater frequency is observed with administration of a single dose of intravertebral corticoid in the treatment of spinal problems.[1,10,23,24,34,58-67]

Patients with Gaucher disease or sickle cell disease are still at risk, as are those with

Table 1 | Frequently Cited Causes of Osteonecrosis

Diagnosis	Possible Mechanisms*
Acquired immuno-deficiency syndrome	5
Alcoholism	4,5
Allograft rejection	5
Aging	5
Aneurysms	3,4,5
Arteritis, atherosclerosis	3
Corticosteroids	4,5
Diabetes mellitus	3
Dysbarism	2
Fracture and dislocation	1,4
Gaucher disease	2,4,5
Hemaglobinopathies	2,4
Lupus erythematosus	2,3
Obesity	2
Pregnancy	4,5
Polycythemia	2,4
Radiation	3
Rheumatoid arthritis	3
Sickle cell anemia	2
Thrombotic thrombocytopenic purpura	2,5

*1:Mechanical interruption
2:Vascular thrombosis or embolism
3:Injury to the vascular wall
4:Chandler's disease
5:Really not sure

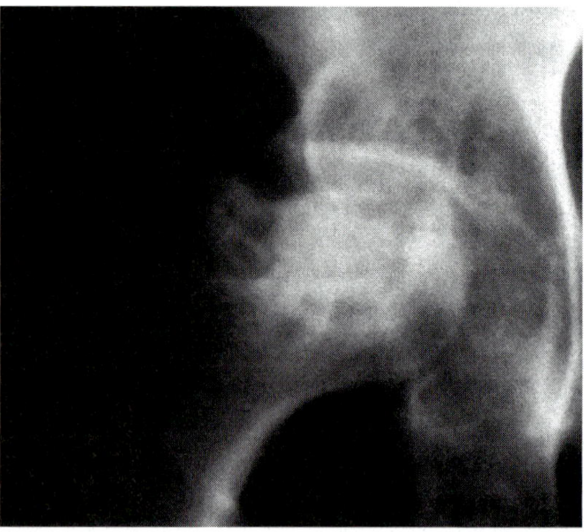

Figure 4
Typical radiographic appearance of extensive osteonecrosis of the femoral head showing the marked increase in bone density and the narrowed joint space.

The one originally proposed in 1979 by a team from the University of Pennsylvania has now been expanded to use not only radiographs but bone scans and magnetic resonance imaging (MRI) as well.[80] The system defines stage 0 as a normal bone and joint on radiograph and bone scan; stage I has a normal radiograph but a positive bone scan. Stage II demonstrates lucent and sclerotic changes on imaging, and stage III shows a subchondral collapse. Stage IV shows flattening of the femoral head; stage V, joint narrowing and acetabular changes; and stage VI, severe degeneration of the joint (Figure 4).

Imaging Studies for Osteonecrosis

In the past, with only radiographs and bone scans to assess the problem, it was sometimes difficult to diagnose osteonecrosis even in the face of complaints of pain and local disability.[81] Many of the bone scans were not positive early in the disease; this was helpful in distinguishing osteonecrotic foci from osteomyelitis lesions, which are almost always positive on bone scan. Scans became positive at some point when local edema and repair processes began to occur, which in some cases took several weeks.[30] Today, computed tomography and especially MRI are very valuable adjuncts in that the site of osteonecrosis can usually be identified almost immediately as a dark focus on both T1 and T2.[11,30,32,81-83] The use of gado-

systemic lupus erythematosus, thrombocytopenic purpura, and more recently AIDS. The mechanism of action of the 20 cited causes is still not clear; in particular, the ways in which obesity, aging, and alcoholism cause osteonecrosis are not fully understood. Furthermore, the entities that occur in special anatomic sites in normal individuals sometimes remain mysterious. These include such disorders as Legg-Calvé-Perthes, Kienböck's, Preiser's, and Friedrich's diseases as well as others, none of which are clearly understood but possibly represent forms of Chandler's disease or subtle posttraumatic osteonecrosis.[7,50,51,76-79]

Staging of Proximal Femoral Corticocancellous Osteonecrotic Foci

Several systems have been proposed for staging of proximal femoral osteonecrosis.

linium will further identify the site as having no or very little blood supply. It is also possible to detect either healing or further progression with the use of serial studies; most treatment protocols suggest that MRI and bone scans be done regularly.

Treatment of Osteonecrosis

Numerous systems have been introduced over the years. There is rarely any reason to treat patients with medullary disease except for those with Gaucher crisis; these patients have been hospitalized, treated with pain medication and intravenous fluids, and even on some occasions been subjected to hyperbaric oxygen therapy.[7,29,30]

For patients with corticocancellous disease, particularly in the hip, the simplest approach is non- or partial weight bearing, and exercises for a period as long as 6 months or more. This system is sometimes successful; although patients may not enjoy the long period of disability, they return to reasonable function as healing of the site occurs without collapse of the joint.[7,51,63,84,85] Core decompression has been advocated and seems to be reasonably successful for some patients with disease in which the femoral head is not collapsed (stages I or II).[63,86] For more advanced disease, vascularized autograft has been advocated; this is reported to be reasonably successful in a high per-

centage of the patients with stage II or III disease.[87] For patients with stage IV, V, or VI disease—particularly if the patient continues to be disabled and complains of pain—there are few options other than total joint replacement.[88] Some have suggested osteotomy, such as that done for Legg-Calvé-Perthes disease, but the problems with this procedure for adults with osteonecrosis are fairly marked; furthermore, if failure occurs, the total joint replacement is more difficult to do.[89] Similar protocols have been proposed for shoulders and sometimes knees. Kienböck's disease and other such problems usually require special approaches, including arthrodesis and replacement of the bony part.

Summary

Osteonecrosis remains an enigma. Although we now understand the pathologic process, the pathogenesis in many cases is mysterious. The rate of progression of the disease is unpredictable, as is the degree of often devastating disability. Despite our knowledge of the syndrome dating back more than 70 years, no simple or uniformly successful treatment protocol has been developed. There are, however, some glimmers of hope and we continue to seek information and learn.

References

1. Assouline-Dayan Y, Chang C, Greenspan A, Shoenfield Y, Gershwin ME: Pathogenesis and natural history of osteonecrosis. *Semin Arthritis Rheum* 2002;32:94-124.

2. Boettcher WG, Bonfiglio M, Hamilton HH, Sheets RF, Smith K: Non-traumatic necrosis of the femoral head: I. Relation of altered hemostasis to etiology. *J Bone Joint Surg Am* 1970;52:312-321.

3. Brookes M: *The Blood Supply of Bone: An Approach to Bone Biology*. London, England, Butterworths , 1971.

4. Hanson ES: Blood flow in the axial and appendicular skeleton, in Urbaniak JR, Jones JP Jr (eds): *Osteonecrosis: Etiology, Diagnosis, and Treatment*. Rosemont, IL, American Academy of Orthopaedic Surgeons, 1997, pp 19-26.

5. Hughes SPF, Corbett SA, Reichert ILH, McCarthy ID: The regulation of blood flow in bone, in Urbaniak JR, Jones JP Jr (eds): *Osteonecrosis: Etiology, Diagnosis, and Treatment*. Rosemont, IL, American Academy of Orthopaedic Surgeons, 1997, pp 11-17.

6. Johnson RW: A physiologic study of the blood supply of the diaphysis. *J Bone Joint Surg* 1927;9:153-184.

7. Mankin HJ: Non-traumatic necrosis of bone (osteonecrosis). *N Engl J Med* 1992;326:1473-1479.

8. Trias A, Fery A: Cortical circulation of long bones. *J Bone Joint Surg Am* 1979;61:1052-1059.

9. Bullough PG: The morbid anatomy of subchondral osteonecrosis, in Urbaniak JR, Jones JP Jr (eds): *Osteonecrosis: Etiology, Diagnosis, and Treatment*. Rosemont, IL, American Academy of Orthopaedic Surgeons, 1997, pp 69-72.

10. Cruess RL: Osteonecrosis of bone: Current concepts as to etiology and pathogenesis. *Clin Orthop Relat Res* 1986;208:30-39.

11. Ecker ML: Spontaneous osteonecrosis of the distal femur. *Instr Course Lect* 2001;50:495-498.

12. Glimcher MJ, Kenzora JE: The biology of osteonecrosis of the human femoral head and its clinical implications: Part I. Tissue biology. *Clin Orthop Relat Res* 1979;138:284-309.

13. Cooper SA: *A Treatise on Fractures and Dislocations of Joints*. London, England, E. Cox and Son, 1822.

14. Phemister DB: Repair of bone in the presence of aseptic necrosis resulting from fractures, transplantations and vascular obstruction. *J Bone Joint Surg* 1930;30:769-787.

15. Kahlstrom SC, Burton CC, Phemister DB: Aseptic necrosis of bone: I. Infarction of bones in Caisson

disease resulting in encapsulated and calcified areas in diaphyses and in arthritis deformans. *Surg Gynecol Obstet* 1939;68:129-146.

16. Kahlstrom SC, Burton CC, Phemister DB: Aseptic necrosis of bone: II. Infarction of bones of undetermined etiology resulting in encapsulated and calcified areas in diaphyses and in arthritis deformans. *Surg Gynecol Obstet* 1939;68:631-641.

17. Phemister DB: Fractures of the neck of the femur, dislocation of hip and obscure vascular disturbances producing aseptic necrosis of the head of the femur. *Surg Gynecol Obstet* 1934;59:415-440.

18. Marcus Aurelius Antoninus Meditations Book IV, in Casaubon M (trans): *The Golden Book of Marcus Aurelius.* New York, NY, EP Dutton, 1906, pp 29-30.

19. Jones JP Jr: Fat embolism and osteonecrosis. *Orthop Clin North Am* 1985;16:593-633.

20. Jones JP Jr: Fat embolism, intravascular coagulation and osteonecrosis. *Clin Orthop Relat Res* 1993;292:294-308.

21. Goodman AH, Sherman MH: Post-irradiation fractures of the femoral neck. *J Bone Joint Surg Am* 1963;45:723-730.

22. Freeman HJ, Owen D, Millan M: Granulomatous osteonecrosis in Crohn's disease. *Can J Gastroenterol* 2000;14:951-954.

23. Klingenstein G, Levy RN, Kornbluth A, Shah AK, Present DH: Inflammatory bowel disease related osteonecrosis: Report of a large series with a review of the literature. *Aliment Pharmacol Ther* 2005;21:243-249.

24. Vakil N, Sparberg M: Steroid-related osteonecrosis in inflammatory bowel disease. *Gastroenterology* 1989;96:62-67.

25. Allison GT, Bostrom MP, Glesby MJ: Osteonecrosis in HIV disease: Epidemiology, etiologies and clinical management. *AIDS* 2003;17:1-9.

26. Miller KD, Masur H, Jones EC, et al: High prevalence of osteonecrosis of the femoral head in HIV-infected adults. *Ann Intern Med* 2002;137:17-25.

27. Mullan RH, Ryan PF: Multiple site osteonecrosis in HIV infection. *Rheumatology (Oxford)* 2002;41:1200-1202.

28. Newman MD: Bone disorders, hypertension and mitochondrial toxicity in HIV disease. *Top HIV Med* 2003;11:10-15.

29. Mankin HJ, Doppelt SH, Rosenberg AE, et al: Metabolic bone disease in patients with Gaucher's disease, in Avioli LV, Krane SM (eds): *Metabolic Bone Disease and Clinically Related Disorders.* Philadelphia, PA, WB Saunders, 1990, pp 730-752.

30. Mankin HJ, Rosenthal DI, Xavier R: Current Concepts Review: Gaucher disease. New approaches to an ancient disease. *J Bone Joint Surg Am* 2001;83:748-762.

31. Rodrigue SW, Rosenthal DI, Barton NW, Zurakowski D, Mankin HJ: Risk factors for osteonecrosis in patients with type 1 Gaucher's disease. *Clin Orthop Relat Res* 1999;362:201-207.

32. Rosenthal DI, Mayo-Smith W, Goodsitt MM, Doppelt S, Mankin HJ: Bone and bone marrow changes in Gaucher disease: Evaluation with quantitative CT. *Radiology* 1989;170:143-146.

33. Langevitz P, Buskila D, Stewart J, Sherrard DJ, Hercz G: Osteonecrosis in patients receiving dialysis: Report of two cases and review of the literature. *J Rheumatol* 1990;17:402-406.

34. Metselaar HJ, van Steenberge EJ, Bijnen AB, Jeekel JJ, van Linge B, Weimar W: Incidence of osteonecrosis after renal transplantation. *Acta Orthop Scand* 1985;56:413-415.

35. Sperschneider H, Stein G: Bone disease after renal transplantation. *Nephrol Dial Transplant* 2003;18:874-877.

36. Gold EW, Cangemi PJ: Incidence and pathogenesis of alcohol-induced osteonecrosis of the femoral head. *Clin Orthop Relat Res* 1979;143:222-226.

37. Hungerford DS, Zizic TM: Alcoholism associated ischemic necrosis of the femoral head: Early diagnosis and treatment. *Clin Orthop Relat Res* 1978;130:144-153.

38. Jones JP Jr, Peltier LF: Alcoholism, hypercortisonism, fat embolism and osseous osteonecrosis (1971). *Clin Orthop Relat Res* 2001;393:4-12.

39. Matsuo K, Hirohata T, Sugioka Y, Ikeda M, Fukuda A: Influence of alcohol intake, cigarette smoking, and occupational status on idiopathic osteonecrosis of the femoral head. *Clin Orthop Relat Res* 1988;234:115-123.

40. Orlic D, Jovanovic S, Anticevic D, Zecivic J: Frequency of idiopathic aseptic necrosis in medically treated alcoholics. *Int Orthop* 1990;14:383-386.

41. Jones JP Jr: Intravascular coagulation and osteonecrosis. *Clin Orthop Relat Res* 1992;277:41-53.

42. Jones JP Jr: Risk factors potentially activating intravascular coagulation and causing nontraumatic osteonecrosis, in Urbaniak JR, Jones JP Jr (eds): *Osteonecrosis: Etiology, Diagnosis, and Treatment.* Rosemont, IL, American Academy of Orthopaedic Surgeons, 1997, pp 89-96.

43. Athanassiou-Metaxa M, Kirkos J, Koussi A, Hatzipantelis E, Tsatra I, Economou M: Avascular necrosis of the femoral head among children and adolescents with sickle cell disease in Greece. *Haematologica* 2002;87:771-772.

44. Johanson NA: Musculoskeletal problems in hemoglobinopathy. *Orthop Clin North Am* 1990;21:191-198.

45. Milner PF, Kraus AO, Sebes JI, et al: Sickle cell disease as a cause of osteonecrosis of the femoral head. *N Engl J Med* 1991;325:1476-1481.

46. Moore J, Coyle L, Isbister J, Roche J: Bilateral knee osteonecrosis in a patient with thrombotic thrombocytopenic purpura. *Aust N Z J Med* 1999;29:88-89.

47. Seiler JG III, Christie MJ, Homra L: Correlation of the findings of magnetic resonance imaging with those of bone biopsy in patients who have stage-I or II ischemic necrosis of the femoral head. *J Bone Joint Surg Am* 1989;71:28-32.

48. Wang T-Y, Avlonitis EG, Relkin R: Systemic necrotizing vasculitis causing bone necrosis. *Am J Med* 1988;84:1085-1086.

49. Montella BJ, Nunley JA, Urbaniak JR: Osteonecrosis of the femoral head associated with pregnancy, in Urbaniak JR, Jones JP Jr (eds): *Osteonecrosis: Etiology, Diagnosis, and Treatment.* Rosemont, IL, American Academy of Orthopaedic Surgeons, 1997, pp 115-130.

50. Pellicci PM, Zolla-Pazner S, Rabhan WN, Wilson PD Jr: Osteonecrosis of the femoral head associated with pregnancy: Report of three cases. *Clin Orthop Relat Res* 1984;185:59-63.

51. Pape D, Seil R, Fritsch E, Rupp S, Kohn D: Prevalence of spontaneous osteonecrosis of the medial femoral condyle in elderly patients. *Knee Surg Sports Traumatol Arthrosc* 2002;10:233-240.

52. Chryssanthou CP: Dysbaric osteonecrosis: Etiologi-

cal and pathogenetic concepts. *Clin Orthop Relat Res* 1978;130:94-108.

53. Hutter CD: Dysbaric osteonecrosis: A reassessment and hypothesis. *Med Hypotheses* 2000;54:585-590.

54. Jacobs B: Alcoholism-induced bone necrosis. *N Y State J Med* 1992;92:334-338.

55. Abu-Shakra M, Buskila D, Shoenfeld Y: Osteonecrosis in patients with SLE. *Clin Rev Allergy Immunol* 2003;25:13-24.

56. Dubois EL, Cozen L: Avascular (aseptic) bone necrosis associated with systemic lupus erythematosus. *JAMA* 1960;174:966-971.

57. Shupak R, Bernier V, Rabinovich S: Avascular necrosis of bone with rheumatoid vasculitis. *J Rheumatol* 1983;10:261-266.

58. Weiner ES, Abeles M: Aseptic necrosis and glucocorticosteroids in systemic lupus erythematosus: A re-evaluation. *J Rheumatol* 1989;16:604-608.

59. Zizic TM, Marcoux C, Hungerford DS, Dansereau JV, Stevens MB: Corticosteroid therapy associated with ischemic necrosis of bone in systemic lupus erythematosus. *Am J Med* 1985;79:596-604.

60. Carlson L: Aseptic necrosis following transplantation. *ANNA J* 1993;20:185-201.

61. Heimann WG, Freiberger RH: Avascular necrosis of the femoral and humeral heads after high-dosage corticosteroid therapy. *N Engl J Med* 1960;263:672-675.

62. Herndon JH, Aufranc OE: Avascular necrosis of the femoral head in the adult: A review of its incidence in a variety of conditions. *Clin Orthop Relat Res* 1972;86:43-62.

63. Jones LC, Hungerford DS: Osteonecrosis: Etiology, diagnosis and treatment. *Curr Opin Rheumatol* 2004;16:443-449.

64. Low K, Mont MA, Hungerford DS: Steroid-associated osteonecrosis of the knee: A comprehensive review. *Instr Course Lect* 2001;50:489-493.

65. Mirzai R, Chang C, Greenspan A, Gershwin ME: The pathogenesis of osteonecrosis and the relationships to corticosteroids. *J Asthma* 1999;36:77-95.

66. Oinuma K, Harada Y, Nawata Y, et al: Osteonecrosis in patients with systemic lupus erythematosus develops very early after starting high dose corticosteroid treatment. *Ann Rheum Dis* 2001;60:1145-1148.

67. Wang GJ, Cui Q, Balian G: The Nicolas Andry award: The pathogenesis and prevention of steroid-induced osteonecrosis. *Clin Orthop Relat Res* 2000;370:295-310.

68. Glimcher MJ, Kenzora JE: The biology of osteonecrosis of the human femoral head and its clinical implications: Part II. The pathological changes in the femoral head as an organ and in the hip joint. *Clin Orthop Relat Res* 1979;139:283-312.

69. Glimcher MJ, Kenzora JE: The biology of osteonecrosis of the human femoral head and its clinical implications: Part III. Discussion of the etiology and genesis of the pathological sequelae; comments on treatment. *Clin Orthop Relat Res* 1979;140:273-312.

70. Jaffe HL, Pomeranz MM: Changes in the bones of the extremities amputated because of arteriovascular disease. *Arch Surg* 1934;29:566-588.

71. Vail TP, Covington DB: The incidence of osteonecrosis, in Urbaniak JR, Jones JP Jr (eds): *Osteonecrosis: Etiology, Diagnosis, and Treatment.* Rosemont, IL, American Academy of Orthopaedic Surgeons, 1997, pp 43-49.

72. Mont MA, Hungerford DS: Non-traumatic avascular necrosis of the femoral head. *J Bone Joint Surg Am* 1995;77:459-474.

73. Hungerford DS, Lennox DW: The importance of increased intraosseous pressure in the development of osteonecrosis of the femoral head: Implications for treatment. *Orthop Clin North Am* 1985;16:635-654.

74. Chandler FA: Coronary disease of the hip. *J Int Coll Surg* 1948;11:34-36.

75. Mankin HJ, Brower TD: Bilateral idiopathic aseptic necrosis of the femur in adults: "Chandler's disease." *Bull Hosp Joint Dis* 1962;23:42-57.

76. Catterall A, Pringle J, Byers PD, et al: A review of the morphology of Perthes' disease. *J Bone Joint Surg Br* 1982;64:269-275.

77. Ferlic DC, Morin P: Idiopathic avascular necrosis of the scaphoid: Preiser's disease? *J Hand Surg (Am)* 1989;14:13-16.

78. Irisarri C: Aetiology of Kienbock's disease. *J Hand Surg (Br)* 2004;29:281-287.

79. Ponseti IV, Maynard JA, Weinstein SI, Ippolito EG, Pous JG: Legg-Calve-Perthes disease: Histochemical and ultrastructural observations of the epiphyseal cartilage and physis. *J Bone Joint Surg Am* 1983;65:797-807.

80. Steinberg ME, Steinberg DR: Classification systems for osteonecrosis: An overview. *Orthop Clin North Am* 2004;35:273-283.

81. Hoffmann S: Kramer J, Plenk H, Kneeland JB: Imaging in osteonecrosis, in Urbaniak JR, Jones JP Jr (eds): *Osteonecrosis: Etiology, Diagnosis, and Treatment.* Rosemont, IL, American Academy of Orthopaedic Surgeons, 1997, pp 213-223.

82. Genez BM, Wilson MR, Houk RW, et al: Early osteonecrosis of the femoral head: Detection in high risk patients with MR imaging. *Radiology* 1988;168:521-524.

83. Pollack MS, Dalinka MK, Kressel HW, Lotke PA, Spritzer CE: Magnetic resonance imaging in the evaluation of suspected osteonecrosis of the knee. *Skeletal Radiol* 1987;16:121-127.

84. Hungerford DS, Jones LC: Asymptomatic osteonecrosis: Should it be treated? *Clin Orthop Relat Res* 2004;429:124-130.

85. Motohashi M, Morii T, Koshino T: Clinical course of roentgenographic changes of osteonecrosis in the femoral condyle under conservative treatment. *Clin Orthop Relat Res* 1991;266:156-161.

86. Hungerford DS, Mont MA: The role of core decompression in the treatment of osteonecrosis of the femoral head, in Urbaniak JR, Jones JP Jr (eds): *Osteonecrosis: Etiology, Diagnosis, and Treatment.* Rosemont, IL, American Academy of Orthopaedic Surgeons, 1997, pp 287-292.

87. Coogan PG, Urbaniak JR: Multicenter experience with free vascularized fibular grafts for osteonecrosis of the femoral head, in Urbaniak JR, Jones JP Jr (eds): *Osteonecrosis: Etiology, Diagnosis, and Treatment.* Rosemont, IL, American Academy of Orthopaedic Surgeons, 1997, pp 327-346.

88. Xenakis TH, Soucacos PN, Beris AE: Total hip arthroplasty in the management of osteonecrosis of the femoral head, in Urbaniak JR, Jones JP Jr (eds): *Osteonecrosis: Etiology, Diagnosis, and Treatment.* Rosemont, IL, American Academy of Orthopaedic Surgeons, 1997, pp 391-396.

89. Gottschalk F: Indications and results of intertrochanteric osteotomy in osteonecrosis of the femoral head. *Clin Orthop Relat Res* 1989;249:219-221.

Chapter 10

Langerhans Cell Histiocytosis

The clinical entity now known as Langerhans cell histiocytosis not only has a long and confusing history, but the causation and clinical characteristics remain enigmatic.[1,2] Dr. Thomas Smith first described it in a 4-year-old child in 1865.[3] The patient died of whooping cough, but at autopsy was found to have an erythematous skin disorder and several destructive lesions in his skull. In 1868, Paul Langerhans[4] described a nonpigmentary dendritic cell in the epidermis; he considered this to be bone marrow-derived and to represent the most peripheral output of the immune system. There is now strong evidence that proliferation of these cells was not only the cause of Dr. Smith's patient's disorder, but also one of a series of three entities known as Langerhans cell histiocytosis.[1,2]

In 1893, Philadelphia physician Alfred Hand[5] described a 3-year-old child with exophthalmos, polyuria, and great thirst. Although Hand's initial impression was that the child had tuberculosis, he corrected that impression in 1921[6] after Artur Schüller described two children with similar findings who had no evidence of tuberculosis.[7] In 1920, Dr. Henry Christian[8] described a 5-year-old child with changes now known as "Christian's triad"—calvarial lesions, diabetes insipidus, and exophthalmos. This complex syndrome, which includes visceromegaly and skin lesions is now known as Hand-Schüller-Christian disease.

In 1924, Erich Letterer[9] described an acute, nonleukemic fatal disorder of the reticuloendothelial system in a 6-month-old child. Nine years later, Sture Siwe[10] described a similar case of a very young child with splenomegaly, hepatomegaly, lymphadenopathy, bone tumors, hemorrhaging, and generalized histocytic hyperplasia. In 1936, Arthur Abt and Edward Denenholz[11] reported another patient with similar findings, but after reviewing the prior literature decided that it was appropriate to name the disease Letterer-Siwe disease.

Otani and Ehrlich[12] from Mount Sinai Hospital in New York and Lichtenstein and Jaffe[13] from the Hospital for Joint Diseases almost simultaneously reported solitary granulomatous histiocytic lesions of bone, which they named eosinophilic granuloma. Unlike the other two forms of the disease, the lesions were considered to be confined to the bone and benign in nature.[14] In 1942, William Green and Sidney Farber[15] linked the eosinophilic granuloma to Letterer-Siwe disease and Hand-Schüller-Christian disease on the basis of almost identical histologic patterns. Jaffe and Lichtenstein[16] concluded the same, and Lichtenstein[17] subsequently suggested that the three entities be named histiocytosis X. However, it was Friedman and Hanoaka[18] in 1969 and Nezelof and associates[19] in 1973 who concluded that the cells that appeared in all three forms of the disease were Langerhans granuloma cells, and proposed that the name be changed to Langerhans cell histiocytosis. What is striking is the fact that the three diseases are totally different in presentation and degree of disability and survival, yet the histology is identical and indistinguishable from one another.

The Cause of the Disease: Still a Mystery

From time to time scientists have tried to define the cause of the three disorders by extensive virologic analyses and genetic studies.[20-34] In favor of an infectious etiology is the disseminated nature of the disease and the almost spontaneous remission of the milder forms. In favor of the neoplastic etiology is the presence of generalized and fatal disease in some patients, not unlike a lymphomatous or leukemic disorder. Based on some virus studies in 1991, Epstein-Barr virus was suggested as the cause.[35] Several authors proposed that the diseases were caused by human herpesvirus (HHV)-6 or HHV-8.[27,29] After a very thorough analysis, however, McClain and associates[30] were unable to find evidence for the presence of HHV, adenovirus, cytomegalovirus, Epstein-Barr virus, herpes simplex, human immunodeficiency virus, t-cell leukemia 1 or 2, or

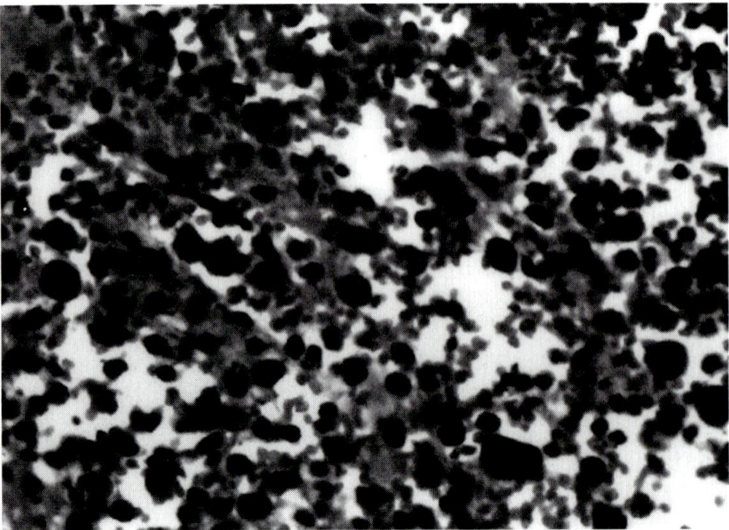

Figure 1
The histologic picture for a typical Langerhans cell histiocytosis bone lesion. The cells are principally monocytic but with a surcharge of eosinophils. Occasional cells show some atypism, and a small number of giant cells may be present. Hematoxylin and eosin × 200.

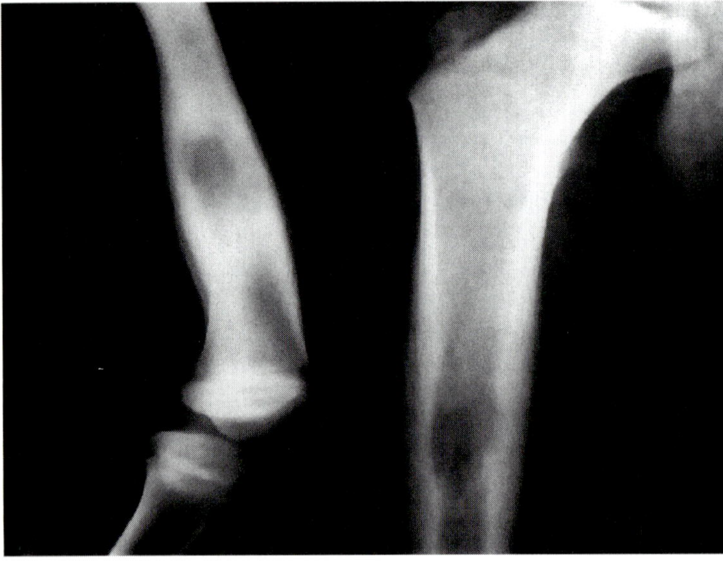

Figure 2
Two classic lesions, both in the femur, illustrate the typical appearance of histiocytosis. The lesions are "punched out," the bone sometimes expanded, the cortices thinned, and internal scalloping is often noted.

finding is rare.[20,37] Exposure to noxious agents has not been identified as a potential cause either. The disease has some similarity to Erdheim-Chester disease, but the differences in appearance of the cells and clinical courses make this less likely.[22,24]

Unusual Histology of Langerhans Cell Histiocytosis

The principal cell present in all three of the lesions that comprise the entity is a monocyte with some unusual characteristics (Figure 1). As described by Langerhans, the cell is a nonpigmentary dendritic cell, which he considered to be bone-marrow–derived and to represent the most peripheral output of the immune system.[1,4,24] The cell resembles other monocytic elements, but has a vesicular nucleus with a groove parallel to the long axis and vacuolated cytoplasm.[24] Occasionally binucleate cells are evident, but cell replication is unusual.[22,24,38] Tiny linear rod-shaped inclusions in the cytoplasm called Birbeck's granules are best seen on electron microscopy.[22,24,39] Most of the Langerhans cells are positive for S-100 protein and CD1a, CD40, CD52, and CD154.[22,24,26,28,36] P53 may be present in some of the cells, but cannot be correlated with outcome.[40] Perhaps the most striking feature of the histology is the presence of eosinophils, which are sometimes so numerous as to dominate the histologic presentation.[22,24,38] The combination of histiocytes and eosinophils is unusual in pathologic specimens. The principal differential for histiocytosis is from Hodgkin's lymphoma, in which eosinophils are often present. However, Hodgkin's lymphoma has another feature (the multinucleated Reed-Sternberg cell) not present in Langerhans histiocytosis.[22,24]

Presentation of the Three Syndromes

Eosinophilic Granuloma

Eosinphilic granuloma is a benign disease located in a bone, occurring most frequently in children under 15 years of age.[21,23,41,42] The lesion presents as a lytic, modestly destructive lesion usually in a long bone (often in the diaphysis). It may occur in the pelvis or spine as well, and on occasion in multiple sites.[22,24,38] Typically, the lesions are located within the bone and produce a "scalloped from within" appearance without a break in

parvovirus. Attempts to identify a genetic error have failed to uncover a consistent abnormality in the gene structure for the three diseases; currently the genetic pattern has not been found to differ significantly from other interdigitating dendritic cells.[21,22,24,26,28,36] Although an occasional positive family history has been reported, the

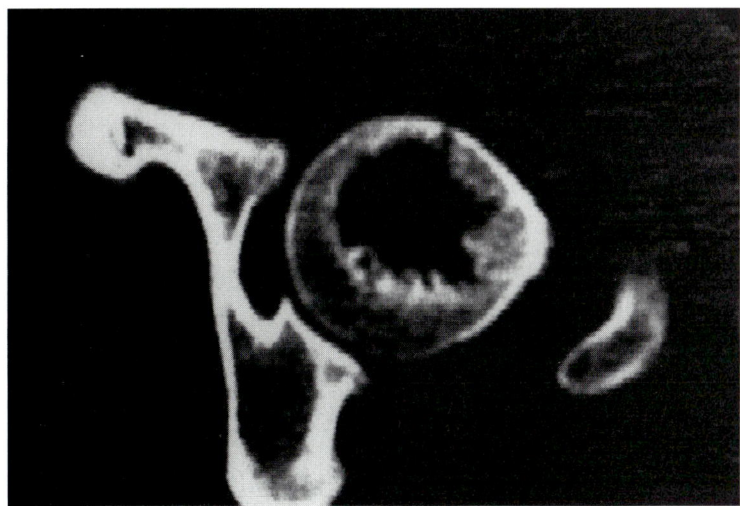

Figure 3
A computed tomography scan showing a lytic lesion in the femoral head with a fracture through the anterior cortex.

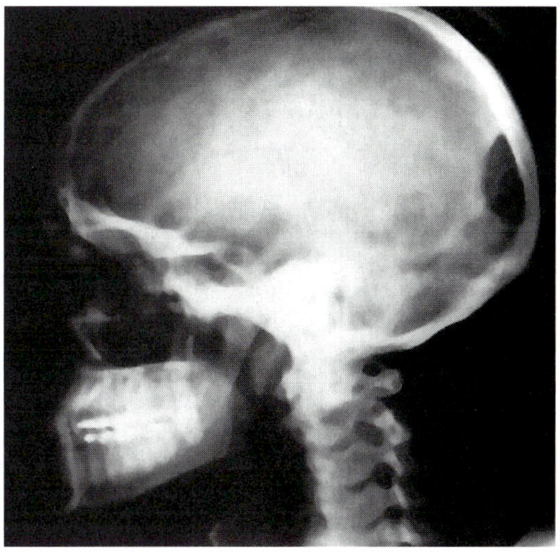

Figure 4
Radiograph of the calvarium of a young person with Hand-Schüller-Christian disease, demonstrating a punched lesion in the occiput. The patient had extensive disease.

the cortex or a soft-tissue mass outside the bone (Figure 2). There is rarely any calcification within the substance of the lesion, and they are seen sometimes as dark on T1 and bright on T2 on magnetic resonance images.[22,24] The lesions are most often asymptomatic but may be the site of a fracture, in which case they are the source of pain, swelling, or deformity (Figure 3). Lesions of the pelvis or scapula may be large and appear destructive; a lesion of a vertebral segment is characteristically described as "vertebra plana," appearing as a symmetrical flattening of the segment, often in a growing child.[16,21-24,38,42] The bone scan is often positive at the site of any of the lesions, and the alkaline phosphatase may be slightly elevated.[22,24] On some occasions, several lesions may be seen in patients with eosinophilic granuloma and they may appear at different times.[22,24]

Hand-Schüller-Christian Disease

Hand-Schüller-Christian disease generally occurs in children under the age of 10 years, but may occasionally appear in patients in their 20s and 30s and more frequently in males.[20,22-24,41-44] Retarded growth and development may be present, and one third of the patients present with diabetes insipidus;[21-23,42,43,45,46] this can sometimes be clearly identified by positron emission to-

mography scanning.[47] Anemia is present in a high percentage of patients, and many have hepatosplenomegaly.[21-24] Patients often present with exophthalmos, which may lead to blindness; hearing loss is frequently present as well.[20,22,23,42,48] Many of the patients develop a progressive cerebellar ataxia after several years.[49,50] Teeth and gum problems are present in approximately 20% of the patients, and mandibular deformity is a common finding.[6] Calvarial lesions are the rule, and are present in over 60% of the patients[21,22,24] (Figure 4). These lesions are frequently multiple and may be sufficiently destructive to cause injury to the underlying neural tissue.[50] Osseous lesions in other sites may be present in almost 50% of patients, and are often much more destructive than the lesions seen in eosinophilic granuloma.[22,24,38,41,50] One of the most distressing findings is a scaly seborrheic skin rash often present at hair lines and hands and feet, which may be the cause of bleeding.[20-24,44] Infiltrative lesions may be present in the lungs and may cause serious pulmonary impairment and even death.[22,50]

Letterer-Siwe Disease

Letterer-Siwe disease is the rarest of the Langerhans histiocytic lesions and the most aggressive. The typical age for patients with Letterer-Siwe disease is usually under 2 years, and males are more often affected than females. After a short period of normal growth and development, the affected children develop visceromegaly and lymphadenopathy.[21,22,24,42] They become severely stunted in growth and lose weight, and their intellectual development becomes severely impaired. Laboratory studies show marked anemia and thrombocytopenia. Most of the children show destructive lesions in the skull associated with brain damage and in the peripheral bones as a cause of frequent fractures.[21,22,24,42] The most evident symptom is a widespread papular crusting hemorrhagic rash, which is associated with a severe neutropenia and thrombocytopenia. Treatment has until recently had little effect, and early demise was the rule for these very ill children.[22,25,50]

Treatment of Patients with Langerhans Cell Histiocytosis

Because the three syndromes are so markedly different, the treatment varies considerably. For eosinophilic granuloma, treatment of a solitary lytic lesion affecting a long bone is best accomplished by curettage of the affected site and implantation of allograft bone chips or polymethylmethacrylate[22,24] or injections of corticoids into the site.[51,52] The lesions rarely recur and most of the patients remain free of disease for a lifetime. Occasionally radiation may be of value; the dose proposed is usually considerably lower than that suggested for more aggressive lesions.[22,24] Spinal vertebra plana lesions are sometimes best treated by observation or occasionally by low-dose radiation to the site.[53,54]

Treatment of Hand-Schüller-Christian and Letterer-Siwe diseases is much more complex and for the most part not very effective. Corticosteroids have been used for the most part; although they seem effective initially, generally they do not reverse the course of the diseases. Methotrexate and vinblastine can help patients with Hand-Schüller-Christian disease, but are of little value for patients with Letterer-Siwe disease.[55] Growth hormone has been useful for patients with Hand-Schüller-Christian disease in terms of increasing their development to a modest extent,[45] and more recently interferon alpha with etoposide has shown some modest success.[56,57] Recent reports suggest that 2-chlorodeoxyadenosine may allow for a complete remission of symptoms for patients with Hand-Schüller-Christian disease and may be useful in maintaining survival for patients with Letterer-Siwe disease.[58-62] Marrow transplant has been tried, and seemed successful in several cases for a relatively short period of time.[63] Extensive bone lesions have been treated with pamidronate with some improvement,[64] and thalidomide appears to help severe skin problems.[65]

It is somewhat distressing to realize that the three disorders known as Langerhans cell histiocytosis, originally described in the 19th century and vastly different in presentation, have thus far resisted attempts to identify a neoplastic, infectious, or genetic cause. The distinctive feature of the three entities is the unique histologic characteristics, which are characterized by the appearance of the Langerhans cells, the Birbeck's granules, and the eosinophils. The treatment protocols, although better than they were 25 years ago, are still problematic for the two more severe disorders; patients with these disorders are at times severely affected and can die of the disease.

References

1. Coppes-Zantinga A, Egeler RM: The Langerhans cell histiocytosis X files revealed. *Br J Haematol* 2002;116:3-9.

2. Komp DM: Historical perspectives of Langerhans cell histiocytosis. *Hematol Oncol Clin North Am* 1987;1:9-21.

3. Smith T: Skull cap showing congenital deficiency of bone. *Trans Path Soc London* 1865;16:224-225.

4. Langerhans P: Uber die nerven der mensclichen haut. *Arch Pathol Anat* 1868;44:325-337.

5. Hand A: Polyuria and tuberculosis. *Arch Pediatr* 1893;10:673-675.

6. Hand A: Defects of membranous bones, exophthalmos and polyuria in childhood: Is it dyspituitarism? *Am J Med Sci* 1921;162:509-515.

7. Schüller A: Uber eigenartige schadeldefekte im jugendalter. *Fortsch Gebiete Roentgenstrahlen* 1915;23:12-18.

8. Christian H: Defects in membranous bones, exophthalmos and diabetes insipidus: An unusual syndrome of dyspituitarism. *Med Clin N Amer* 1920;3:849-871.

9. Letterer E: Aleukamische retikulose (ein beitrag zu den proliferativen erkrankungen des retikuloendot-

helialapparates). *Frankfurt Zeitsch Pathol* 1924;30:377-394.

10. Siwe S: Die reticuloendotheliose: Ein neues krankheitsbild unter den hepatosplenomegalien. *Zeitsch Kinderheilkunde* 1933;55:212-247.

11. Abt A, Denenholz E: Letterer-Siwe's disease: Spleno-hepatomegaly, associated with widespread hyperplasia of non-lipoid-storing macrophages: Discussion of the so-called reticulo-endotheliosis. *Am J Dis Child* 1936;51:499-522.

12. Otani S, Ehrlich J: Solitary granuloma of bone simulating primary neoplasm. *Am J Pathol* 1940;16:479-490.

13. Lichtenstein L, Jaffe HL: Eosinophilic granuloma of bone. *Am J Pathol* 1940;16:595-604.

14. Farber S: The nature of "solitary or eosinophilic granuloma" of bone. *Am J Pathol* 1941;17:625-629.

15. Green W, Farber S: Eosinophilic or solitary granuloma of bone. *J Bone Joint Surg* 1942;24:499-526.

16. Jaffe HL, Lichtenstein L: Eosinophilic granuloma of bone: A condition affecting one, several or many bones but apparently limited to the skeleton, and representing the mildest clinical expresson of the peculiar inflammatory histiocytosis also underlying Letterer-Siwe disease and Schuller-Christian disease. *Arch Pathol* 1944;37:99-118.

17. Lichtenstein L: Histiocytosis X: Integration of eosinophilic granuloma of bone, Letterer-Siwe disease and Schuller-Christian disease as related manifestations of a single nosologic entity. *AMA Arch Pathol* 1953;56:84-102.

18. Friedman B, Hanaoka H: Langerhans cell granules in eosinophilic granuloma of bone. *J Bone Joint Surg Am* 1969;51:367-374.

19. Nezelof C, Bassett F, Rousseau MF: Histiocytosis X histogenic arguments for a Langerhans cell origin. *Biomedicine* 1973;18:365-371.

20. Arico M, Girshikofsky M, Genereau T, et al: Langerhans cell histiocytosis in adults: Report from the International Registry of the Histiocyte Society. *Eur J Cancer* 2003;39:2341-2348.

21. Broadbent V, Gadner H, Komp DM, Ladisch S: Histiocytosis syndromes in children: II. Approach to the clinical and laboratory evaluation of children with Langerhans cell histiocytosis. *Med Pediatr Oncol* 1989;17:492-495.

22. Campanacci M: *Bone and Soft Tissue Tumors*, ed 2. New York, NY, Springer Verlag, 1999, pp 857-876.

23. Chu T, D'Angio GJ, Favara B, Ladisch S, Nesbit M, Pritchard J: Histiocytosis syndromes in children. *Lancet* 1987;2:41-42.

24. Dorfman HD, Czerniak B: *Bone Tumors*. St Louis, MO, Mosby, Inc, 1997, pp 690-701.

25. Egeler RM, D'Angio GJ: Langerhans cell histiocytosis. *J Pediatr* 1995;127:1-11.

26. Egeler RM, Favara BE, Laman JD, Claasen E: Abundant expression of CD40 and CD40 ligand (CD154) in paediatric Langerhans cell histiocytosis lesions. *Eur J Cancer* 2000;36:2105-2110.

27. Jenson HB, McClain KL, Leach CT, Deng GH, Gao SJ: Evaluation of human herpesvirus type 8 infection in childhood Langerhans cell histiocytosis. *Am J Hematol* 2000;64:237-241.

28. Jordan MB, McClain KL, Yan X, Hicks J, Jaffe R: Anti-CD52 antibody, alemtuzumab, binds to Langerhans cells in Langerhans cell histiocytosis. *Pediatr Blood Cancer* 2005;44:251-254.

29. Leahy MA, Krejci SM, Friednash M, et al: Human herpesvirus 6 is present in lesions of Langerhans cell histiocytosis. *J Invest Dermatol* 1993;101:642-645.

30. McClain K, Jin H, Gresik V, Favara B: Langerhans cell histiocytosis: Lack of a viral etiology. *Am J Hematol* 1994;47:16-20.

31. McClain K, Ramsay NK, Robison L, Sundberg RD, Nesbit M Jr: Bone marrow involvement in histiocytosis X. *Med Pediatr Oncol* 1983;11:167-171.

32. Scappaticci S, Danesino C, Rossi E, et al: Cytogenetic abnormalities in PHA-stimulated lymphocytes from patients with Langerhans cell histiocytosis. *Br J Haematol* 2000;111:258-262.

33. Willman CL, Busque L, Grith BB, et al: Langerhans' cell histiocytosis (histiocytosis X): A clonal proliferative disease. *N Engl J Med* 1994;331:154-160.

34. Willman CL, McClain KL: An update on clonality, cytokines and viral etiology in Langerhans cell histiocytosis. *Hematol Oncol Clin North Am* 1998;12:407-416.

35. Dreyer ZE, Dowell BL, Chen H, Hawkins E, McClain KL: Infection-associated hemophagocytic syndrome: Evidence for Epstein-Barr virus gene expression. *Am J Pediatr Hematol Oncol* 1991;13:476-481.

36. Betts DR, Leibundgut KF, Feldges A, Pluss HJ, Niggli FK: Cytogenetic abnormalities in Langerhans cell histiocytosis. *Br J Cancer* 1998;77:552-555.

37. Shahla A, Parvaneh V, Hossein HD: Langerhans cells histiocytosis in one family. *Pediatr Hematol Oncol* 2004;21:313-320.

38. Jaffe HL: *Metabolic, Degenerative and Inflammatory Diseases of Bones and Joints*. Philadelphia, PA, Lea and Febiger, 1972, pp 875-906.

39. Breathnach AS, Birbeck MS, Everall JD: Observations bearing on the relationship between Langerhans cells and melanocytes. *Ann NY Acad Sci* 1963;100:223-238.

40. Bank MI, Rengtved P, Carstensen H, Petersen BL: P53 expression in biopsies from children with Langerhans cell histiocytosis. *J Pediatr Hematol Oncol* 2002;24:733-736.

41. Ghanem I, Tolo VT, D'Ambra P, Malgalowkin MH: Langerhans cell hstiocytosis of bone in children and adolescents. *J Pediatr Orthop* 2003;23:124-130.

42. Kilpatrick SE, Wenger DE, Gilchrist GS, Shives TC, Wollan PC, Unni KK: Langerhans' cell histiocytosis (histiocytosis X) of bone: A clinicopathologic analysis of 263 pediatric and adult cases. *Cancer* 1995;76:2471-2484.

43. Dunger DB, Broadbent V, Yeoman E, et al: The frequency and natural history of diabetes insipidus in children with Langerhans-cell histiocytosis. *N Engl J Med* 1989;321:1157-1162.

44. Gotz G, Fichter J: Langerhans cell histiocytosis in 58 adults. *Eur J Med Res* 2004;9:510-514.

45. Donadieu J, Rolon MA, Pion I, et al: Incidence of growth hormone deficiency in pediatric-onset Langerhans cell histiocytosis: Efficacy and safety of growth hormone treatment. *J Clin Endocrinol Metab* 2004;89:604-609.

46. Maghnie M, Cosi G, Genovese E, et al: Central diabetes insipidus in children. *N Engl J Med* 2000;343:998-1007.

47. Calming U, Bemstrand C, Mosskin M, et al: Brain 18-FDG PET scan in central nervous system Langerhans'- cell histiocytosis. *J Pediatr* 2002;141:435-440.

48. Eckardt A, Schultze A: Maxillofacial manifestations of Langerhans cell histiocytosis: A clinical and therapeutic analysis of 10 patients. *Oral Oncol* 2003;39:687-694.

49. Imashuku S, Ishida S, Koike K, et al: Cerebellar ataxia in pediatric patients with Langerhans cell histiocytosis. *J Pediatr Hematol Oncol* 2004;26:735-739.

50. Kusumakumary P, James FV: Permanent disabilities in childhood survivors of Langerhans cell histiocytosis. *Pediatr Hematol Oncol* 2000;17:375-381.

51. Capanna R, Springfield DS, Ruggieri P, et al: Direct cortisone injection in eosinophilic granuloma of bone: A preliminary report on 11 patients. *J Pediatr Orthop* 1985;5:339-342.

52. Cohen M, Zornoza J, Cangir A, Murray JA, Wallace S: Direct injection of methylprednisolone sodium succinate in the treatment of solitary eosinophilic granuloma of bone: A report of 9 cases. *Radiology* 1980;136:289-293.

53. Bavbek M, Atalay B, Altinors N, Caner H: Spontaneous resolution of lumbar vertebral eosinophilic granuloma. *Acta Neurochir (Wien)* 2004;146:165-167.

54. Nesbit ME, Kieffer S, D'Angio GJ: Reconstitution of vertebral height in histiocytosis X: A long term follow-up. *J Bone Joint Surg Am* 1969;51:1360-1368.

55. Steen AE, Steen KH, Bauer R, Bieber T: Successful treatment of cutaneous Langerhans cell histiocytosis with low-dose methotrexate. *Br J Dermatol* 2001;145:137-140.

56. Culic S, Jakobson A, Culic V, et al: Etoposide as a basic and interferon-alpha as the maintenance therapy for Langerhans cell histiocytosis: A RTC. *Pediatr Hematol Oncol* 2001;18:291-294.

57. Ladisch S, Gadner H, Arico M, et al: LCH-I: A randomized trial of etoposide vs vinblastine in disseminated Langerhans cell histiocytosis. *Med Pediatr Oncol* 1994;23:107-110.

58. Goh NS, McDonald CE, MacGregor DP, Pretto JJ, Brodie GN: Successful treatment of Langerhans cell histiocytosis with 2-chlorodeoxyadenosine. *Respirology* 2003;8:91-94.

59. Ottaviano F, Finlay JL: Diabetes insipidus and Langerhans cell histiocytosis: A case report of reversibility with 2-chlorodeoxyadenosine. *J Pediatr Hematol Oncol* 2003;25:575-577.

60. Pardanani A, Phyliky RL, Li CY, Tefferi A: 2-chlorodeoxyadenosine therapy for disseminated Langerhans cell histiocytosis. *Mayo Clin Proc* 2003;78:301-306.

61. Rodriguez-Galindo C, Kelly P, Jeng M, Presbury GG, Rieman M, Wang W: Treatment of children with Langerhans cell histiocytosis with 2-chlorodeoxyadenosine. *Am J Hematol* 2002;69:179-184.

62. Stine KC, Saylors RL, Saccente S, McClain KL, Becton DL: Efficacy of continuous infusion 2-CDA (cladribine) in pediatric patients with Langerhans cell histiocytosis. *Pediatr Blood Cancer* 2004;43:81-84.

63. Nagarajan R, Neglia J, Ramsay N, Baker KS: Successful treatment of refractory Langerhans cell histiocytosis with unrelated cord blood transplantation. *J Pediatr Hematol Oncol* 2001;23:629-632.

64. Farran RP, Zaretski E, Egeler RM: Treatment of Langerhans cell histiocytosis with pamidronate. *J Pediatr Hematol Oncol* 2001;23:54-56.

65. Sander CS, Kaatz M, Elsner P: Successful treatment of cutaneous Langerhans cell histiocytosis with thalidomide. *Dermatology* 2004;208:149-152.

Chapter 11

Paget's Disease of Bone

Introduction

Paget's disease of bone is a mysterious entity with no readily identifiable cause and an array of different presentations. The disorder is common, with an incidence of approximately 3% in the population over the age of 50 years. Many of those affected have no knowledge of the presence of the disease. The disease rarely occurs in patients younger than 50 years and increases in frequency as people age. Males and females appear to be equally affected, but there is a strong difference in ethnic frequency. Caucasians and particularly persons of English, Australian, or New Zealand origin have a much higher incidence rate than native Americans, Eskimos, Africans, Indians, or Asians. Although there have been some suggestions regarding a slow virus or conceivably genetic errors as a cause, there is still no clear definition as to the origin of the disease. Specifically, there is no concrete knowledge of the cause of the distribution of solitary bone disease to various bones and why these patients are often asymptomatic. There is also no understanding of the causes of extensive disease and why these patients are often severely affected and disabled. Perhaps the most disturbing unknown is why up to 10% of patients with extensive Paget's disease develop and very frequently die with Paget's sarcoma.

History

Paget's disease is not of recent origin. Findings suggestive of Paget's disease were found in Anglo-Saxon skulls,[1,2] Egyptian mummies,[3] and American Indian skeletons.[4] The first description of the disease in the medical literature was by Sir Samuel Wilks in 1869; Wilks reported a case of a 60-year-old man who died after a 20-year history of leg pain.[5] Initially the patient's tibiae became enlarged, and then many other bones increased in size, including his clavicles, humeri, and cranium; the latter required increasing hat sizes. At autopsy, his bones were found to be enlarged and very thick; however, when cut through, they were softer than usual. Wilks assigned the name "osteoporosis or spongy hypertrophy of the bones" to describe the findings. A similar case was described by Czerny in 1873.[6] In 1876, at a meeting of the Royal Medical Chirurgical Society of London, Sir James Paget described a male patient he had treated for 20 years for a bone structural disorder.[7] After the patient died, the material Paget and his pathologist, Sir Henry Butlin, obtained at autopsy showed changes similar to those reported by Wilks. The case is not only famous for the extraordinary clarity of the description and illustrations, but also because of the reported increase in size of the patient's "shako" from 22.5 inches inside diameter in 1844 to 28.5 inches at the time of the patient's death. Paget became intrigued by the syndrome, and in a signal presentation in 1882 he described 11 cases of the same disease that he called "osteitis deformans."[8] In Paget's words, "It begins in middle age and later, is very slow in progress, may continue for many years without influence on the general health, and may give no trouble other than those which are due to the changes of shape, size and direction of the diseased bones. Even when the skull is hugely thickened, and all of its bone exceedingly altered in structure, the mind remains unaffected." In 1888, Jonathan Hutchinson declared in *Illustrative Medical News* that the name osteitis deformans should be changed to "Paget's Disease of Bone."[3] Paget had an illustrious career in British surgery and served as the long-time chairperson and principal force at St. Bartholomew's Hospital and the physician to Queen Victoria.[9-12] After a long and prolific career in which he defined many additional pathologic disorders, Paget died in 1899 at the age of 86.[9,10,13,14]

Many physicians subsequently described patients with Paget's disease, often with only one bone involved. In 1932, Schmorl of Dresden reported that of 4,614 randomly selected autopsies, 138 cases (3%) were found to have solitary Paget's disease.[15] Subsequent studies published in the

1950s by Rosenkrantz and associates,[16] Collins,[17] and Pygott[18] confirmed this incidence rate.

The clinical and histologic findings in patients with Paget's disease are well documented in subsequent publications, as are the methods of therapy proposed for the entity. In addition, neoplasms arising in relation to Paget's bone has been defined by a number of studies. In Paget's original article published in 1877,[7] he wrote that two of the five patients died of sarcomatous metastases; in his subsequent report in 1882,[8] five of the 23 patients had the same affliction. In 1901, Packard and associates[19] reported a sarcoma rate of 7.5% in 67 patients with Paget's disease; Bird[20] reviewed 64 cases, reporting 7 with metastases. Pike[21] later defined the rate as 7.5%, and Rosenkrantz and associates[16] reported 7.2%. In 1969, Barry reviewed the world literature and decided that the frequency of Paget's sarcoma was less than 1% for all patients, and less than 10% for patients with extensive disease.[10,22] As noted by Barry[10] and Jaffe,[23] patients with Paget's disease may also develop aggressive but benign giant cell tumors in the affected bones.

Epidemiology and Putative Causation Factors for Paget's Disease of Bone

The causes of Paget's disease of bone have always been somewhat obscure. Because the disease appeared to occur in patients usually after reaching the age of 50 years, genetic causes initially seemed unacceptable and a slow virus etiology was postulated. One of the most intriguing suggestions was a possible relationship to parvomyxoviruses such as parainfluenza, mumps, and measles.[9,14,24-26] One of the more popular considerations was that respiratory syncytial virus may be the cause, but studies of the tissues by electron microscopy and immunologic techniques failed to support this concept.[9] The possibility of animal-related infection seemed possible because many of the patients had dogs, but this also was not borne out by additional studies.[9,14,25,26] In relation to genetics, the racial and ethnic distribution seemed to strongly support the occurrence of the disease in patients of British origin. Several authors have noted the frequency of the disease in En-

gland, Australia, and New Zealand[10,26-34] and its relative rarity in individuals from Sweden, the Netherlands, Africa, India, Japan, and China.[13,26-28,35-38]

Familial Paget's disease is occasionally encountered; the patients so afflicted seem to be younger than those without a family history.[9,14,32,39-41] The documented frequency of familial history suggests that the disease is transmitted as an autosomal dominant, with as many as four siblings and several aunts and uncles presenting with usually minor forms of the disease.[30,42,43] The familial occurrence also seems to support the virus etiology, but the evidence is too sparse to endorse this concept.[24,25,32]

Recently, a number of investigators have proposed the existence of one of several genetic errors as the cause of Paget's disease of bone.[9,13,44,45] These include modifications of the sequestosome 1 gene (also known as p62);[40,46-48] modifications in the RANKL, RANK, and osteoprotegerin systems with alterations in Bcl-2,[49-51] an apoptotic suppressor; or findings of alterations in chromosome 9p13.3-p12, 18g21.1-q22, or 6p21.3.[41,43,52,53] Investigations are still in progress, particularly among familial cases of the disease, but at this time there is no evidence to support a single chromosomal or genetic cause for the disease.

Nature and Histology of the Disease

Paget's disease is a disorder in which bone is both synthesized and destroyed at extremely rapid rates, but generally equally so that synthesis and degradation are essentially equivalent, described as "coupling."[9,10,13,14,23,54] Osteoblastic and osteoclastic activities are both much more rapid than in normal bone, but are nearly identical to each other in the Pagetoid bone. Because of this rapid turnover, the affected bone seems to lose control of its structure; does not obey Wolff's law ("Every change in the form and function of a bone, or its function alone is followed by certain definite changes in its internal architecture and equally definite secondary alterations in its mathematical laws."[55]); and generally becomes markedly enlarged with very thick cortices, coarse but purposeful trabeculae, and irregular lytic areas in some parts of the bone.[9,10,13,14,23,54] Bowing of the affected bone is common. Because of the significant increase in synthetic activity, the bone scan is almost always intensely positive over the site,[56] and the alkaline phosphatase and the hydroxyproline peptides become markedly higher.[9,10,13,14]

Histologically, in active sites one sees an extraordinary vascularity and an enormous collection of osteoclasts making irregular columns of mature bone, which are simultaneously being destroyed by an equal number of osteoclasts (Figure 1). The effect is one of irregularity of contour of the new trabeculae and cortices, vascular malformations, microfractures, gross enlargement of the bone, and frequently bowing deformities. The normal marrow is often suppressed based on the collection of abnormal osteoblasts and osteoclasts and blood vessels in the space between the trabeculae.[9,10,13,14,23,54]

The pattern described above and shown in Figure 1 is characteristic of what Henry Jaffe[23] referred to as "hot" Paget's. With time, at various sites the process becomes "cooled off" (but never "cold"); under these circumstances, the bone that is formed appears to be enlarged, has osteoid seams separating the columns of cells and segments of bone, and presents an appearance that according to several authors resembles Roman bath tiles ("brecchiae") (Figure 2).[23] In patients with Paget's disease, uninvolved bone sites are normal in appearance, consistent with the patient's age and level of disability.

Imaging Studies of Paget's Disease

The diagnosis of Paget's disease on plain radiographs, computed tomography, or even magnetic resonance imaging is not difficult.[9,10,13,14,17,23,29,36,57-63] Four findings clearly distinguish Paget's disease from almost all other disorders (Figure 3): (1) the bone is greater in width (and often in length) than normal; (2) the cortices are wider than normal; (3) the trabeculae in the medullary cavity are coarse but purposeful; and (4) the medullary bone often contains lytic areas, sometimes quite large.

In addition, several changes are sometimes present. These include:
- The "advancing wedge." Paget's disease may start at one end of the bone and progress to the other; this provides a segment of Paget's disease at one end of the bone that extends to a site where

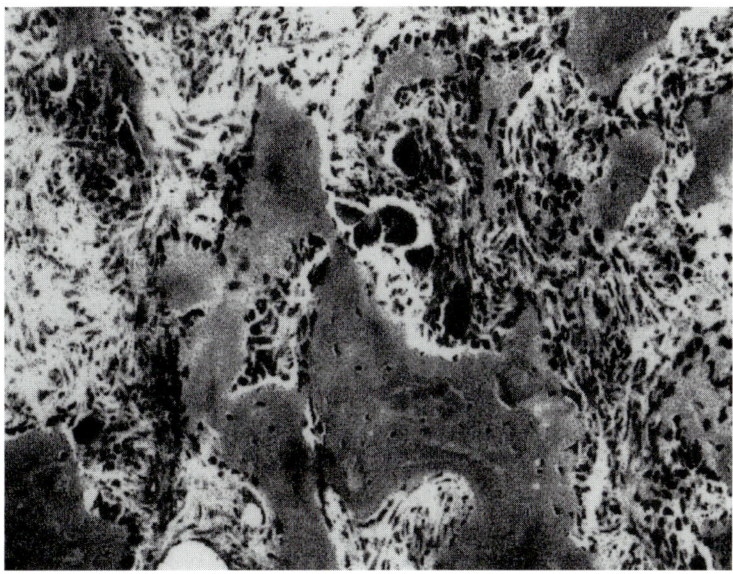

Figure 1
Histologic picture of the bone showing "hot" Paget's disease. There are numerous osteoblasts making mature bone, and many osteoclasts destroying the trabeculae. The marrow space is impaired and the bone shows irregular structure. Hematoxylin and eosin × 100.

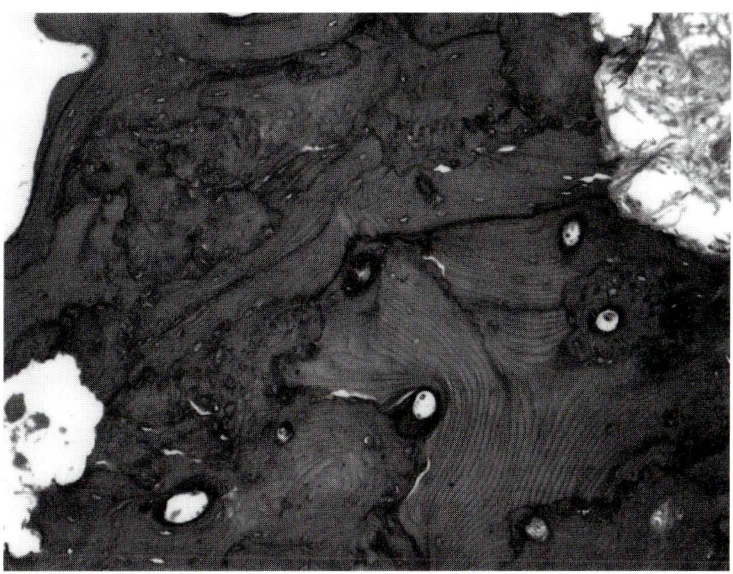

Figure 2
This histologic picture shows the "cooling off" Paget's disease described by Jaffe. The bone consists of sheets of dense bone with osteoid seams, which create a resemblance to Roman bath tiles ("brecchiae").

the bone is normal. The advancing wedge is often oblique, and the Pagetoid bone immediately behind it is usually expanded but somewhat more lytic.[9,10,13,14,23]

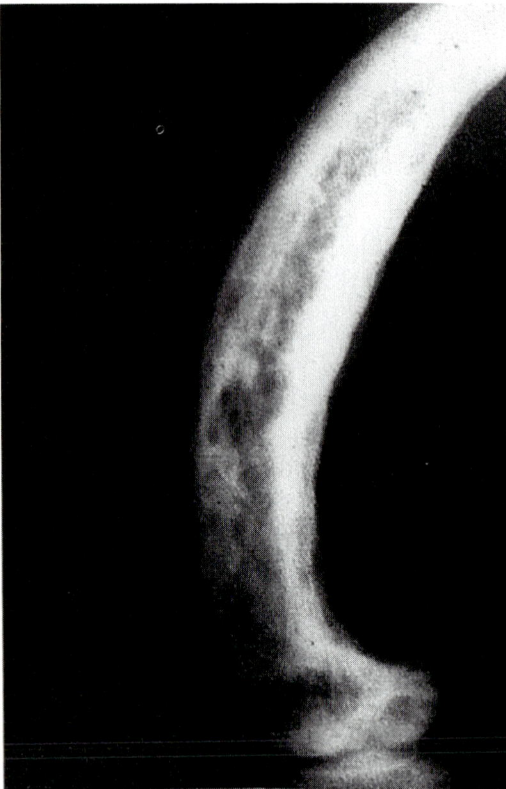

Figure 3
Radiograph of an anteriorly bowed femur of a patient with severe Paget's disease. Note the increased width of the bone, the markedly thickened cortices, the coarse but purposeful trabeculae, and the lytic areas within the medullary cavity.

- "Stress lines" are thin lytic incomplete lines at right angles to the longitudinal structure of the bone present on the convex side of the bone (to be distinguished from Looser's lines, which occur in patients with rickets or osteomalacia and are frequently on the concave sides of the bones). The stress lines sometimes lead to fractures of the bone through the site.[9,13,14]
- "Osteoporosis circumscripta cranii" is the term applied to what probably is the advancing wedge, but in the calvarium. The bones are initially lytic in appearance and then slowly and sometimes irregularly develop the classic appearance of Paget's disease changes, with marked enlargement of the bone, thickening of the cortices, coarse but purposeful trabeculae, and lytic areas[9,10,23,61] (Figure 4).

- "Large ivory vertebrae" describes the changes seen in the affected spinal segments.[9,10,14,34,58,62,63] The vertebrae are larger than normal (in particular, wider than normal), have coarse trabeculae, and thick and often very dense cortices, hence the designation "ivory" (Figure 5). These lesions must be distinguished from the normal-sized ivory vertebrae, which is characteristic of Hodgkin's lymphoma.[62]
- Jaw and teeth changes may sometimes be severe and impair dietary and speech activities. The jaw may become enlarged, sometimes more so on one side than the other, and the teeth loosened, producing a characteristic appearance of "floating teeth" on imaging studies. This finding is not diagnostic for Paget's disease but can occur in Langerhans cell histiocytosis, polyostotic fibrous dysplasia, or non-Hodgkin's lymphoma of bone.[9,61,64]

All lesions of Paget's disease are most often extremely dense on a bone scan, and sometimes even bones that do not appear affected may show increased activity.[56] This is particularly true for the calvarium. Positron emission tomography scans are also very active over sites of Paget's disease.

Complications of Paget's Disease

Because many patients with Paget's disease at a single site are asymptomatic, the diagnosis is made on the basis of an imaging study for some other problem. This is particularly true for the spine, where it is estimated that roughly 3% of the population over the age of 50 years have a solitary involvement of one vertebra. It is often the complications of the disease that produce symptoms and cause the patient to seek medical attention. Complications include:

- Bone pain may be mild or severe and can occur even when the disease is mild and localized. The pain is over the site of the lesion and may be associated not only with tenderness of the bony segment with pressure but skin discomfort, particularly over the tibiae, clavicles, or ulnae, where the bone lies in close proximity to the skin.[9,10,13,14]
- Deformities of the bone can be striking and are, in Paget's original case, the site of sometimes severe disabili-

ty.[4,9,10,13,14,23,33,65] Bowing of the tibiae and femora are common, but enlargement of these and other bones such as the clavicles may cause disturbances in function possibly related to nerve or vascular damage. Patients often become shorter in stature, related to bowing of their extremities and flexion or scoliosis of the spine.

- Osteoarthritis can frequently be a presenting problem for patients with hip, knee, or spinal Paget's disease. The classic form is in the hip, where the femoral head and the acetabulum have different rates of structural alteration, even when both sides are involved. The cartilage damage and the joint structural change lead to sometimes severe and incapacitating osteoarthritis. The temporomandibular joint may also be involved; this can cause considerable pain and limitation of jaw movement.[9,10,13,14,61,64]

- Foraminal encroachment is one of the most severe complications of skull and spinal Paget's diseases. Patients with even mild calvarial disease may become deaf, lose visual acuity, or possibly develop Bell's palsy. Patients with spinal Paget's disease frequently develop narrowing of the central canal, leading to nerve deficits in the upper or lower extremities; the individual root canals may be equally impaired.[9,13,57,58,60,62,66]

- Pathologic fractures of the bones can cause serious damage to the limb or spinal structures. The femur or tibia may fracture with minimal trauma, and the fracture is often related to the stress lines. Fractures of the vertebrae can cause paraplegia or even tetraplegia. Fractures may heal poorly despite the increased osteoblastic activity present in the tissue, and nonunion is common. Use of standard treatment techniques such as rodding or applying plates and screws is difficult because the bone, although more dense than normal, cannot be expected to hold metallic devices.[9,13,33,34,58,64,66,67]

- High-output left heart cardiac failure is one of the most serious problems with extensive Paget's disease. The cause of this problem is related to the increased blood supply of the bones, which can

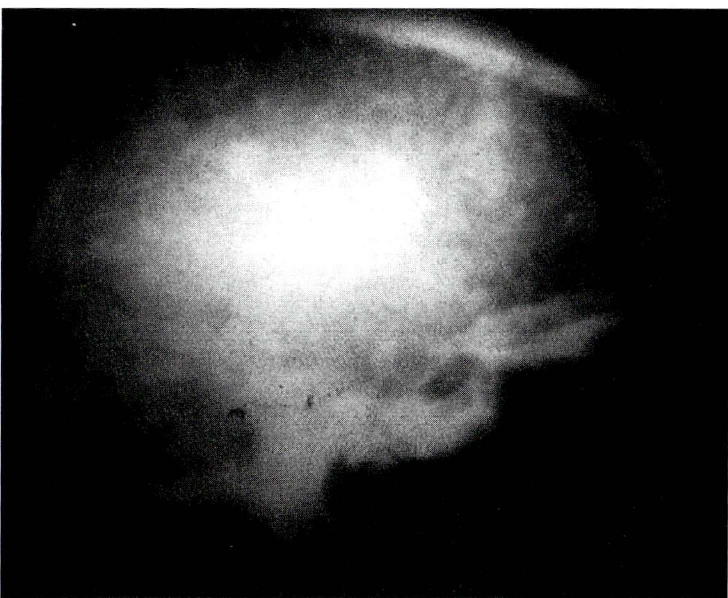

Figure 4

Calvarial changes in a patient with extensive Paget's disease. The disorder, known as "osteoporosis circumscripta cranii," ultimately results in a marked increase in bone density, loss of hearing, and sometimes severe neurologic changes.

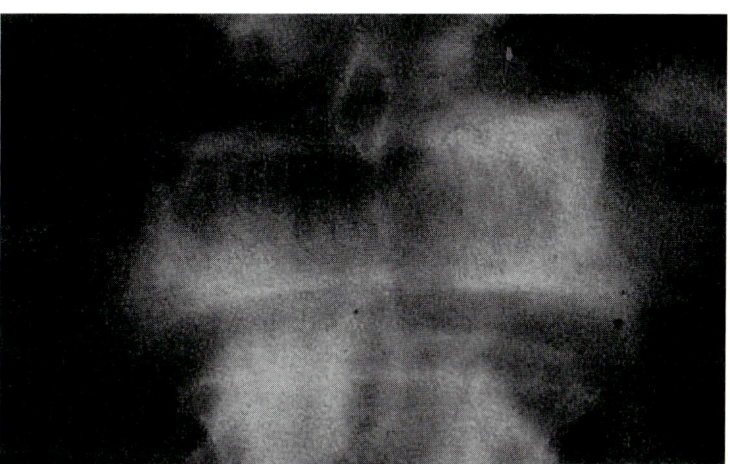

Figure 5

Radiograph showing a classic "large ivory vertebra" characteristic of Paget's disease. The changes may cause canal narrowing and neurologic problems.

sequester large amounts of the cardiac output in the bones and thus impair left heart function. The heart becomes enlarged, and the patient becomes short of breath and develops high-output failure; if untreated, this can lead to death.[9,13,14]

- Nephrocalcinosis occurring with bed rest is related to release of calcium from the bones during prolonged periods of rest and is also associated with the alteration in the vascular system. The syndrome, first described in the early literature, was a serious problem for the patients, who were sometimes confined to bed for weeks at a time. With modern treatment technology and methods of managing calcium metabolic disorders, this problem is now quite uncommon.[9]

- Paget's sarcoma of bone is without a doubt the worst complication of all, for both patient and physician. It occurs in less than 1% of the patients with single bone disease. In Barry's[10] extensive 1969 review, which included not only patients from Australia but a literature review for other parts of the world, the rate of Paget's sarcoma for all patients with any Pagetoid change was less than 1%; the value for extensive disease was under 10%. A comprehensive review of the literature on Paget's sarcoma suggests that the disease is twice as frequent in males as females, and that it is rare in African Americans and Asians.[20-22,31,56,68-77] The mean age for appearance of the disease is 75 years, and it is most frequently located in the femur, pelvis, humerus, and skull.[10,22,31,34,68,70,72,76] Paget's sarcoma of the spine is uncommon.[10,22,62,70]

Treatment of Paget's Disease

Until relatively recently, very little treatment was available for patients with Paget's disease. Those patients who have a solitary focus with little or no discomfort or deformity may be watched periodically with serial radiographs, bone scans, and assays for serum alkaline phosphatase. There is no reason to treat these patients unless they develop more extensive disease.[9,10,13,14] Bone pain should be controllable with medication, and bracing and exercise programs may be helpful in restoring the patient with more extensive disease to a higher level of activity.

Patients who develop osteoarthritis or fractures may need to be treated by appropriate surgery. This is sometimes difficult because of the potential complications of excessive blood loss; difficulty getting hardware to work effectively; high-output cardiac disease, making anesthesia complicat-

ed; or possible renal failure with bed rest.[13,60,62,66,67] Although the cardiac and hypercalcemic aspects of the surgical procedures should not be a problem with modern medical management, considering the age of the patient and the marked degree of impairment of function that the patient may present with, restoration may represent a major challenge.

The newest systems of treatment for patients with extensive Paget's disease are based on medications that markedly diminish the bone turnover and thus decrease the bone pain. Perhaps more importantly, the agents are thought likely to reduce the probability of fracture, cardiac problems, and possibly the rate at which sarcoma arises. One of the principal agents at present is calcitonin, which demonstrates dramatic effectiveness in the therapy of patients with Paget's disease.[9,78,79] The drug lowers alkaline phosphatase and plasma calcium concentration, and markedly inhibits osteoclastic bone resorption. Study of the bone from patients treated with calcitonin disclose a reduction in the number and size of the osteoclasts, a decrease in bone density, and an increase in more normal appearing lamellar bone.[9,13,78,79] In addition, hearing loss is reduced in severity and the cardiac index generally falls toward normal. The drug has in the past been administered parenterally. Recently, synthetic calcitonin has been given by nasal spray; this reduces some of the problems for elderly patients, who find it difficult to administer intramuscular agents.[9,13]

The second group of agents that appear to be extraordinarily effective in the management of patients with extensive Paget's disease are the bisphosphonates.[9,13,14,65,80-82] These agents act principally by altering calcium metabolism and, more importantly, inhibiting osteoclastic activity to an extraordinary degree. Studies have shown that patients treated with these agents intravenously at intervals of 1 to 2 months for pamidronate and less frequently for zolendronate have a "remission" in their symptoms and a marked change in their bone pain, cardiac index, arthritis difficulty, spinal canal narrowing, hearing loss, and fracture rate.[9,10,13,26,45,60,62]

The treatment of Paget's sarcoma remains a major issue in relation to this puzzling disorder. It is interesting to speculate why the results for Paget's sarcoma are no different today then they were long ago, considering the advances that have been made in the treatment of other tumors such as osteosarcoma or Ewing's sarcoma. There are several possible explanations for these findings. First, the Paget's sarcoma tumor is probably more malignant than other connective tissue tumors, and in fact the percentage of patients with high-grade disease with metastases at the time of presentation is well over 25%. A second issue is the excessive vascularity in the Pagetoid bone, which far exceeds that of other disorders, including most connective tissue tumors. It is possible that metastatic disease is not only present in a higher percentage of patients at the outset, but may occur much more rapidly than with other tumors, even when the patient is treated with appropriate additional therapy. The third issue is that the age and general health of patients with disseminated Paget's disease may markedly limit the use of chemotherapy. Patients with widespread Paget's disease are prone to high-output left ventricular failure, and are considered by many to be poor risks not only for chemotherapy but also for extensive surgery. The fourth issue is the location of the tumors. Most of the Paget's sarcomas are located in the pelvis, proximal femur, and proximal humerus rather than the distal femur and proximal tibia as in younger patients with osteosarcoma. Finally, patients with widespread Paget's disease may be less aware of the development of a malignant tumor, based on their limited physical and sometimes mental capacity, high degree of disability, and skeletal deformity; together with their chronic pain pattern, this makes the development of a sarcoma harder to detect. Because of these issues, the lesions may grow to very large volumes and metastasize prior to discovery.

Conclusions

The medical community has come a very long way over the 130 years since Sir James Paget first described his patient. Our understanding of the genesis of the disease and its manifestations, consequences, and treatment have changed radically, surely to the happiness of our patients and their treating physicians. Regrettably, our knowledge and capacity to care for patients with Paget's disease has not really improved to the extent it has for other disorders. We still do not know the cause or why the disease presents in the forms that it does. Although treatment with calcitonin and bisphosphonates have improved the situation, we still are unable to really eradicate the disease. Furthermore, the Paget's sarcoma still represents a true curse on the patients with the problem, with virtually no successful method of treatment. Paget's disease remains a genuine challenge for the orthopaedic profession.

References

1. Rogers J, Jeffrey DR, Watt I: Paget's disease in an archeological population. *J Bone Miner Res* 2002;17:1127-1134.

2. Wells C, Woodhouse N: Paget's disease in an Anglo Saxon. *Med Hist* 1975;19:396-400.

3. Hutchinson J: On osteitis deformans. *Illus Med News* 1889;2:169.

4. Bett WR: Osteitis deformans before and after Paget. *Ann R Coll Surg Engl* 1956;19:390-393.

5. Wilks S: Case of osteoporosis, or spongy hypertrophy of the bones (calvaria, clavicles, os femoris and rib). *Trans Path Soc Lond* 1869;20:273-277.

6. Czerny V: Eine lakale maladie des unterschenkels. *Wien Med Wochenschr* 1873;23:895-925.

7. Paget J: On a form of chronic inflammation of bone (osteitis deformans). *Med Chir Trans* 1877;60:37-63.

8. Paget J: Additional cases of osteitis deformans. *Med Chir Trans* 1882;65:225-236.

9. Altman RD: Paget's disease of bone, in Coe FL, Favus MJ (eds): *Disorders of Bone and Mineral Metabolism*. New York, NY, Raven Press, 1992, pp 1027-1064.

10. Barry HC: *Paget's Disease of Bone*. Baltimore, MD, William and Wilkins Co, 1969.

11. Colman E: Sir James Paget: The man and the eponym. *Calcif Tissue Int* 2002;70:430-431.

12. Coppes-Zantinga AR, Coppes MJ: Sir James Page (1814-1889): A great academic Victorian. *J Am Coll Surg* 2000;191:70-74.

13. Singer FR, Krane SM: Paget's disease of bone, in Avioli LV, Krane SM (eds): *Metabolic Bone Disease and Clinically Related Disorders*, ed 3. Boston, MA, Boston Academic Press, 1998, pp 545-605.

14. Singer FR: *Paget's Disease of Bone*. New York, NY, Plenum Publishing Company, 1977.

15. Schmorl G: Uber ostitis deformans Paget. *Virchows Arch Path Anat Physiol* 1932;283:694-751.

16. Rosenkrantz JA, Wolf J, Kaicher JJ: Paget's disease (osteitis deformans): Review of one hundred eleven cases. *Arch Intern Med* 1952;90:610-633.

17. Collins DH: Paget's disease of bone: Incidence and subclinical forms. *Lancet* 1956;2:51-57.

18. Pygott FL: Paget's disease of bone: The radiological incidence. *Lancet* 1957;1:1170-1171.

19. Packard FA, Steele JD, Kirkbride TS Jr: Osteitis deformans. *Am J Med Sci* 1901;122:552-569.

20. Bird CE: Sarcoma complicating Paget's disease of bone: Report of 9 cases, 5 with pathologic verifica-

tion. *Arch Surg* 1927;14:1187-1208.

21. Pike MM: Paget's disease with associated osteogenic sarcoma: Report of three cases. *Arch Surg* 1943;46:750-754.

22. Barry HC: Sarcoma in Paget's disease of bone in Australia. *J Bone Joint Surg Am* 1961;43:1122-1133.

23. Jaffe HL: *Metabolic, Degenerative and Inflammatory Diseases of Bone and Joints.* Philadelphia, PA, Lea and Febiger, 1972, pp 240-271.

24. Barry HC: The cause of Paget's disease of bone. *J Bone Joint Surg Br* 1982;64:126-127.

25. Seton M, Choi HK, Hansen MF, Sebaldt RJ, Cooper C: Analysis of environmental factors in familial versus sporadic Paget's disease of bone: The New England Registry for Paget's Disease of Bone. *J Bone Miner Res* 2003;18:1519-1524.

26. Sissons HA: Epidemiology of Paget's disease. *Clin Orthop Relat Res* 1966;45:73-79.

27. Detheridge PM, Guyer PB, Barker DJP: European distribution of Paget's disease of bone. *Br Med J (Clin Res Ed)* 1982;285:1005-1008.

28. Eekhoff ME, van der Kilift M, Kroon HM: Paget's disease of bone in the Netherlands: A population-based radiological and biochemical survey: The Rotterdam Study. *J Bone Miner Res* 2004;19:566-570.

29. Gardner MJ, Guyer PB, Barker DJB: Radiologic prevalence of Paget's disease of bone in British migrants to Australia. *Br Med J* 1978;1:1655-1657.

30. Morales-Piga AA, Rey-Rey JS, Corres-Gonzales J, Garcia-Sagredo JM, Lopez-Abente G: Frequency and characteristics of familial aggregation of Paget's disease of bone. *J Bone Miner Res* 1995;10:663-670.

31. Price CHG, Goldie W: Paget's sarcoma of bone: A study of eighty cases from the Bristol and Leeds bone tumour registries. *J Bone Joint Surg Br* 1969;51:205-224.

32. Sofaer JA, Holloway SM, Emery AEH: A family study of Paget's disease of bone. *J Epidemiol Community Health* 1983;37:226-231.

33. Van Staa TP, Selby P, Leufkens HG: Incidence and natural history of Paget's disease of bone in England and Wales. *J Bone Miner Res* 2002;17:465-471.

34. Whitehouse RW: Paget's disease of bone. *Semin Musculoskelet Radiol* 2002;6:313-322.

35. Rosenbaum HD, Hanson DJ: Geographic variation in the prevalence of Paget's disease of bone. *Radiology* 1969;92:959-963.

36. Rousiere M, Michou L, Cornelis F, Orcel P: Paget's disease of bone. *Best Pract Res Clin Rheumatol* 2003;17:1019-1041.

37. Thogo O, Ito K, Takeda H, et al: Paget's disease of bone. *Orthop Traum Surg* 1984;27:525-530.

38. Pompe Van Meerdervoort HF, Richter GG: Paget's disease in South African Blacks. *S Afr Med J* 1976;50:1897-1899.

39. Choma TJ, Kuklo TR, Islinger RB, Murphey MD, Temple HT: Paget's disease of bone in patients younger than 40 years. *Clin Orthop Relat Res* 2004;418:202-204.

40. Eekhoff EW, Karperien M, Houtsma D, et al: Familial Paget's disease in The Netherlands: Occurrence, identification of new mutations in the sequestosome 1 gene, and their clinical associations. *Arthritis Rheum* 2004;50:1650-1654.

41. Hocking L, Slee F, Haslam SI, et al: Familial Paget's disease of bone: Patterns of inheritance and

42. Jones JV, Reed MF: Paget's disease in a family with six cases. *Br Med J* 1967;4:90-95.

43. Kimonis VE, Kovach JJ, Waggoner B, et al: Clinical and molecular studies in a unique family with autosomal dominant limb-girdle muscular dystrophy and Paget disease of bone. *Genet Med* 2000;2:232-241.

44. Nance MA, Nuttall FQ, Econs MJ, et al: Heterogeneity in Paget disease of the bone. *Am J Med Genet* 2000;92:303-307.

45. Takata S, Yasui N, Nakatsuka K, Ralston SH: Evolution of understanding of genetics of Paget's disease of bone and related diseases. *J Bone Miner Metab* 2004;22:519-523.

46. Hofbauer LC, Heufelder AE: Role of receptor activator of nuclear factor-kappaB ligand and osteoprotegerin in bone cell biology. *J Mol Med* 2001;79:243-253.

47. Layfield R, Ciani B, Ralston SH, et al: Structural and functional studies of mutation affecting the UA domain of SQSTM1 (p62) which cause Paget's disease of bone. *Biochem Soc Trans* 2004;32:728-730.

48. Layfield R, Hocking LJ: SQSTM1 and Paget's disease of bone. *Calcif Tissue Int* 2004;75:347-357.

49. Brandwood CP, Hoyland JA, Hillarby MC, et al: Apoptotic gene expression in Paget's disease: A possible role for Bcl-2. *J Pathol* 2003;201:504-512.

50. Sparks AB, Peterson SN, Bell C, et al: Mutation screening of the TNFRSF11A gene encoding receptor activator of NF kappa B (RANK) in familial and sporadic Paget's disease of bone and osteosarcoma. *Calcif Tissue Int* 2001;68:151-155.

51. Wuyts W, Van Wesenbeeck L, Morales–Piga A, et al: Evaluation of the role of RANK and OPG genes in Paget's disease of bone. *Bone* 2001;28:104-107.

52. Good D, Busfield F, Duffy D, et al: Familial Paget's disease of bone: Nonlinkage to the PDB1 and PDB2 loci on chromosomes 6p and 18q in a large pedigree. *J Bone Miner Res* 2001;16:33-38.

53. Kovach MJ, Waggoner B, Leal SM, et al: Clinical delineation and localization to chromosome 9p13.3-p12 of a unique dominant disorder in four families: Hereditary inclusion body myopathy, Paget disease of bone, and frontotemporal dementia. *Mol Genet Metab* 2001;74:458-475.

54. Helfrich MH: Osteoclast diseases. *Microsc Res Tech* 2003;61:514-532.

55. Wolff J: *Das Gesetz der Transformation der Knochen.* Berlin, Germany, A. Hirschwald, 1892.

56. Hain SF, Fogelman I: Nuclear medicine studies in metabolic bone disease. *Semin Musculoskelet Radiol* 2002;6:323-329.

57. Campbell E, Whitfield RD: Osteogenic sarcoma of vertebrae secondary to Paget's disease: Report of three cases with compression of spinal cord and cauda equina. *N Y State J Med* 1943;43:931-938.

58. Carpineta L, Gagne M: The ivory vertebra: An approach to investigation and management base on two case studies. *Spine* 2002;27:E242-E247.

59. Golding C: Museum pages: IV On the differential diagnosis of Paget's disease. *J Bone Joint Surg Br* 1960;42:641-643.

60. Hadjipavlou AG, Gaitanis LN, Katonis PG, Lander P: Paget's disease of the spine and its management. *Eur Spine J* 2001;10:370-384.

61. Hullar TE, Lustig LR: Paget's disease and fibrous

dysplasia. *Otolaryngol Clin North Am* 2003;36:707-732.

62. Saifuddin A, Hassan A: Paget's disease of the spine: Unusual features and complications. *Clin Radiol* 2003;58:102-111.

63. Whitten CR, Saifuddin A: MRI of Paget's disease of bone. *Clin Radiol* 2003;58:763-769.

64. Bender IB: Paget's disease. *J Endod* 2003;29:720-723.

65. Wang LM, Au-Yeong ML, McKenna MJ: Paget's disease of bone: Presentation, extent and response to bisphosphonates. *Ir Med J* 2002;95:244-246.

66. Langston AL, Ralston SH: Management of Paget's disease of bone. *Rheumatology (Oxford)* 2004;43:955-959.

67. Lewallen DG: Hip arthroplasty in patients with Paget's disease. *Clin Orthop Relat Res* 1999;369:243-250.

68. Goldenberg RR: Neoplasia in Paget's disease of bone. *Bull Hosp Joint Dis* 1961;22:1-38.

69. Giunti A, Laus M: Sarcoma in Paget's disease (11 cases). *Ital J Orthop Traumatol* 1979;5:311-320.

70. Haibach H, Farrell C, Dittrich PJ: Neoplasms arising in Paget's disease of bone: A study of 85 patients. *Am J Clin Pathol* 1985;83:594-600.

71. Huvos AG, Butler A, Bretsky SS: Osteogenic sarcoma associated with Paget's disease. *Cancer* 1983;52:1489-1495.

72. Miner IE: Sarcoma in Paget's disease of bone. *Bull Hosp Joint Dis* 1950;11:26-42.

73. Moore TE, King AR, Kathol MH, el-Khoury GY, Palmer R, Downey PR: Sarcoma in Paget's disease of bone: Clinical, radiologic, and pathologic features in 22 cases. *AJR Am J Roentgenol* 1991;156:1199-1203.

74. Porretta CA, Dahlin DC, Janes JM: Sarcoma in Paget's disease of bone. *J Bone Joint Surg Am* 1957;39:1314-1329.

75. Schajowicz F, Santini Araujo E, Berenstein M: Sarcoma complicating Paget's disease of bone: A clinicopathological study of 62 cases. *J Bone Joint Surg Br* 1983;65:299-307.

76. Summey TJ, Presley CL: Sarcoma complicating Paget's disease of bone. *Ann Surg* 1946;123:135-153.

77. Wick MR, Siegal GP, Unni GP, McLeod RA, Greditzer HG III: Sarcomas of bone complicating osteitis deformans (Paget's disease): Fifty years' experience. *Am J Surg Pathol* 1981;5:47-59.

78. DeRose J, Singer FR, Avramides A, et al: Response of Paget's disease to porcine and salmon calcitonin: Effects of long-term treatment. *Am J Med* 1974;56:858-866.

79. Ziegler R, Holz G, Raue F, et al: Therapeutic studies with human calcitonin, in MacIntyre I (ed): *Human Calcitonin and Paget's Disease*. Bern, Switzerland, H Huber, 1977, pp 167-178.

80. Devogelaer JP: Modern therapy for Paget's disease of bone: Focus on bisphosphonates. *Treat Endocrinol* 2002;1:241-257.

81. Garnero P, Christgau S, Delmas PD: The bisphosphonate zoledronate decreases type II collagen breakdown in patients with Paget's disease of bone. *Bone* 2001;28:461-464.

82. Theriault RL: Zolendronic acid (Zometa) use in bone disease. *Expert Rev Anticancer Ther* 2003;3:157-166.

Chapter 12

Fibrous Dysplasia

Fibrous dysplasia is a common disorder characterized by lesions of the bones containing a distinctive pathologic fibrous tissue, which produces irregular gracile, poorly ossified trabeculae.[1-4] The lesions may be monostotic, with little effect on the patient's general status or bone structure, or polyostotic, which may in some cases be associated with bizarre additional syndromes and major functional impairments.[1,2] There is little doubt that both forms of the disease are congenital; some children are born with the abnormalities, but neither form appears to be familial or hereditary.[1,5] Despite a great deal of research effort, both forms of the disease remain of unknown cause. Gene errors have been described for the multiple forms of the disease, but not for the solitary or monostotic process.[2] With some exceptions, the monostotic form is relatively simple to eradicate; however, the polyostotic form may be impossible to effectively eliminate and sometimes causes bizarre and distressing abnormalities, which can be associated with severe disabilities.[1,2,4-9]

Nomenclature and History of Fibrous Dysplasia

Although it is highly likely that the lesions of fibrous dysplasia were seen, histologically studied, and treated for many years prior to the definition of the disease by Lichtenstein,[10] they were not considered to be a separate entity; in fact, considerable confusion still exists in nomenclature of fibrous lesions within the bone. Jaffe and Lichtenstein[11] reported on nonosteogenic fibroma of bone in 1942, and Ponseti and Friedman[12] described metaphyseal fibrous defects in 1949. Marcove, working with Jaffe and others, reported on a disorder called fibromyxoma of bone in 1964,[13] and Cohen and Goldenberg[14] introduced the term desmoplastic fibroma of bone the following year. In 1982, Mirra and associates[3] reported a series of fibrous tumors of bone associated with skin lesions, which they called Jaffe-Campanacci syndrome. The term benign fibrous histiocytoma was proposed by Bertoni

and associates[15] in 1986 to describe a lesion containing fibroblasts within the bone. The terms ossifying fibroma or osteofibrous dysplasia, although originally considered to describe fibrous dysplasia, have now been applied to lesions of the tibia that closely resemble adamantinomas but are more benign and occur in younger children.[2,15-17] It is also likely that the term low-grade fibrosarcoma of bone, rarely used today, may have served to describe the lesions of fibrous dysplasia in the past.[1,2]

The first recognized report regarding "true" fibrous dysplasia was the 1931 article by Hunter and Turnbull[18] in the *British Journal of Surgery* on the subject of hyperparathyroidism, in which they described localized solitary osteofibrous lesions of bone. They stated, "Of much more common occurrence than the generalized disease is focal osteitis fibrosa. This is a condition affecting one or more bones; usually not disabling; of slow progress and symptomless until spontaneous fracture occurs. The figures for serum calcium and phosphorous are invariably normal."[18] In 1936, McCune[19] described a 9-year-old girl with lesions of the bone that he termed "osteitis fibrocystica." The patient also had precocious puberty, skin lesions, and hyperthyroidism. Albright and associates[20] then described the polyostotic fibrous dysplasia syndrome in five patients with emphasis on the hormonal and dermal lesions. This rare and extraordinary syndrome became known as McCune-Albright or Albright-Butler disease. In 1938, Lichtenstein[10] described patients with multiple bone lesions and introduced the term polyostotic fibrous dysplasia. Several years later, he and Jaffe used the term "fibrous dysplasia" for both the monostotic and polyostotic syndromes.[11,21] A syndrome known as leontiasis ossea was attributed to fibrous dysplasia, and numerous other reports have further defined not only the long bone disease, but the spinal, calvarial, mandibular, and scapular disorders associated with both forms of the disease.[7,21-31] Harris and his coworkers[7] from the Massachusetts General

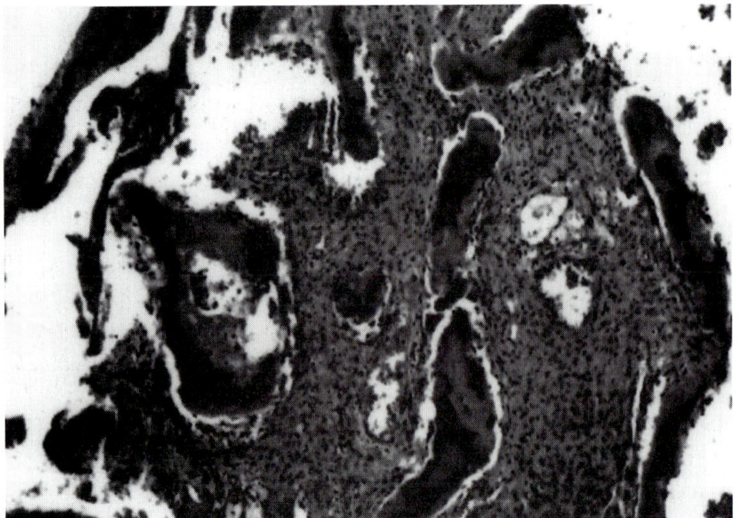

Figure 1

Classic histologic pattern for fibrous dysplasia. The marrow is replaced by small fibrous elements that show little evidence of atypism or aggressive structural behavior. The bone segments formed are small, seemingly purposeless, and poorly mineralized, with irregular osteoid seams within the bone. Hematoxylin and eosin x 40.

Hospital, Van Horn and his Mayo Clinic colleagues,[32] and a number of additional authors[6,12,23-25,33,34] provided clinical descriptions of large series of patients with both monostotic and polyostotic disease. In 1967, Mazabraud and associates[35] described several patients with classic fibrous dysplasia of bone who also had sometimes large benign myxomas in multiple sites within their musculature—a syndrome now known eponymically as Mazabraud's disease.

Histologic Findings for Both Monostotic and Polyostotic Fibrous Dysplasia

Regardless of the type of disease (monostotic, polyostotic, or McCune-Albright syndrome), the histologic pattern is virtually identical, suggesting that despite the rather marked variation in presentation and extent of disease, the three disorders are related.[2,4-8,22,27,31,36,37] The "parent tissue" type is a fibrocyte or fibroblast, and the cells are arranged in an irregular pattern with only limited areas of columnation. The cells rarely show any atypia or pleomorphism, and mitotic figures are rarely seen. The fibroblasts make tiny spicules of gracile woven bone, which are structurally atypical and sometimes poorly calcified.[1,2,7,36] The patterns of the cells are in the form of irregular commas, sometimes elongated thin struc-

tures or solitary round elements that look like alphabet figures (Figure 1). The pattern has no resemblance to normal medullary bone structure. Of considerable importance is that the bone appears to be synthesized by the fibroblasts; true osteoblasts and osteoclasts are rarely seen. The bone that is formed does not respond to Wolff's law ("Every change in the form and function of a bone, or its function alone is followed by certain definite changes in its internal architecture and equally definite secondary alterations in its mathematical laws."[38]) Although the cortices are often markedly thinned and expanded by the fibrous tissue within the lesion, they are histologically consistent with normal cortical bone; however, they may have small islands of stress fracture repair.[2,39]

Causation and Genetic Abnormalities in the Forms of Fibrous Dysplasia

No consistent errors have been identified in monostotic fibrous dysplasia, but polyostotic and especially McCune-Albright syndrome have been found to have patterns of genetic alteration.[2,22] The concern related to this discovery is that a single consistently present error is not what causes the disease, and familial transmission is quite unusual.[40] In the past, the error has been attributed to the gene 20q13.2; however, this is not consistent, and another study has suggested that the error lies in gene 12.[2,22,41] More recent studies have described an error in the alpha subunit of the cell membrane-bound G protein (Gs alpha).[5,42-47] These data suggest a missense point mutation at the arginine codon, resulting in a substitution of arginine for histidine or arginine for cysteine. Adenyl cyclase is excessive, increasing the concentrations of cyclic adenosine monophosphate.[5,42,44,45] The second proposal related to the genetics of the disease is the increased production of the proto-oncogene c-fos, which is believed to alter cellular differentiation, particularly for the cells that form bone.[5,48,49] Another feature in the disease is the increase in the secretion of interleukin-6, which may be responsible for the resorptive activity. The disease is sometimes markedly activated during pregnancy, suggesting a relationship to estrogen activity.[50] Some patients with both polyostotic fibrous dysplasia and McCune-Albright syn-

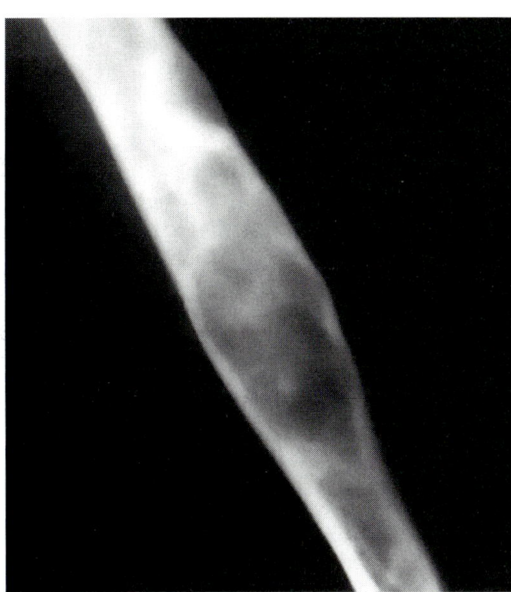

Figure 2
Classic radiographic depiction of fibrous dysplasia. The lesions are lytic and expansile, have a ground glass appearance in the medullary cavity, and show scallops from within.

drome have no identifiable genetic or Gs alpha abnormality, which makes the problem somewhat confusing.[2,5,51]

The Clinical Syndromes
Monostotic Fibrous Dysplasia
Monostotic fibrous dysplasia is a relatively common entity, which more often affects children and usually appears prior to 15 years of age.[2,5,22,24,37,52] A family history of such lesions rarely exists, and only occasional reports suggest that it may occur in siblings. The disorder is equally present in males and females and most often occurs in the diaphysis or metaphysis of the long bones. The femur, tibia, humerus, pelvis, and less commonly the jaws, ribs, and spine are affected. The lesions are often asymptomatic until a fracture occurs through the thinned bony segment and is revealed by imaging studies.[5,36,52] Patients with monostotic disease may actually have more than one lesional site, but this is unusual.[2,22]

Imaging studies of monostotic fibrous dysplasia usually show an expanded lesion often eccentrically located in the midshaft of a long bone, with fairly marked thinning of the cortex and some "scalloping" from within[2,5,7,22,24,52] (Figure 2). Soft-tissue masses are rarely present unless a fracture has occurred or an aneurysmal bone cyst develops

at the site. The bone shows a "ground glass" appearance on radiograph and computed tomography,[53] and magnetic resonance imaging (MRI) usually shows that the lesions are dark on T1 and brighter on T2.[2,5,54] Gadolinium shows a modestly increased vascular supply, and the bone scan is often moderately positive over the site.[54] Despite the fact that the tissue is forming bone, there is little evidence for active bone formation on either MRI or bone scan.[2,5,22,54]

Polyostotic Fibrous Dysplasia
Patients with polyostotic disease usually have multiple bony sites involved, with large and destructive fibrous dysplastic lesions.[2,5,7,10,22,25,36,37,52] The patient may be severely disabled by the disease. The lesions may become much larger with time, markedly expanding the bone and at times undergoing cystic degeneration.[55] The bones may be bowed and shortened, and cause considerable functional loss in ambulation and use of the extremities. Bone lesions are more frequently located on one side in both upper and lower extremities.[2] Of equally great concern is the presence of calvarial and mandibular deformity; classically, the patients have a syndrome of "hemihypertrophy cranii," with damage to the cranial nerves and marked facial abnormality.[26,29,30,56] Fractures are common, particularly in the proximal femur, resulting in increasing coxa vara and ultimately the "shepherd's crook deformity".[5,39,52,57,58] Patients with polyostotic disease may display skin abnormalities consisting of irregularly marginated café-au-lait spots ("coast of Maine").[5]

McCune-Albright Syndrome
McCune-Albright syndrome is a very uncommon disorder with a very broad pattern of effect on patients that can under some circumstances dominate their lives. Most of these patients have polyostotic fibrous dysplasia with multiple sites involved. The deformities of the head and face are often prominent, related to marked hemihypertrophy cranii, with facial "cherubism," deafness, visual disturbances, dental problems, and sometimes altered vocal cord function and respiratory difficulties.[2,5,26,27,29,30,56,59] Women are more frequently affected than men, and precocious puberty is present in about 50% of them.[2,5,22] Menstrual periods starting at 1 to 7 years of age are not un-

usual, and early secondary sexual development is frequently present. Most of the patients are of short stature and have sometimes very large, irregularly marginated café-au-lait skin lesions resembling the coast of Maine rather than the smooth coast of California (present in patients with neurofibromatosis type1).[5] A small number of these patients have additional problems. Male patients with McCune-Albright syndrome may very infrequently develop precocious puberty and even more rarely testicular microlithiasis.[60] Patients may also present with hyperparathyroidism, hypophosphatemic vitamin D-resistant rickets, acromegaly, gynecomastia, hyperthyroidism, or Cushing's syndrome.[5,8,59,61-63] A rare event is left heart failure, such as occurs with Paget's disease.[2,5] Female patients with precocious puberty also have an increased frequency of breast cancer, possibly related to the high levels of estrogen starting at an early age.[1,5,50,64]

The bone lesions observed in these patients resemble those from polyostotic fibrous dysplasia in that they are often much more deforming than those in patients with monostotic disease.[2,4,5,22,59] Bones are short, distorted in shape and structure, and have frequent stress fractures; patients may present or develop severe coxa vara.[39,59] As noted above, the facial distortion is sometimes marked and dominates the patient's course and status.

Laboratory studies for patients with McCune-Albright syndrome may show increased blood alkaline phosphatase, osteocalcin, and urinary pyridinolines.[2,5] Patients with precocious puberty usually show increased estrogen levels.[5,50,64]

Mazabraud's Disease

Patients with either polyostotic fibrous dysplasia or McCune-Albright syndrome may have multiple benign myxomatous tumors often in the thighs, buttocks, or shoulders.[35,65-70] They may be close to the fibrous dysplastic lesions but are physically not associated with them. The lesions may be tender and painful. Malignancies may rarely occur in Mazabraud's disease, and are most frequently osteosarcomas of the bone lesion involved with fibrous dysplasia.[71,72] The lesions are best seen on MRI, where they appear as light on both T1 and T2 and with gadolinium enhancement.[67]

Other Bone Neoplasms Occurring With Fibrous Dysplasias

Bone neoplasms in the site of fibrous dysplastic tumors are rare.[2,5,22] Several reports have suggested that aneurysmal bone cysts may be present at the site of the bone lesions and are sometimes difficult to distinguish from the primary process.[73-75] Osteosarcoma and less commonly chondrosarcoma can occur more often with polyostotic disease or with McCune-Albright syndrome.[1,76-80] As mentioned above, breast cancer frequency is increased in females who develop precocious puberty.[64,78] The myxomas in Mazabraud's do not become malignant, but osteosarcomas may occur in the underlying bone.[71,72] Fibrosarcoma of bone has been reported in patients who have received radiation to control skull deformities or severe structural changes in the extremities.[2,5]

Treatment of the Fibrous Dysplastic Syndromes

Treatment of a solitary lesion in monostotic fibrous dysplasia may vary depending on the size of the lesion, its location, and the likelihood of fracture.[7,24,52,81] Many of the lesions can be treated by observation alone and need no surgical procedures. As a child grows older, the lesions may actually become smaller and occasionally disappear. If concern exists regarding the diagnosis, biopsy and curettage and implantation of allograft chips or polymethylmethacrylate are logical choices for treatment; the recurrence rate is low.[2,5,22] Special concern exists for fibrous dysplastic lesions arising in the proximal femur because fractures may occur and a shepherd's crook deformity may eventually develop, which is difficult to treat. These lesions should be treated more aggressively than those in other locations.[5,36,39,52,57,58,81,82] Fibrous dysplastic lesions of the jaw or skull may require special and sometimes difficult surgery to restore the function of the teeth or improve hearing or visual problems.[29,30,56] Radiation should be avoided for these lesions because of the risk of fibrosarcoma in later years.[2,5]

A variety of treatment options are available for patients with polyostotic disease or those with McCune-Albright syndrome. Surgery is indicated for fractures or for lesions that look like they are likely to fracture, particularly in the region of the proximal femur.[36,39,52,81,82] Prophylactic rodding of the long bones often seems appropriate, as does the introduction of intercalary allograft segments, either to replace the diseased tissue or be placed within the expanded cortex to strengthen the bone.[57,58] Recently patients have been treated with intravenous pamidronate and other forms of bisphosphonate, which appears to be successful in improving the quality of the bone and reducing the risk of fracture.[83-86] For females with precocious puberty, tamoxifen lowers the estrogen level and reduces the bony lesion activity; more recently testolactone has also been used to accomplish this.[2,5,64]

Summary

The three syndromes and Mazabraud's disease, which are all included in the generic title fibrous dysplasia, remain puzzling, enigmatic, and at times difficult to treat. Fortunately, the simplest form (monostotic disease) is the most common and presents the least difficulty for the patient; however, the polyostotic form, Mazabraud's disease, and especially McCune-Albright syndrome remain difficult in terms of defining the cause, establishing the nature of the clinical presentations, and developing a competent and clearly effective treatment protocol.

References

1. Campanacci M, Bertoni F, Capanna R: Malignant degeneration in fibrous dysplasia: Report of 6 cases and review of the literature. *Ital J Orthop Traumatol* 1979;5:373-381.

2. Dorfman HD, Czerniak B: *Bone Tumors.* St. Louis, MO, Mosby Co, 1998, pp 441-477.

3. Mirra JM, Gold RH, Rand F: Disseminated non-ossifying fibromas in association with cafe-au-lait spots (Jaffe-Campanacci syndrome). *Clin Orthop Relat Res* 1982;168:192-205.

4. Unni KK: *Dahlin's Bone Tumors.* Philadelphia, PA, Lippincott Raven, 1996, pp 367-376.

5. Parekh SG, Donthineni-Rao R, Ricchetti E, Lackman RD: Fibrous dysplasia. *J Am Acad Orthop Surg* 2004;12:305-313.

6. Grabias SL, Campbell CJ: Fibrous dysplasia. *Orthop Clin North Am* 1977;8:771-783.

7. Harris WH, Dudley R Jr, Barry RJ: The natural history of fibrous dysplasia: An orthopaedic, pathological and roentgenographic study. *J Bone Joint Surg Am* 1962;44:207-233.

8. Mirra JM, Gold RH, Picci P: Osseous tumors of intramedullary origin, in *Bone Tumors: Clinical, Radiologic and Pathological Correlations.* Philadelphia, PA, Lea and Febiger, 1989, pp143-148.

9. Smith SE, Kransdorf MJ: Primary musculoskeletal tumors of fibrous origin. *Semin Musculoskelet Radiol* 2000;4:73-88.

10. Lichtenstein L: Polyostotic fibrous dysplasia. *Arch Surg* 1938;36:874-898.

11. Jaffe HL, Lichtenstein L: Non-osteogenic fibroma of bone. *Am J Pathol* 1942;18:205-221.

12. Ponseti IV, Friedman B: Evolution of metaphyseal fibrous defects. *J Bone Joint Surg Am* 1949;31:582-585.

13. Marcove RC, Kambolis C, Bullough PG, Jaffe HL: Fibromyxoma of bone: A report of three cases. *Cancer* 1964;17:1209-1213.

14. Cohen P, Goldenberg RR: Desmoplastic fibroma of bone. *J Bone Joint Surg Am* 1965;47:1620-1625.

15. Bertoni F, Caldroni P, Bacchini P, et al: Benign fibrous histiocytoma of bone. *J Bone Joint Surg Am* 1986;68:1225-1230.

16. Campanacci M, Laus M: Osteofibrous dysplasia of the tibia and fibula. *J Bone Joint Surg Am* 1981;63:367-375.

17. Springfield DS, Rosenberg AE, Mankin HJ, Mindell ER: Relationship between osteofibrous dysplasia and adamantinoma. *Clin Orthop Relat Res* 1994;309:234-244.

18. Hunter D, Turnbull HM: Hyperparathyroidism: Generalized osteitis fibrosa. *Br J Surg* 1931;19:203.

19. McCune DJ: Osteitis fibrocystica: The case of a nine year old girl who also exhibits precocious puberty, multiple pigmentation of the skin and hyperthyroidism. *Am J Dis Child* 1936;52:743-744.

20. Albright F, Butler AM, Hampton AO, Smith P: Syndrome characterized by osteitis fibrosa disseminata, areas of pigmentation and endocrine dysfunction with precocious puberty in females: Report of five cases. *N Engl J Med* 1937;216:727-746.

21. Lichtenstein L, Jaffe HL: Fibrous dysplasia of bone: A condition affecting one, several or many bones, graver cases of which may present abnormal pigmentation of skin, premature sexual development, hyperthyroidism or still other extraskeletal abnormalities. *Arch Pathol* 1942;33:777-816.

22. Campanacci M: *Bone and Soft Tissue Tumors*, ed 2. New York, NY, Springer Verlag, 1999, pp 435-461.

23. Hatcher CH: The pathogenesis of localized fibrous lesions in the metaphyses of long bones. *Ann Surg* 1945;122:1016-1033.

24. Henry A: Monostotic fibrous dysplasia. *J Bone Joint Surg Br* 1969;51:300-306.

25. Henry AN: Polyostotic fibrous dysplasia. *J Bone Joint Surg Br* 1963;45:803.

26. Jaffe HL: Giant cell reparative granuloma, traumatic bone cyst and fibrous (fibro-osseous) dysplasia of the jaw bones. *Oral Surg* 1953;36:159-175.

27. Jaffe HL: *Tumors and Tumorous Conditions of Bones and Joints.* Philadelphia, PA, Lea and Febiger, 1958, pp 117-142.

28. Leet AI, Magur E, Lee JS, Wientroub S, Robey PG, Collins MT: Fibrous dysplasia in the spine: Prevalence of lesions and association with scoliosis. *J Bone Joint Surg Am* 2004;86:531-537.

29. Nager GT, Kennedy DW, Kopstein E: Fibrous dysplasia: A review of the disease and its manifestations in the temporal bone. *Ann Otol Rhinol Laryngol Suppl* 1982;92:1-52.

30. Pierce AM, Wilson DF, Goss AN: Inherited craniofacial fibrous dysplasia. *Oral Surg Oral Med Oral Pathol* 1985;60:403-409.

31. Wright JF, Stoker DJ: Fibrous dysplasia of the spine. *Clin Radiol* 1988;39:523-527.

32. Van Horn PE Jr, Dahlin DC, Bickel WH: Fibrous dysplasia: A clinical pathologic study of orthopedic surgical cases. *Mayo Clin Proc* 1963;38:175-189.

33. Pritchard JE: Fibrous dysplasia of the bones. *Am J Med Sci* 1951;222:313-332.

34. Reed RJ: Fibrous dysplasia of bone: A review of 25 cases. *Arch Pathol* 1963;75:480-495.

35. Mazabraud A, Semat P, Roze R: A propos d'association de fibromyxomes des tissue mous a la dysplasie fibreuse des os. *Presse Med* 1967;75:2223-2228.

36. Keijser LC, Van Tienen TG, Schreuder HW, Lemmens JA, Pruszczynski M, Veth RP: Fibrous dysplasia of bone: Management and outcome of 20 cases. *J Surg Oncol* 2001;76:157-166.

37. Marks KE, Bauer TW: Fibrous tumors of bone. *Orthop Clin North Am* 1989;20:377-393.

38. Wolff J: *Das Gesetz der Transformation der Knochen.* Berlin, Germany, A. Hirschwald, 1892.

39. Leet AI, Chebli C, Kushner H, et al: Fracture incidence in polyostotic fibrous dysplasia and the McCune-Albright syndrome. *J Bone Miner Res* 2004;19:571-577.

40. Endo M, Yamada Y, Matsuura N, Niikawa N: Monozygotic twins discordant for the major signs of McCune-Albright syndrome. *Am J Med Genet* 1991;41:216-220.

41. Dal Cin P, Bertoni F, Bacchini P, Hagemeijer A, Van den Berghe H: Fibrous dysplasia and the short arm of chromosome 12. *Histopathology* 1999;34:279-280.

42. Akintoye SO, Chebli C, Booher S, et al: Characterization of gsp-mediated growth hormone excess in the context of McCune-Albright syndrome. *J Clin Endocrinol Metab* 2002;87:5104-5112.

43. Lumbroso S, Paris F, Sultan C: Activating Gsalpha mutations: Analysis of 113 patients with signs of McCune-Albright syndrome. A European Collaborative Study. *J Clin Endocrinol Metab* 2004;89:2107-2113.

44. Mantovani G, Bondioni S, Lania AG, et al: Parental origin of Gsalpha mutations in the McCune-Albright syndrome and in isolated endocrine tumors. *J Clin Endocrinol Metab* 2004;89:3007-3009.

45. Okamoto S, Hisaoka M, Ushijima M, Nakahara S, Toyoshima S, Hashimoto H: Activating Gs(alpha) mutation in intramuscular myxomas with and without fibrous dysplasia of bone. *Virchows Arch* 2000;437:133-137.

46. Perdigao PF, Pimenta FJ, Castro WH, DeMarco L, Gomez RS: Investigation of the GSalpha gene in the diagnosis of fibrous dysplasia. *Int J Oral Maxillofac Surg* 2004;33:498-501.

47. Song HD, Chen FL, Shi WJ, et al: A novel, complex heterozygous mutation with Gsalpha gene in patients with McCune-Albright syndrome. *Endocrine* 2002;18:121-128.

48. Candeliere GA, Glorieux FH, Prudhomme J, St-Arnaud R: Increased expression of c-fos proto-oncogene in bone from patients with fibrous dysplasia. *N Engl J Med* 1995;332:1546-1551.

49. Weisstein JS, Majeska RJ, Klein MJ, Einhorn TA: Detection of c-fos expression in benign and malignant musculoskeletal lesions. *J Orthop Res* 2001;19:339-345.

50. Kaplan FS, Fallon MD, Boden SD, Schmidt R, Senior M, Haddad JG: Estrogen receptors in bone in a patient with polyostotic fibrous dysplasia (McCune-Albright syndrome). *N Engl J Med* 1988;319:421-425.

51. Parham DM, Bridge JA, Lukacs JL, Ding Y, Tryka AF, Sawyer JR: Cytogenetic distinction among benign fibro-osseous lesions of bone in children and adolescents: Value of karyotypic finds in differential diagnosis. *Pediatr Dev Pathol* 2004;7:148-158.

52. Ippolito E, Bray EW, Corsi A, et al: Natural history and treatment of fibrous dysplasia of bone: A multicenter clinicopathologic study promoted by the European Pediatric Orthopaedic Society. *J Pediatr Orthop B* 2003;12:155-177.

53. MacDonald-Jankowski DS, Yeng R, Li TK, Lee KM: Computed tomography of fibrous dysplasia. *Dentomaxillofac Radiol* 2004;33:114-118.

54. Utz JA, Kransdorf MJ, Jelinek JS, Moser RP Jr, Berrey BH: MR appearance of fibrous dysplasia. *J Comput Assist Tomogr* 1989;13:845-851.

55. Simpson AH, Creasy TS, Williamson DM, Wilson DJ, Spivey JS: Cystic degeneration of fibrous dysplasia masquerading as sarcoma. *J Bone Joint Surg Br* 1989;71:434-436.

56. Akintoye SO, Lees JS, Feimster T, et al: Dental characteristics of fibrous dysplasia and McCune-Albright syndrome. *Oral Surg Oral Med Oral Pathol Oral Radiol Endod* 2003;96:275-282.

57. Enneking WF, Gearen PF: Fibrous dysplasia of the femoral neck: Treatment by cortical bone grafting. *J Bone Joint Surg Am* 1986;68:1415-1422.

58. Guille JT, Kumar SJ, MacEwen GD: Fibrous dysplasia of the proximal part of the femur: Long-term results of curettage and bone grafting and mechanical realignment. *J Bone Joint Surg Am* 1998;80:648-658.

59. Lee PA, Van Dop C, Migeon CJ: McCune-Albright syndrome: Long-term follow-up. *JAMA* 1986;256:2980-2984.

60. Wasniewska M, DeLuca F, Bertelloni S, et al: Testicular microlithiasis: An unreported feature of McCune-Albright syndrome in males. *J Pediatr* 2004;145:670-672.

61. Chattopadhyay A, Bhansali A, Mohanty SK, Khandelwal N, Mathur SK, Dash RJ: Hypophosphatemic rickets and osteomalacia in polyostotic fibrous dysplasia. *J Pediatr Endocrinol Metab* 2003;16:893-896.

62. Corsi A, Collins MT, Riminucci M, et al: Osteomalacic and hyperparathyroid changes in fibrous dysplasia of bone: Core biopsy studies and clinical correlations. *J Bone Miner Res* 2003;18:1235-1246.

63. Riminucci M, Collins MD, Fedarko NS, et al: FGF-23 in fibrous dysplasia of bone and its relationship to renal phosphate wasting. *J Clin Invest* 2003;112:683-692.

64. Eugster EA, Rubin SD, Reiter EO, et al: Tamoxifen treatment for precocious puberty in McCune-Albright syndrome: A multicenter trial. *J Pediatr* 2003;143:60-66.

65. Gober GA, Nicholas RW: Case report 800: Skeletal fibrous dysplasia associated with intramuscular myxoma (Mazabraud's syndrome). *Skeletal Radiol* 1993;22:452-455.

66. Ireland DCR, Soule EH, Ivins JC: Myxoma of somatic soft tissues: A report of 58 patients, 3 with multiple tumors and fibrous dysplasia of bone. *Mayo Clin Proc* 1973;48:401-410.

67. Iwasko N, Steinback LS, Disler D, et al: Imaging findings in Mazabraud's syndrome: Seven new cases. *Skeletal Radiol* 2002;31:81-87.

68. Kabukcuoglu F, Kabukcuoglu Y, Yilmaz B, Erdem Y, Evren I: Mazabraud's syndrome: Intramuscular myxoma associated with fibrous dysplasia. *Pathol Oncol Res* 2004;10:121-123.

69. Logel RJ: Recurrent intramuscular myxoma associated with Albright's syndrome: Case report and review of the literature. *J Bone Joint Surg Am* 1976;58:565-568.

70. Prayson MA, Leeson MC: Soft tissue myxoma and fibrous dysplasia of bone. *Clin Orthop Relat Res* 1993;291:222-228.

71. Jhala DN, Eltoum I, Carroll AJ, et al: Osteosarcoma in a patient with McCune-Albright syndrome and Mazabraud's syndrome: A case report emphasizing the cytological and cytogenetic findings. *Hum Pathol* 2003;34:1354-1357.

72. Lopez-Ben R, Pitt MJ, Jaffe KA, Siegal GP: Osteosarcoma in a patient with McCune-Albright syndrome and Mazabraud's syndrome. *Skeletal Radiol* 1999;28:522-526.

73. Diercks RL, Sauter AJ, Mallens WM: Aneurysmal bone cyst in association with fibrous dysplasia. *J Bone Joint Surg Br* 1986;68:144-146.

74. Lin WC, Wu HT, Wei CJ, Chang CY: Aneurysmal bone cyst arising from fibrous dysplasia of the frontal bone. *Eur Radiol* 2004;14:930-932.

75. Lomasney LM, Basu A, Demos TC, Laskin W: Fibrous dysplasia complicated by aneurysmal bone cyst formation affecting multiple cervical vertebrae. *Skeletal Radiol* 2003;32:533-536.

76. Huvos AG, Higinbotham NL, Miller TR: Bone sarcomas arising in fibrous dysplasia. *J Bone Joint Surg Am* 1972;54:1047-1056.

77. Milgram JW: Malignant degeneration of polyostotic fibrous dysplasia of bone. *Bull Hosp Joint Dis* 1975;36:137-149.

78. Ruggieri P, Sim FH, Bond JR, Unni KK: Malignancies in fibrous dysplasia. *Cancer* 1994;73:1411-1424.

79. Taconis WK: Osteosarcoma in fibrous dysplasia. *Skeletal Radiol* 1988;17:163-170.

80. Yabut SM Jr, Kenan S, Sissons HA, Lewis MM: Malignant transformation of fibrous dysplasia: A case report and review of the literature. *Clin Orthop Relat Res* 1988;228:281-289.

81. Stephenson RB, London MD, Hankin FM, Kaufer H: Fibrous dysplasia: An analysis of options for treatment. *J Bone Joint Surg Am* 1987;69:400-409.

82. O'Sullivan M, Zacharin M: Intramedullary rodding and bisphosphonate treatment of polyostotic fibrous dysplasia associated with the McCune-Albright syndrome. *J Pediatr Orthop* 2002;22:255-260.

83. Chapurlat RD, Delmas PD, Lierns D, Meujnier PJ: Long-term effects of intravenous pamidronate in fibrous dysplasia of bone. *J Bone Miner Res* 1997;12:1746-1752.

84. Lane JM, Khan SN, O'Connor WJ, et al: Bisphosphonate therapy in fibrous dysplasia. *Clin Orthop Relat Res* 2001;382:6-12.

85. Plotkin H, Rauch F, Zeitlin L, et al: Effect of pamidronate treatment in children with polyostotic fibrous dysplasia of bone. *J Clin Endocrinol Metab* 2003;88:4569-4575.

86. Zacharin M, O'Sullivan M: Intravenous pamidronate treatment of polyostotic fibrous dysplasia associated with the McCune-Albright syndrome. *J Pediatr* 2000;137:403-449.

Chapter 13

Sarcoidosis

Sarcoidosis is a granulomatous disease of unknown origin that affects multiple organ systems. In some respects, the disease is similar to tuberculosis; however, it has some specific histologic and immunologic characteristics and does not seem to be infectious by respiratory contact. Although virus infection has been suggested as a cause, no organism has been consistently discovered in patients or tissues. Instead, it appears to represent a disorder associated with excessive T helper lymphocyte abnormalities of unknown cause. The disease principally affects the lungs; lymph nodes; eyes; skin; neurologic system; viscera; and, in 10% to 50% of the patients, the bones and joints, especially of the hands and feet. The disease is relatively mild, with spontaneous regression of symptoms commonly observed. The osseous findings may be a puzzling feature because of the resemblance to other disorders.

History of Sarcoidosis

Sarcoid disease was first described by Sir Jonathan Hutchinson[1] in 1877, in a book in which he provided illustrations of an array of clinical skin conditions. In 1889, Ernest Besnier[2] further described the skin alterations and suggested the name "lupus pernio" for the unusual features. Caesar P. Moeller Boeck,[3] a Norwegian dermatologist, further clarified the syndrome and the skin aspects of the disease in 1899. In 1917, Jorgën Schaumann[4] described the additional nondermatologic features of the disease. On the basis of these three contributions, the eponym for sarcoidosis became Besnier-Boeck-Schaumann's disease (more easily defined as Boeck's sarcoidosis). The pulmonary characteristics as well as the histologic features strongly resembled tuberculosis, but additional studies by Löfgren[5] and descriptions of the bone changes by Otto Jüngling[6] separated the disorder from the infectious diseases. The changes in the wrist are now known as Jüngling's syndrome, also called pseudotuberculosis cystica of the carpus.[7] The granulation tissue seen in the lungs, lymph nodes, skin, and bone have no caseation; although giant cells that resemble Langhans cells are present, they often contain structures known as Schaumann granules that are not seen in tuberculosis.[8-11]

The Nature of the Disease

Sarcoidosis is a peculiar entity of unknown etiology.[9,10,12-18] It is defined in *Harrison's Principles of Internal Medicine* as a "chronic multi-system disorder of unknown etiology characterized in affected organs by an accumulation of lymphocytes and mononuclear phagocytes, non-caseating epitheliod granulomas and derangement of the normal tissue architecture."[14] The incidence varies significantly by geographic area, ranging from 6% of the population in Scandinavia and parts of Africa to well below 1% in Caucasian Americans.[10,12,16,19,20] The average age of onset is 20 to 40 years, but some very young children have been diagnosed with the disease.[8,10,12-16,21] Although males and females are affected equally, women seem to have more problems with bone and joint disease.[5,6,13,16,22-25] Approximately 90% of the patients have lung lesions with alveolar involvement and subsequent granuloma formation.[12,14,15,26-28] Erythema nodosum (tender erythematous nodules on the extremities, commonly the leg) with arthralgia and hilar adenopathy (Löfgren's syndrome) is present in about 30% of the patients,[5,9,12,13,23,25,29,30] and ocular problems (anterior uveitis) occur in approximately 25%.[14,15,21,25,29,31] Cardiac findings, liver involvement, lupus pernio (hyperpigmented papules on the face and neck), and neurologic findings are less frequent although potentially life-threatening and disabling.[12-14,25,29,32,33] Articular and osseous findings are present in approximately 40% of patients and in some cases are not reported because the patients may be relatively asymptomatic.[13,14,17,22-25,29,30,34-37] Muscle pain is present in as many as 80% of the patients and is a source of major complaint when symptoms first appear.[14,23,25,29,36] The muscles are tender and joint movement is somewhat limited.

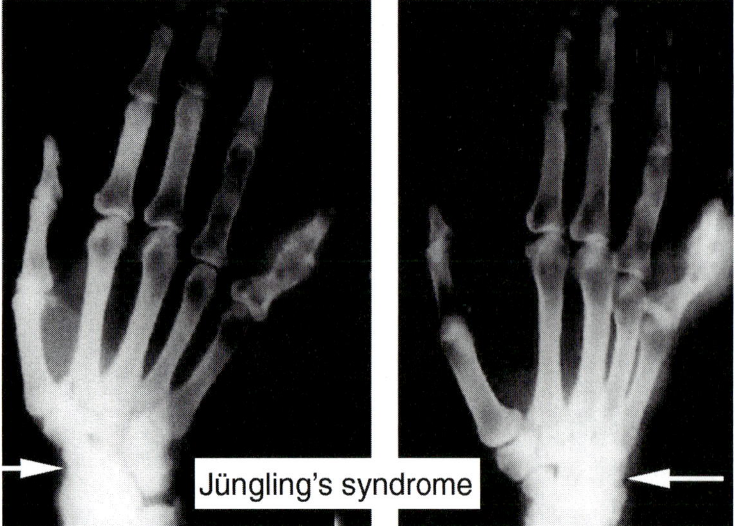

Figure 1
Characteristic bone lesions in the hand and wrist of a patient with sarcoidosis. The lytic lesions are in many of the small bones, and the carpus may show pseudotuberculosis of Jüngling, which is characterized by loss of joint space and irregular structural change in the bones.

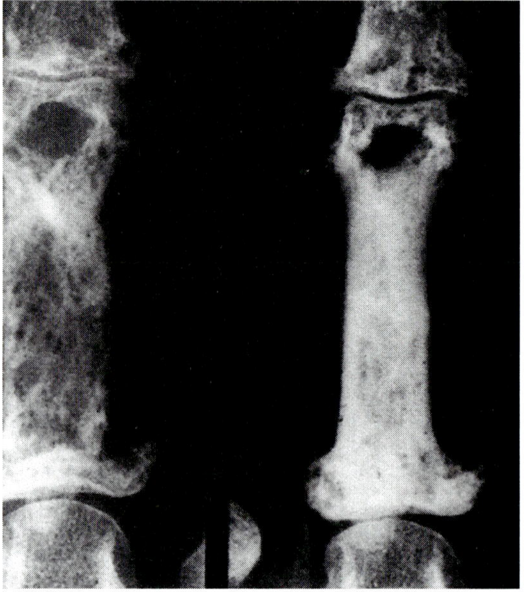

Figure 2
Striking changes in the phalanges in a patient with sarcoidosis.

Patients may walk poorly or limp because of pain in the muscles, often with associated joint problems. Acute sarcoid arthropathy often exists in multiple sites and presents with effusion and joint tenderness.[14,17,23,29,30,38] If the joint lesions are not treated, they may lead to a chronic arthropathy and slow destruction of the joint.[17,24,30,39] The bone lesions, principally located in the hands and feet, can be a major problem[8,35,36,40] (Figure 1). The presence of limitation of motion and tenderness over the bones in the carpus may be evidence of the presence of Jüngling's syndrome[7,37] (Figure 2). Long bones are less commonly involved, but sometimes become osteopenic and develop a pathologic fracture.[8,22,34-38,40]

Many patients with sarcoidosis are ill with their disease but appear stable at first because the disease does not progress. These patients then improve and their complaints become limited. The lung lesions may disappear in several months or years and leave only scars at the site of involvement. Patients of African or Scandinavian origin do not fare as well; progression of the disease for these patients is more rapid and the death rate, ordinarily low, is considerably higher in these populations, particularly for older patients.[14,16,19-21,32,33]

Pathology and Causation of the Disease

Sarcoidosis was originally thought to be a form of tuberculosis, particularly because the histologic picture is similar. The patient develops granulomas with collections of epitheliod types of macrophagic cells, and within the structure giant cell tumors that resemble Langhans giant cells appear, typical of the tuberculous granuloma[8,11,14-16,27] (Figures 3 and 4). The problem with this assumption is that cultures have never shown an organism, there is no caseation in the granuloma, and the tuberculin test is almost always negative. Furthermore, the presence of Schaumann granules in the cells and more specifically in the giant cells is typical for sarcoidosis (and some other disorders) but does not occur in tuberculosis.[8] The collection of cells, and particularly the T cell constituency, strongly suggest an infectious agent; human herpesvirus-8 DNA sequences have been found in the tissue of some patients with sarcoidosis, but not consistently.[12,13,15]

The principal manifestation of the disease is an accumulation of mononuclear inflammatory cells, mostly T helper lymphocytes and mononuclear phagocytes.[11-15,18,41] T cell accumulation appears to be principally related to release of interleukin-2. The cells also release fibronectin, which promotes adherence of macrophages to extracellular matrix and stimulates production of fibrous matrix. An increase in KL-6, a glycoprotein secreted by type II alveolar cells in the lungs, has also been reported.[13,14,31]

As far as genetic studies are concerned, there is no gene error reported for sarcoidosis; however, the increased incidence and severity in the Scandinavian and African populations seem to suggest that some alterations in the genetic structure for these people make them more susceptible to the disease.[19,20] Several human leukocyte antigen (HLA)-alleles have been reported, including HLA-B8 in patients with erythema nodosum and HLA-DR3 in patients with chronic arthritis and bone disease.[12,13,18,42] The disease has been reported to occur in monozygotic but not in polyzygotic twins.[13]

A specific test for sarcoidosis is the Kveim test, in which tissue from the spleen or a lymph node of the patient is administered intradermally. At 6 weeks, a biopsy should show noncaseating granuloma formation.[8,13,14] The test is difficult to do and is now rarely performed.

Orthopaedic Manifestations of Sarcoidosis

The principal findings in patients with sarcoidosis are pulmonary diseases—alveolitis, lymph node involvement, and at times extensive diffuse pulmonary nodular disease associated with fibrosis.[26] Skin manifestions include erythema nodosum (reddened swelling of the skin), lupus pernio (raised pigmented skin lesions on the head and neck), and occasionally such disorders as abnormal fingernails.[13,15,25,27,43]

The joint complaints of patients with sarcoidosis include arthralgia, arthritis, and periarthritis.[12-14,17,23,29] The arthritis frequently presents with synovitis.[30] The most common sites are the knees, ankles, wrists, elbows, and proximal interphalangeal joints.[30] The carpus is frequently involved and is defined as Jüngling's syndrome.[6,7] The disorder rarely involves the disk spaces and the adjacent vertebrae.[44,45]

Lesions of bone are principally in the hands and feet; they consist of cystic lesions sometimes associated with expansion and fractures of the small bony segments, creating a deformed hand or foot.[8,22,36,40,46] Syn-

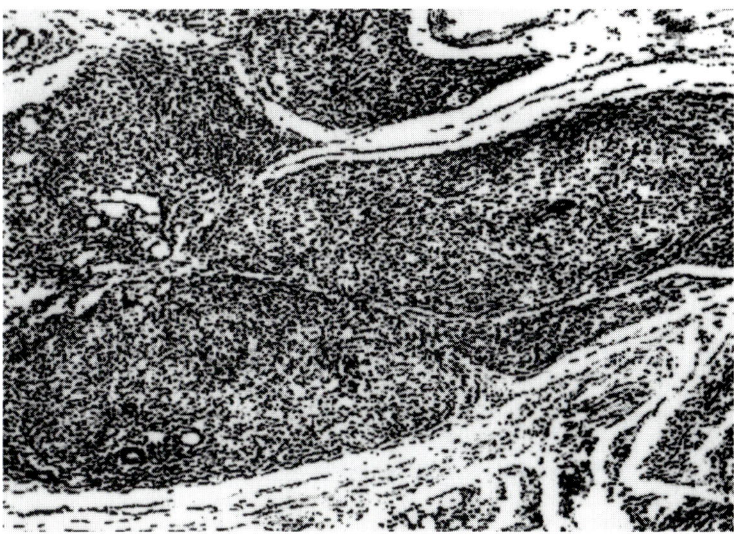

Figure 3
Histologic feature of sarcoidosis showing the collections of monocytic elements somewhat resembling tuberculosis. Hematoxylin and eosin × 40.

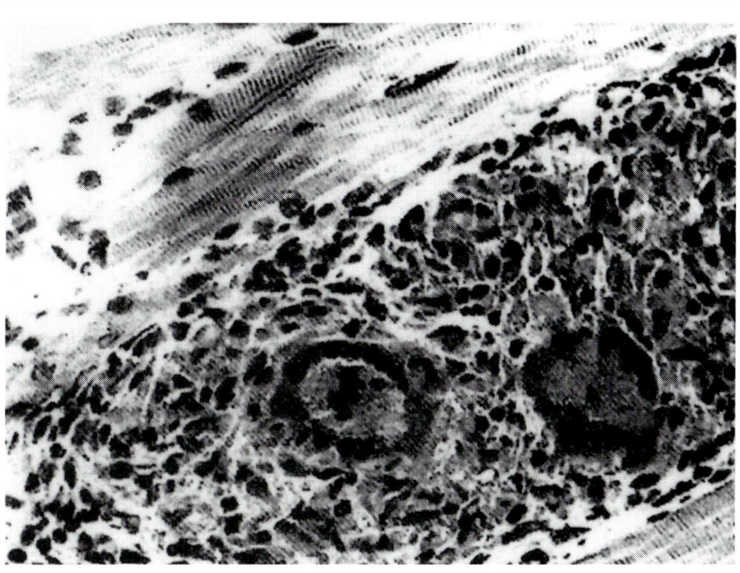

Figure 4
High-powered magnification of giant cells from a lesion of a patient with sarcoidosis. The cells may resemble the Langhans giant cells. Hematoxylin and eosin × 350.

ovial and tendon sheath granulomatous masses may occur in the hand, foot, or forearm and can be disabling.[39] Muscle enlargement and tenderness may indicate the presence of lesions within the muscle of the forearm or calf. Bone scan, magnetic resonance imaging, and most recently positron emission tomography scanning seem to provide more recognition of bone and joint disease in patients with sarcoidosis.[45,47-49]

In some patients with sarcoidosis, hypercalcemia and hypercalcuria may occur in association with increased production of 1,25 dihydroxy vitamin D and parathyroid hormone.[12,50] The cause of these changes is unknown; however, there is a risk involved related to the sarcoid changes in the heart, which may be severely aggravated by a calcium abnormality.[32] Laboratory findings for patients with sarcoidosis include the presence of a rapid sedimentation rate and increased angiotensin converting enzyme (ACE) and 1,25 dihydroxy vitamin D;[12-14] unfortunately, none of these studies are specific. Increased concentrations of ACE are present in tuberculosis, Gaucher disease, and some other chronic disorders that affect the bones.

Treatment of Sarcoidosis

For many patients, treatment is unnecessary because the disease is mild and disappears over time. Corticosteroids have been used in many patients with some success.[13] In recent years, methotrexate at weekly intervals and daily doses of tetracyline have seemed to be successful.[13,14,21] Thalidomide and chloroquine have been shown to be effective for patients with bone and joint complaints.[37,51,52] Calcitonin and alendronate may be helpful for patients with osteopenia related to metabolic bone disease; thalidomide and infliximab, a monoclonal antibody against tumor necrosis factor, seem to have increased curative effect on skin problems.[13,30,51] Surgical correction of hand and foot deformities may be necessary for patients with severe rheumatic and orthopaedic abnormalities. Pain may be reduced and function improved by appropriate surgical procedures.

Sarcoidosis remains a disease of unknown cause. Many patients who develop the disease are troubled initially and then clinically improve with time. Although the difficulties with lungs, uveitis, and severe skin involvement may require more vigorous treatment, for the most part the orthopaedist is not involved in the management of these patients. Of critical importance is that the clinician considers the possibility of sarcoidosis in the patient with arthralgia, chest problems, bone pain, weight loss, etc. As orthopaedic clinicians, we should be prepared to perform the necessary physical examination, laboratory tests, and appropriate imaging studies to define the presence of this mysterious entity. Although the bone and joint disease is not life-threatening, it may be incapacitating and may require medication and at times somewhat complicated surgical procedures.

References

1. Hutchinson J: *Illustrations of Clinical Surgery.* London, England, JA Churchill, 1877, p 42.

2. Besnier E: Lupus pernio de la face: Synovite fongueses (scrofulotuberculeuses). *Ann Dermatol Syphiligr* 1889;10:333-396.

3. Boeck CP: Multipeltl benignt hud-sarcoid. *Norsk Mag Laegevid* 1899;60:1321-1334.

4. Schaumann J: Etude sur le lupus pernio et ses rapports avec les sarcoides et la tuberculose. *Ann Ederm Syp* 1917;6:357-373.

5. Löfgren SH: Erythema nodosum: Studies on the etiology and pathogenesis in 185 women. *Act Med Scand Suppl* 1946;124:1-197.

6. Jüngling O: Ostitits tuberculosa mutiplex cystica (eine eigenartige form der knochentuberkulose). *Forsch Roentgen* 1919;27:375-383.

7. Baltzer G, Behrend H, Domkrowski H: On the relative importance of Jungling's disease in sarcoidosis, in *Proceedings of the Fifth International Conference on Sarcoidosis.* Prague, University of Karlova Press, 1971, pp 601-603.

8. Jaffe HL: *Metabolic, Degenerative and Inflammatory Diseases of Bones and Joints.* Philadelphia, PA, Lea and Febiger, 1972, pp 1004-1014.

9. James DG: Historical background: Sarcoidosis and other granulomatous disorders. *Lung Biol Health Dis* 1994;73:1-18.

10. James DG, Neville E, Siltzbach LE: A worldwide review of sarcoidosis. *Ann N Y Acad Sci* 1976;278:321-334.

11. Sheffield EA: Pathology of sarcoidosis. *Clin Chest Med* 1997;18:741-754.

12. Bell NH: Sarcoidosis and related disorders, in Avioli LV, Krane SM (eds): *Metabolic Bone Disease and Related Disorders,* ed 3. San Diego, CA, Academic Press, 1998, pp 607-619.

13. Chatham WW: Sarcoidosis, in Ruddy S, Harris ED, Sledge CS (eds): *Kelley's Textbook of Rheumatology,* ed 6. Philadelphia, PA, WB Saunders Company, 2001, pp 1551-1557.

14. Crystal RG: Sarcoidosis, in Isselbacher KJ, Braunwald E, Wilson JD, Martin JB, Fauci AS, Kasper DL (eds): *Harrison's Principles of Internal Medicine,* ed 13. New York, NY, McGraw Hill, 1994, pp 1679-1684.

15. Newman LS, Rose CS, Maier LA: Sarcoidosis. *N Engl J Med* 1997;336:1224-1234.

16. Siltzbach LE, Jamesz DG, Neville E, et al: Course and prognosis of sarcoidosis around the world. *Am J Med* 1974;57:847-852.

17. Sokoloff LK, Bunim JJ: Clinical and pathological studies of joint involvement in sarcoidosis. *N Engl J Med* 1959;260:841-847.

18. Thomas PD, Hunninghake GW: Current concepts

on the pathogenesis of sarcoidosis. *Am Rev Respir Dis* 1987;135:747-760.

19. Rybicki BA, Major M, Popovich J Jr, Maliarik MJ, Iannuzzi MC: Racial differences in sarcoidosis incidence: A 5-year study in a health maintenance organization. *Am J Epidemiol* 1997;145:234-241.

20. Sartwell PE: Racial differences in sarcoidosis. *Ann N Y Acad Sci* 1976;278:368-370.

21. Johns CJ, Michele TM: Clinical management of sarcoidosis: A 50-year experience at the Johns Hopkins Hospital. *Medicine (Baltimore)* 1999;78:65-111.

22. Neville E, Carstairs L, James D: Sarcoidosis of bone. *Q J Med* 1977;46:215-227.

23. Pettersson T: Rheumatic features of sarcoidosis. *Curr Opin Rheumatol* 1998;10:73-78.

24. Rahbar M, Sharma O: Hypertrophic osteoarthropathy in sarcoidosis. *Sarcoidosis* 1990;7:125-127.

25. Roberts SD, Mirowski GW, Wilkes D, Kwo PY, Knox KS: Sarcoidosis Part II: Extrapulmonary and systemic manifestations. *J Am Acad Dermatol* 2004;51:628-630.

26. Roberts SD, Mirowski GW, Wilkes D, Teague SD, Knox KS: Sarcoidosis Part I: Pulmonary manifestations. *J Am Acad Dermatol* 2004;51:448-451.

27. Schwarz MI: Diagnosis of sarcoidosis. *Clin Dermatol* 1986;4:165-167.

28. Siltzbach LE: Sarcoidosis: Clinical features and management. *Med Clin North Am* 1967;51:483-502.

29. Lynch JP III, Sharma OP, Baughman RP: Extrapulmonary sarcoidosis. *Semin Respir Infect* 1998;13:229-254.

30. Torralba KD, Quismorio FP Jr: Sarcoid arthritis: A review of clinical features, pathology and therapy. *Sarcoidosis Vasc Diffuse Lung Dis* 2003;20:95-103.

31. Kitaichi N, Kotake S, Shibuya H, et al: Increase of KL-6 in sera of uveitis patients with sarcoidosis. *Graefes Arch Clin Exp Ophthalmol* 2003;241:879-883.

32. Bargout R, Kelly RF: Sarcoid heart disease: Clinical course and treatment. *Int J Cardiol* 2004;97:173-182.

33. Gullapalli D, Phillips LK II: Neurosarcoidosis. *Curr Neurol Neurosci Rep* 2004;4:441-447.

34. Fallon MD, Perry HM III, Teitelbaum S: Skeletal sarcoidosis with osteopenia. *Metab Bone Dis Relat Res* 1981;3:171-174.

35. Rohatgi PK: Osseous sarcoidosis seminar. *Respir Med* 1992;13:468-488.

36. Shorr AF, Murphy FT, Gilliland WR, Hnatiuk W: Osseous disease in patients with pulmonary sarcoidosis and musculoskeletal symptoms. *Respir Med* 2000;94:228-232.

37. Wilcox A, Bhaaradwaj P, Sharma O: Bone sarcoidosis. *Curr Opin Rheumatol* 2000;12:321-330.

38. Blank NM, Steininger H, Kalden JR, Burhardt H: Symptomatic bone lesion of the tibial head as onset manifestation of sarcoidosis. *J Rheumatol* 1999;26:936-937.

39. Terzioglu A, Bingul F, Tuncali D, Sahin F, Aslan G: Osseous destruction and rupture of the extensor tendon caused by sarcoidosis of the finger. *Scand J Plast Reconstr Surg Hand Surg* 2004;38:317-319.

40. Allanore Y, Perrot S, Menkes CJ, Kahan A: Management of a patient with sarcoid calcaneitis and dactylitis. *Joint Bone Spine* 2001;68:175-177.

41. Hunninghake GW, Bedell GN, Zavala DC, Monick M, Brady M: Role of interleukin-2 release by lung T-cells in active pulmonary sarcoidosis. *Am Rev Respir Dis* 1983;128:634-638.

42. Amoli MM, Thomson W, Hajeer AH, et al: HLA-DRB1 associations in biopsy proven erythema nodosum. *J Rheumatol* 2001;28:2660-2662.

43. Cohen PD, Lester RS: Sarcoidosis presenting as nail dystrophy. *J Cutan Med Surg* 1999;3:302-305.

44. Jelinek JS, Mark AS, Barth WF: Sclerotic lesions of the cervical spine in sarcoidosis. *Skeletal Radiol* 1998;27:702-704.

45. Lisle D, Mitchell K, Crouch ZM, Windsor M: Sarcoidosis of the thoracic and lumbar spine: Imaging findings with an emphasis on magnetic resonance imaging. *Australas Radiol* 2004;48:404-407.

46. Yanardag H, Pamuk ON: Bone cysts in sarcoidosis: What is their clinical significance? *Rheumatol Int* 2004;24:294-296.

47. Kobayashi A, Shinozaki T, Shinjyo Y, et al: FDG PET in clinical evaluation of sarcoidosis with bone lesions. *Ann Nucl Med* 2000;14:311-313.

48. Milman N, Lund JO, Graudal N, Enevoldsen H, Evald T, Norgard P: Diagnostic value of routine radioisotope bone scanning in a series of 63 patients with pulmonary sarcoidosis. *Sarcoidosis Vasc Diffuse Lung Dis* 2000;17:67-70.

49. Rayner CK, Burnet SP, McNeil JD: Osseous sarcoidosis: A magnetic resonance imaging diagnosis. *Clin Exp Rheumatol* 2002;20:546-548.

50. Rizzato G: Clinical impact of bone and calcium metabolism changes in sarcoidosis. *Thorax* 1998;53:425-429.

51. Baughman RP, Lower EE: Newer therapies for cutaneous sarcoidosis: The role of thalidomide and other agents. *Am J Clin Dermatol* 2004;5:385-394.

52. O'Leary TJ, Jones G, Yip A, Lohnes D, Cohanim M, Yendt ER: The effects of chloroquine on serum 1,25 dihydroxyvitamin D and calcium metabolism in sarcoidosis. *N Engl J Med* 1986;315:727-730.

Chapter 14

Fracture Healing

The healing of fractures is a great and crucial benefit for all creatures with osseous structures in their bodies. Healing is not only a restorative process to a damaged being, but also provides a means of dealing with bone and soft-tissue diseases that require skeletal structure repair for a return to health and necessary body functions. Bone healing is not a simple process; a variety of systems interact both at the cellular and mechanical levels to provide for restoration of a skeletal part after injury. Physicians and scientists often take the process for granted because of long history and observation of sometimes remarkable restorative events; however, it is definitely not simple nor is it always easily achieved. This chapter is in essence a tribute to the biologists, engineers, and clinicians who have over the centuries provided us with knowledge that has allowed us to understand and restore the damaged skeletal system.

History of Fracture Healing

The history of fracture healing and treatment is a very long story that runs from ancient times to modern days, and from amputation to traction, splints, casts, and most recently to metallic plates, rods, and even bone substitutes.[1,2] The medical profession has evolved in many aspects over the centuries in our ability to care for a broken bone. The additions include improved diagnostic and imaging techniques, better immobilization systems, competent antibiotics, new metals and sometimes spectacular metallic devices, improved operative capability, and now systems for rehabilitation and restoration to a productive life.[2,3]

The earliest records of fracture occurrences are paleopathologic studies of dinosaur bones that have shown evidence of fractures, fracture healing, and nonunion, particularly in the tail bones that were at greatest risk.[4,5] Fractures were common in prehistoric Egyptian mummies, with multiple sites and types involved.[1,6,7] Fracture of the left ulna was particularly frequent, presumably as a result of raising the arm in defense during an attack. Egyptians used splints made of bamboo, reeds, wood, or bark that were found attached to the fractured part and were thought to be the first attempts at fracture immobilization to achieve healing.[1,6,7] In ancient India, the physicians who cared for fractures classified them as spiral, oblique, comminuted, and transverse, a language virtually identical to modern day descriptions.[8,9] Treatment consisted of closed reduction, and splinting with bark covered with ghee-soaked cloths and bandages.[8,9] Homer's *Iliad* of ancient Greece includes a section intended as a textbook of traumatology and military surgery, in which methods of dealing with open and closed fractures are described.[1,10,11] In addition to his stature as an astute clinician interested in cancer and other disorders, Hippocrates was also concerned with fractures and dislocations; he wrote a text known as Corpus on Fractures, which describes methods of dealing with trauma to the skeleton and joints.[1,2,12,13] His bandaging methods were quite competent, and were adopted by many other treating physicians in the early days in Greece and Rome. Even more interesting, they were also used virtually without change by trauma clinicians in the late 19th and early 20th centuries. Texts on the closed treatment of fractures written by medical icons such as Hugh Owen Thomas,[14] Sir Robert Jones,[15] Henry Bigelow,[16] Earnest William Hey Groves[17] and Charles Scudder[18] advocated closed reduction and application of braces, and subsequently introduced a great addition in the form of plaster casting. Open fractures were a problem that sometimes resulted in amputation or patient death,[1,14,15] but solutions were approached by many individuals, including Pierre Desault who introduced the term "débridement" and described a technique for the management of these difficult problems long before antibiotics were available.[19]

The introduction of metallic fixation devices in the management of fractures in the early part of the 20th century radically changed the treatment protocol systems. Hey Groves[17] and Lane[20] were two of the pioneers in the development of intramedullary nailing, and stimulated Küntscher[21] and Rush[22] to devise systems that are still in use today. Marius Smith-Petersen and associates[23] developed a nail for the fractured hip in the 1930s that is not structurally different from internal devices available today. Plates and screws were introduced by William O'Neill Sherman;[24] after multiple improvements in design and application technique, they were subsequently modified to provide rigid compressive immobilization by Müller and his AO[25] group in Switzerland. The addition of modular prostheses, Ilizarov techniques for external immobilization, and tremendous changes in physiotherapeutic restoration have truly changed the outlook for trauma patients and happily for their physicians.[1,26]

Normal Bone Structure and Development

Normal bone is a compound structure, consisting mostly of large-sized bundles of type I collagen that are impregnated with calcium salts in the form of crystals of calcium hydroxyapatite.[27-30] Attached to the collagen fibers are some small segments of noncollagenous protein and glycosaminoglycans, including chondroitin sulfate, decorin, biglycan, and heparin, which are in part responsible for the deposit and maintenance of the crystalline calcium salts.[28-31] Osteonectin, fibronectin, thrombospondin, vitronectin, osteopontin, and bone sialoprotein are all locally synthesized agents that seem to be necessary for the crystals to bind to collagen.[27,28,30,31] The cells of bone are under the influence of transforming growth factor-beta (TGF-β), an array of bone morphogenetic proteins (BMPs), and insulin-like growth factors (IGFs).[28-33]

Osteoblasts make the bone. The cells arise from osteoprogenitor cells, which appear in relation to bony surfaces possibly as a result of osteopontin production. Parathyroid hormone, prostaglandins, TGF-β, BMPs, fibroblast growth factor, and IGF all act on these cells to convert them to osteoblasts, which can make bone.[27,30,31] The osteoblast produces the collagen structure and then, under the influence of the agents described above, causes the calcium hydroxy-

apatite crystals to develop both on the surface and within the collagen fibers.[27,28,30,31] The osteoblasts produce bone and ultimately surround themselves with bone. By a system of development of elongated cell projections, they then become osteocytes and relate to the adjacent cells by the processes, which allow the transport of nutrients from an osteonal vascular channel. Osteocytes maintain the bone.

Osteoclasts destroy bone. They arise from macrophages and other mononuclear cells from the blood stream and are activated by interleukin-1, -6 and -17; RANKL; and prostaglandins.[28,29,31] They attach themselves to the surface of the bone in Howship's lacunae, and destroy bone by eroding the collagen structure and releasing the calcific salts.[27]

Markers for bone formation in serum are alkaline phosphatase, bone-specific alkaline phosphatase, osteocalcin, and type I collagen carboxypropeptides. Markers for bone destruction include plasma tartrate-resistant acid phosphatase and urinary hydroxyproline, collagen peptides, and pyrodinolines.[28,29,31]

Response of the Body Tissues and Bone to Injury

There are a number of injury-related types of fractures. These include nondisplaced, transverse, oblique, spiral comminuted, pathologic, and segmental fractures.[3] One form of nondisplaced fracture is known as a "stress fracture," in which forces of low magnitude are cyclically repeated over a period of time. This injury is related to cortical bone susceptibility, collagen orientation, and fatigue injury, which cause progressive accumulation of injury to the bone, starting in cortical cement lines and ultimately resulting in minor displacement and a repair process.[3,27,28]

Regardless of the type of injury, the result is a four-phase response that ultimately results in healing of the fracture. The first phase is avascular, and consists of a variable degree and extent of tissue necrosis. This phase is characterized by bone and soft-tissue necrosis. The second phase is also vascular, consisting of inflammation, vascular dilatation, transudation, exhudation, and clot formation. The fibrin clot containing the other materials serves as a vascular

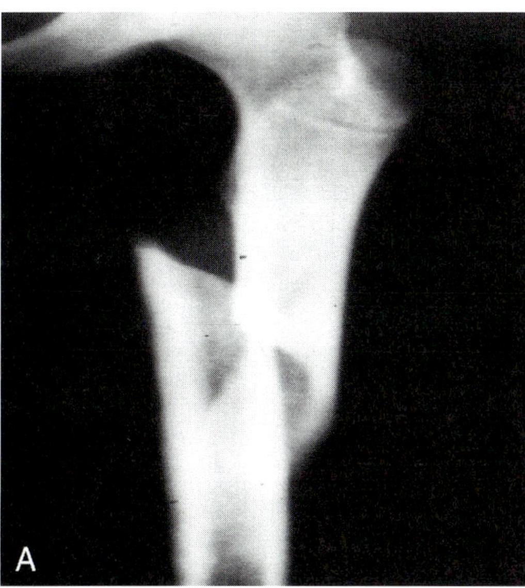
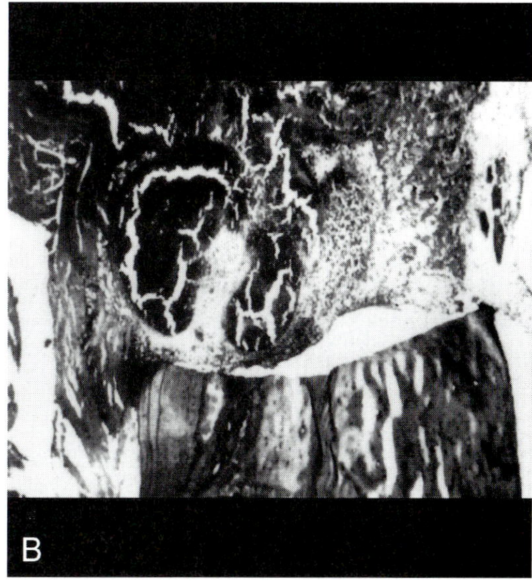

Figure 1
A, Femoral shaft fracture shortly after injury. **B,** Histologic picture of the junction of the two parts of the fracture. Hemorrhage, fibrin clot formation, and inflammation are evident. Hematoxylin and eosin × 20.

granulation tissue. The third phase is another vascular one that consists of beginning and progressive osseous repair, organization and osteogenesis of the granulation tissue, and bone formation. The fourth phase is one of bone remodeling.[3,27,28,34]

It should be evident that the first phase has a major impact on the process of fracture healing.[3,27] In order to fracture a bone, considerable energy is required; usually, both medullary and periosteal blood systems are damaged and vascularity seriously impaired. Cell death occurs not only in these sites but in the adjacent periosteum and muscular attachment sites. Medullary and cortical osteonecrosis occur at the fracture site and, depending on the extent of the injury, farther up and down the damaged bone. The second phase involves the development of a fibrin clot in the site, with considerable transudation and exudation of cellular elements and, as a result, a significant inflammatory response[3,27,28,34] (Figure 1). At this point, the patient has pain, shows swelling, and exhibits marked tenderness and sometimes vascular abnormalities in the extremity. The third phase is one of healing. The lifted periosteum on the shaft responds in standard fashion by producing bone adjacent to the cortex. Osteoprogenitor cells appear in the cambium layer and, under the influence of the cytokines described above, begin to lay down

bone (Figure 2). At the same time, the region of the fracture site also undergoes a productive process, but because the oxygen content is low and the blood supply poor, the cells produced are cartilaginous rather than osseous. The tissue resembles a markedly disordered epiphyseal plate.[27,28,34] The cells proliferate and produce a frequently enormous amount of cartilaginous callus at the fracture site, which then slowly undergoes endochondral ossification[3,29,34] (Figure 3). The mass converts to bone as the blood supply increases; at the same time, the dead tissue within the bone at the fracture site also begins to lay down bone. Soon the fracture is united. Phase 4 demands that the bone be restored in shape and structure to not only allow the patient to function, but to respond to the needs expressed in Wolff's law ("Every change in the form and function of a bone, or its function alone is followed by certain definite changes in its internal architecture and equally definite secondary alterations in its mathematical laws.").[35] This remodeling of the fracture callus is not always rapid, particularly in older individuals. It requires the invasion of the dead bone by the "cutting cones," bringing osteoclasts in to destroy the dead bone and following with osteoblasts to restore the bone structure. Healing of fractures is sometimes slow; phase 4 remodeling may take years, and the bony structure may never return to a normal contour or alignment.[34,36]

Just as noted in the description of bone formation, biochemical systems play a major role in the response to fractures. New collagen is formed that is mostly type I, except in the cartilaginous parts, where type II plays a role.[37,38] Type III can be found along

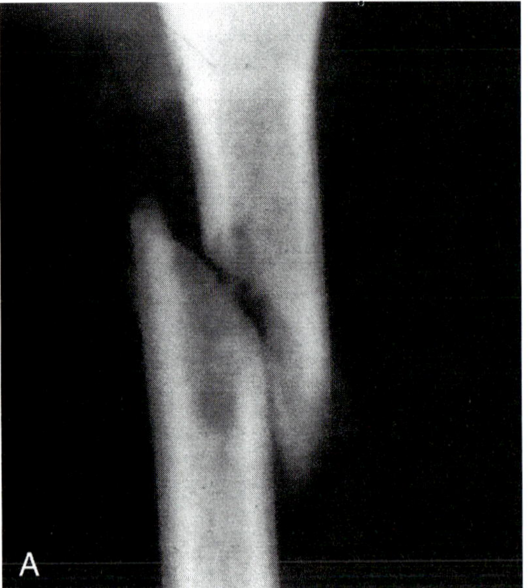

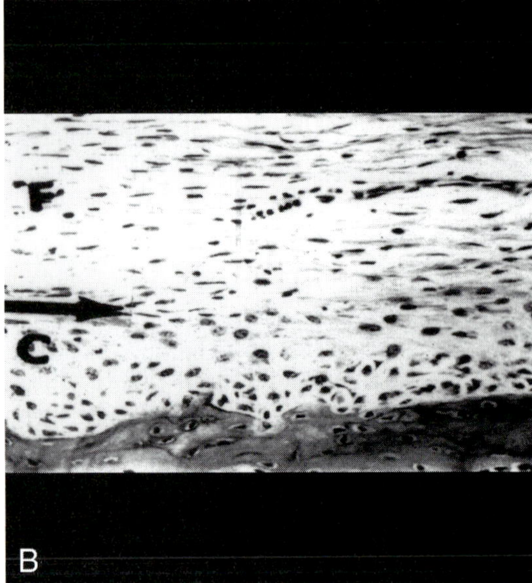

Figure 2
A, The fracture begins to heal, with periosteal new bone formation and beginning organization at the fracture site, usually with cartilaginous tissue that goes on to form bone. **B,** The cambium layer of the periosteum laying down bone adjacent to the cortex. F = fibrous layer; C = cambium layer. Hematoxylin and eosin × 60.

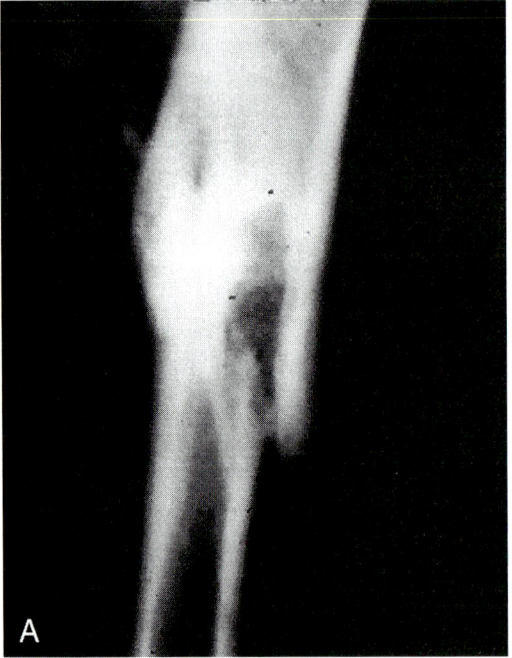

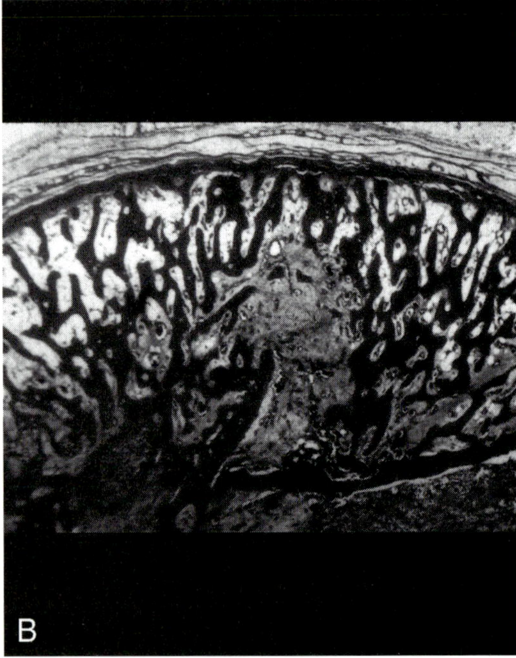

Figure 3
A, The fracture is now almost healed, with a considerable amount of external bony callus resulting from endochondral ossification. **B,** Histologic pattern shows evidence of cartilage in the tissue along with the bone, both of which serve to unite the fracture. Hematoxylin and eosin × 20.

periosteal surfaces, along with small amounts of type V and type XI.[37,38] Increased concentrations of proteoglycans appear, and may have a role in facilitating osteoblastic activity.[39] Osteonectin, osteopontin, osteocalcin, and fibronectin are involved in the development of osteoprogenitor cells and functional osteoblasts.[37,40,41] The healing phase is materially aided by TGF-β, glycosaminoglycans, and BMPs.[37,40,42,43] An increase in alkaline phosphatase and bone-specific alkaline phosphatase are frequently noted.[27,30,40]

Nonunion of Fractures

There are many explanations for fractures healing slowly or at times not at all. These include an inadequate or badly damaged blood supply; anemia; elderly or chronically ill patients with osteoporosis or osteonecrosis at the fracture site; patients with diabetes or with an array of genetic disturbances affecting bone strength and healing; malnutrition, steroid, and anticoagulant use; cigarette smoking and alcoholism; excessive movement at the fracture site; excessive damage to soft tissue and/or bone; wound infection; prior radiation treatment; and immune failures, such as with medications, autoimmune deficiency syndrome, etc.[3,25,27,28,42]

Nonunion may result in bone lying adjacent to bone without continuity, despite large amounts of callus. Another form of nonunion is referred to as pseudarthrosis, in which cartilage appears between or around the fracture fragments. The cartilage is usually not hyaline cartilage and often has a markedly increased concentration of type I collagen rather than type II.[27,28,34]

The Use of Metallic Implants in Fractures

The great advantages of metallic devices in relation to fracture healing are that they prevent excessive movement at the fracture site and more rapidly restore the patient to improved function. The problem with them, however, is that they require surgery, which may introduce problems in wound healing or infection and, more importantly, may further impair an already damaged blood supply. Intramedullary rods interfere with and may destroy the medullary blood supply; plates and screws require scraping off the periosteum, which is the site of the cortical blood supply. Surgery should be rapid, carefully performed without excessive wound exposure or damage, and the skin should be carefully observed and treated with grafting or appropriate alternatives if necessary. The advantage of the compression devices is that they markedly decrease excessive motion at the fracture site and enhance the more rapid osteonal repair, rather than the slower and sometimes more capricious cartilaginous system. The patient may be restored to function more rapidly using such systems.[3,25,27-29,34,36,42]

Bone Substitutes and Their Use in Fracture Treatment

Over the past 100 or more years, it has become apparent that adding materials to the site of a segment of healing or defective bone may enhance repair and decrease the rate of nonunion and disability. The initial materials included allografts, autografts, and in rare cases xenografts.[1-3,6,36,42,44-46] Over the last few decades, we have learned that there are three types of materials—osteogenetic, osteoinductive, and osteoconductive—available as additions to the fracture site to improve healing.[36,40,42,47,48]

Osteogenetic materials can actually grow bone, and usually consist of living osseous tissue or marrow elements. Thus vascularized fibular grafts are of the highest order, but fresh autografts from the iliac crest or another bony site introduced as soon as they are obtained remain the gold standard. Success rates for such grafts are usually high and can promote healing for sometimes very large defects.[28,36,42,45-47,49]

Osteoinductive materials do not actually form bone but serve to stimulate bone healing. The classic form of these materials is the demineralized bone matrix (DBM), originally described and introduced by Marshall Urist[50,51] in 1965. The advantages of the DBMs are that they continue to induce bone formation for the life of the product and are biocompatible.[52] Furthermore, they can be introduced in minimally invasive fashion.[51,53-55] The DBMs are probably not directly osteoinductive but are responsible for the synthesis of BMPs, which can stimulate bone formation.[30,32,33,36,40,42,45,53,56,57] The BMPs currently thought to serve as inductive materials include BMP-2A, BMP-2B,

BMP-3 (osteogenin), BMP-4, BMP-7 (osteogenic protein [OP]-1); BMP-10, BMP-15, and BMP-16.[33,57,58] In addition, TGF-β serves as a coactivator in this system.[27,30,42,59]

The area of greatest potential for the future in the inductive system is the use of stem cells to increase bone synthesis and improve fracture healing. Mesenchymal stem cells from the periosteum, muscle, bone marrow, or even fat can convert to osteoprogenitor cells under appropriate circumstances.[44,60-62] The difficulty at this point is defining the type of stimulating material that will convert these cells to osteoblasts rather than chondroblasts or fibroblasts. Furthermore, in order to use these materials, an appropriate scaffold such as polylactic acid, tricalcium phosphate, or a collagen structure must first be introduced to prevent cell loss. It also seems necessary to introduce BMPs such as TGF-β, BMP-7, or OP-1 to activate the cells.[60-62] The system has been tried in several settings and seems to be effective. The use of genetic materials may well represent the next major advance in fracture healing.[63]

Osteoconductive materials are those agents that serve as a passive trellis to allow blood vessels and new bone to enter the fracture site. These materials do not actually stimulate bone formation, but are often helpful in serving as a scaffold and maintaining the position of the fragments while vascular invasion and bone formation take place. Typical osteoconductive materials include coral hydroxyapatite composite (derived from marine madreporic corals), calcium phosphate injectable paste, calcium sulfate, and special materials including a substance consisting of hydroxyapatite, tricalcium phosphate, and bovine collagen.[27,36,42,47,49,53,59,64]

The final type of material that is used to enhance fracture repair and more importantly to fill major defects in the bone is cadaveric allografts. Allografts probably do not play any role in fracture healing and may produce additional problems at the site that further compromise the healing process. The principal applications for these agents are in patients with tumors or other such lesions where a large defect is present in the bone. The defect can be filled with allograft chips, which is now considered an acceptable solution for benign lesions such as a unicameral bone cyst or a giant cell tumor. Allograft seg-

ments have also been used in the repair of the shaft of a femur following bone failure of a total joint replacement.[65,66] Frozen osteoarticular and intercalary cadaveric allograft segments have had a long history in the field of orthopaedic oncology and are generally considered acceptable for the treatment of tumor sites after resection.[16,67-69] Allografts, however, represent "loci resistentiae minoris" in that infection, fracture, and nonunion are frequent occurrences and additional surgery is often required to improve the status of the limb.[68,70-73] The overall success rate for most of these is approximately 75%; with matches in the human leukocyte class 2 antigen, the success rate is increased.[73] Banking remains a major issue with these materials, however; currently, considerable effort is being expended to improve the quality of the bank systems to avoid transmission of diseases.[74]

Conclusions

There is little doubt that orthopaedics has come a long way throughout fracture history; now most or at least many fractures heal, restoring the structure of the bone. The difficulty is that not all of them do, and there are now many new problems with increased patient longevity, greater severity of wartime and peacetime injuries, infections or skin damage as a result of fracture or fracture treatment, and sometimes incomplete understanding of the process of healing. Orthopaedic surgeons are the principal players in this complex field and really must know as much about bone structure and formation as possible and understand the cytokine activities that control the process. We must become thoroughly familiar with the four phases of fracture healing. We must fully understand the role of blood distribution in bone and the dangers associated with extensive operations to treat the fracture, which may interfere with the hematologic structure of the bone. We need to understand the appropriate applications for osteogenetic, osteoinductive, and osteoconductive materials that are used to improve fracture healing. We must know as much as possible about the DBM, BMPs, TGF-β, and the materials that provide scaffolds for these important contributions. Allograft materials are still important, particularly for healing of damaged joint devices and for the treatment of tumors by curettage or resection. Understanding the process of fracture healing and carrying out quality care for fracture patients are difficult tasks but important ones that can restore patients to a good life despite injury and impairment.

References

1. Court-Brown CM: History of orthopaedic trauma, in Klenerman L (ed): *The Evolution of Orthopaedic Surgery*. London, England, Royal Society of Medicine Press, 2002, pp 49-64.

2. Peltier LF: *Fractures: A History and Iconography of Their Treatment*. San Francisco, CA, Norman, 1990.

3. Hayes WC, Lane JM: Fracture, etiology and outcome, in Brighton CT, Friedlaender G, Lane JM (eds): *Bone Formation and Repair*. Rosemont, IL, American Academy of Orthopaedic Surgeons, 1994, pp 471-533.

4. Moodie RI: *Palaeopathology*. Champaign, IL, University of Illinois Press, 1923.

5. Petersen K, Isakson JI, Madsen JH: Preliminary study of palaeopathologies in the Cleveland-Lloyd dinosaur collection. *Utah Acad Proc* 1972;49:44-50.

6. Bick E: *Source Book of Orthopaedics*. New York, NY, Hafner Publishing Company, 1968.

7. Breasted JH: *The Edwin Smith Papyrus*. Chicago, IL, The University of Chicago Press, 1930.

8. Duraiswami PK, Tuli SM: 5000 years of orthopaedics in India. *Clin Orthop Relat Res* 1971;75:269-280.

9. Hamada G, Rida A: Orthopaedics and orthopaedic diseases in ancient and modern Egypt. *Clin Orthop Relat Res* 1972;89:253-268.

10. Beasley AW: Homer and orthopaedics. *Clin Orthop Relat Res* 1972;89:10-16.

11. Hartofilakidis-Garofalidi G, Papthanassiou BT: Orthopaedics in ancient Greece. *Clin Orthop Relat Res* 1972;88:308-312.

12. Adams F: *Hippocrates: The Genuine Works of Hippocrates*. Baltimore, MD, William and Wilkins, 1939.

13. *Loeb Edition of Hippocrates*. Cambridge, MA, Harvard University Press, 1928.

14. Thomas HO: *Fractures, Dislocations, Deformities and Diseases of the Lower Extremities in Contributions to Surgery and Medicine*. London, England, HK Lewis, 1890.

15. Jones R: *Orthopaedic Surgery of Injuries*. London, England, Oxford University Press, 1921.

16. Bigelow HJ: *The Mechanism of Dislocations and Fractures of the Hip*. Boston, MA, Little Brown and Company, 1894.

17. Hey Groves EW: *On Modern Methods of Treating Fractures*, ed 2. Bristol, England, John Wright, 1921.

18. Scudder CL: *The Treatment of Fractures*. Philadelphia, PA, WB Saunders Company, 1916.

19. Desault PJ: *Treatise on Fractures, Luxations and other Affections of the Bones*. Philadelphia, PA, C. Caldwell, 1805.

20. Lane WA: *Operative Treatment of Fractures*. London, England, Medical Rutheday Co. Ltd, 1905.

21. Küntscher G: *The Practice of Intramedullary Nailing*. Springfield, IL, Charles C. Thomas, 1967.

22. Rush LV: Atlas of Rush pin techniques. *Miss Doct* 1953;31:1-13.

23. Smith-Petersen MN, Cave EF, van Gorder GW: Treatment of fractures of the neck of the femur by internal fixation. *Arch Surg* 1931;23:715-759.

24. Sherman WO: Vanadium steel bone plates and screws. *J Bone Joint Surg* 1926;8:494-503.

25. Müller MF, Allgöwer M, Willinegger H: *Techniques of Internal Fixation*. Berlin, Germany, Springer Verlag, 1965.

26. Venable CS, Stuck WG: *The Internal Fixation of Fractures*. Springfield, IL, Charles C. Thomas, 1947.

27. Brighton CT, Rodan GA: Bone regeneration and repair, in Brighton CT, Friedlaender G, Lane JM (eds): *Bone Formation and Repair*. Rosemont, IL, American Academy of Orthopaedic Surgeons, 1994, pp 115-239.

28. Brighton CT, Friedlaender G, Lane JM (eds): *Bone Formation and Repair*. Rosemont, IL, American Academy of Orthopaedic Surgeons, 1994.

29. Buckwalter JA, Einhorn TA, Simon SR (eds): *Orthopaedic Basic Science: Biology and Biomechanics of the Musculoskeletal System*, ed 2. Rosemont, IL, American Academy of Orthopaedic Surgeons, 2000.

30. Mohan S, Baylink DJ: Bone growth factors. *Clin Orthop Relat Res* 1991;263:30-48.

31. Robey PG: Normal bone formation: Structure, in Brighton CT, Friedlaender G, Lane JM (eds): *Bone Formation and Repair*. Rosemont, IL, American Academy of Orthopaedic Surgeons, 1994, pp 3-10.

32. Riley EH, Lane JM, Urist MR, Lyons KM, Lieberman JR: Bone morphogenetic protein-2: Biology and applications. *Clin Orthop Relat Res* 1996;324: 39-46.

33. Rosen V, Wozney JM: *Bone Morphogenetic Proteins: Principles of Bone Biology*, ed 2. San Diego, CA, Academic Press, 2002, pp 919-928.

34. Brighton CT: Fracture callus metabolism, in Brighton CT, Friedlaender G, Lane JM (eds): *Bone Formation and Repair*. Rosemont, IL, American Academy of Orthopaedic Surgeons, 1994, pp 167-183.

35. Wolff J: *Das Gesetz der Transformation der Knochen*. Berlin, Germany, A. Hirschwald, 1892.

36. Perry CR: Bone repair techniques, bone graft and bone graft substitutes. *Clin Orthop Relat Res* 1999;360:71-86.

37. Einhorn TA, Majeska RJ, Rush EB, Levine PM, Horowitz MC: The expression of cytokine activity by fracture callus. *J Bone Miner Res* 1995;10:1272-1281.

38. Liu SH, Yang RS, al-Shaikh R, Lane JM: Collagen in tendon, ligament and bone healing: A current review. *Clin Orthop Relat Res* 1995;318:265-278.

39. Kopman CR, Boskey AL, Lane JM, Pita JC, Eaton B II: Biochemical characterization of fracture callus proteoglycans. *J Orthop Res* 1987;5:7-13.

40. Lieberman JR, Daluiski A, Einhorn TA: The role of growth factors in the repair of bone: Biology and clinical applications. *J Bone Joint Surg Am* 2002;84:1032-1044.

41. Yamazaki M, Majaeska RJ, Moriya H, Einhorn TA: Role of osteonectin during fracture healing. *Trans Orthop Res Soc* 1997;22:254.

42. Einhorn TA: Enhancement of fracture-healing. *J Bone Joint Surg Am* 1995;77:940-956.

43. Joyce ME, Kingushi S, Bolander ME: Transforming growth factor-beta in the regulation of fracture repair. *Orthop Clin North Am* 1990;21:199-209.

44. Connolly JF: Injectable bone marrow preparations to stimulate osteogenic repair. *Clin Orthop Relat Res* 1995;313:8-16.

45. Gazdag AR, Lane JM, Glaser D, Forster RA: Alternatives to autogenous bone graft: Efficacy and indications. *J Am Acad Orthop Surg* 1995;3:1-8.

46. Goldberg V, Stevenson S, Shaffer J: Biology of autografts and allografts, in Friedlaender GE, Goldberg VM: *Bone and Cartilage Allografts: Biology and Clinical Applications*. Park Ridge, IL, American Academy of Orthopaedic Surgeons, 1991.

47. Bucholz RW: Clinical issues in the development of bone graft substitutes in orthopedic trauma care, in Laurencin CT (ed): *Bone Graft Substitutes*. Conshohocken, PA, American Society for Testing and Materials, 2003, pp 289-297.

48. Yoon ST, Boden SD: Osteoinductive molecules in orthopaedics: Basic science and preclinical studies. *Clin Orthop Relat Res* 2002;395:33-43.

49. Hollinger JO, Brekke J, Gruskin E, Lee D: Role of bone substitutes. *Clin Orthop Relat Res* 1996;324:55-65.

50. Urist MR: Bone: Formation by autoinduction. *Science* 1965;150:893-899.

51. Urist MR, Silverman BF, Buring K, Dubuc FL, Rosenberg JM: The bone induction principle. *Clin Orthop Relat Res* 1967;53:243-283.

52. Killian JT, Wilkinson L, White S, Brassard M: Treatment of unicameral bone cyst with demineralized bone matrix. *J Pediatr Orthop* 1998;18:621-624.

53. Border M: The development of bone graft materials using various formulations of demineralized bone matrix, in Laurencin CT (ed): *Bone Graft Substitutes*. Conshohocken, PA, American Society for Testing and Materials, 2003, pp 96-112.

54. Russell JL, Block JE: Clinical utility of demineralized bone matrix for osseous defects, arthrodesis and reconstruction: Impact of processing techniques and study methodology. *Orthopedics* 1999;22:524-531.

55. Tiedeman JJ, Garvin KL, Kile TA, Connolly JF: The role of a composite, demineralized bone matrix and bone marrow in the treatment of osseous defects. *Orthopedics* 1995;18:1153-1158.

56. Friedlaender GE, Perry CR, Cole JD, et al: Osteogenic protein-1 (bone morphogenetic protein-7) in the treatment of tibial non-unions. *J Bone Joint Surg Am* 2001;83(suppl 1):S151-S158.

57. Sampath TK, Reddi AH: Bone morphogenetic protein (BMP) implants as bone graft substitutes: Promises and challenges, in Laurencin CT (ed): *Bone Graft Substitutes*. Conshohocken, PA, American Society for Testing and Materials, 2003, pp 194-213.

58. Yasko A, Lane JM, Fellinger EJ, Rosen V, Wozney JM, Wang EA: The healing of segmental bone defects, induced by recombinant human bone morphogenetic protein (rhBMP-2): A radiographic, histological and biomechanical study in rats. *J Bone Joint Surg Am* 1992;74:659-670.

59. Boyan BD, McMillan J, Lohmann CH, et al: Bone graft substitutes: Basic information for successful clinical use with special focus on synthetic graft substitutes, in Laurencin CT (ed): *Bone Graft Substitutes*. Conshohocken, PA, American Society for Testing and Materials, 2003, pp 231-259.

60. Bosch P, Musgrave DS, Lee JY, et al: Osteoprogenitor cells within skeletal muscle. *J Orthop Res* 2000;18:933-944.

61. Bruder SP, Kurth AA, Shea M, Hayes WC, Jaiswal N, Kadiyala S: Bone regeneration by implantation of purified, culture-expanded human mesenchymal stem cells. *J Orthop Res* 1998;16:155-162.

62. Whang PG, Lieberman JR: Clinical issues in the development of cellular systems for use as bone graft substitutes, in Laurencin CT (ed): *Bone Graft Substitutes*. Conshohocken, PA, American Society for Testing and Materials, 2003, pp 142-163.

63. Scaduto AA, Lieberman JR: Gene therapy for osteoinduction. *Orthop Clin North Am* 1999;30:625-633.

64. Haggard WO, Richelsoph KC, Parr JE: Calcium sulfate-based bvone void substitutes, in Laurencin CT (ed): *Bone Graft Substitutes*. Conshohocken, PA, American Society for Testing and Materials, 2003, pp 260-270.

65. Emerson RH Jr, Head WC, Berklacich FM, Malinin TI: Noncemented acetabular revision arthroplasty using allograft bone. *Clin Orthop Relat Res* 1989;249:30-43.

66. Engh GA, Herzwurm PJ, Parks NL: Treatment of major defects of bone with bulk allografts and stemmed components during total knee arthroplasty. *J Bone Joint Surg Am* 1997;79:1030-1039.

67. Clohisy DR, Mankin HJ: Osteoarticular allografts for reconstruction after resection of a musculoskeletal tumor in the proximal end of the tibia. *J Bone Joint Surg Am* 1994;76:549-554.

68. Mankin HJ, Gebhardt MC, Jennings LC, Springfield DS, Tomford WW: Long-term results of allograft replacement in the management of bone tumors. *Clin Orthop Relat Res* 1996;324:86-97.

69. Ortiz-Cruz E, Gebhardt MC, Jennings LC, Springfield DS, Mankin HJ: The results of transplantation of intercalary allografts after resection of tumors: A long-term follow-up study. *J Bone Joint Surg Am* 1997;79:97-106.

70. Hornicek FJ, Gebhardt MC, Tomford WW, et al: Factors affecting nonunion of the allograft-host junction. *Clin Orthop Relat Res* 2001;382:87-98.

71. Mankin HJ: Major limb reconstruction using massive cadaveric allografts, in Phillips GO (ed): *Advances in Tissue Banking*. Singapore, World Scientific Publishing, 2004, vol 7, pp 389-415.

72. Sorger JI, Hornicek FJ, Zavatta M, et al: Allograft fractures revisited. *Clin Orthop Relat Res* 2001;382:66-74.

73. Strong DM, Friedlaender GE, Tomford WW, et al: Immunologic responses in human recipients of osseous and osteochondral allografts. *Clin Orthop Relat Res* 1996;326:107-114.

74. Tomford WW, Mankin HJ: Massive bone allografts, in Urist MR, O'Connor BR, Burwell RG (eds): *Bone Grafts, Derivatives and Substitutes*. Oxford, England, Butterworth Heinemann, 1994, pp 187-192.

Chapter 15

Osteogenesis Imperfecta

Introduction

Osteogenesis imperfecta (OI) has been known for centuries as a severe and disabling disease affecting children. Until fairly recently, OI has continued to be an uncommon but terribly devastating and frequently fatal disorder. The disease is genetic and is most often transmitted as an autosomal dominant disorder. It sometimes causes fractures and death in utero. Fractures, severe bony distortion, and extraordinary alterations of the skull, teeth, and sclerae are present in very young children with "osteogenesis imperfecta congenita," now classified as type II disease. Less severe forms occur in older patients (osteogenesis imperfecta tarda, now known as either type I or type IV); another less severe form in children is known as type III. Of recent interest is the identification of the gene errors associated with the synthesis of type I collagen. Of equal importance is the response of the disease to bisphosphonates. Attempts at genetic engineering and stem cell treatment are currently underway, but are limited by the marked fragility of the patients, particularly those with OI types II and III.

History and Language of Osteogenesis Imperfecta

The earliest literary description of a possible case of OI is that of "Ivar the Boneless," who led the Scandinavians on their invasion of England in the 9th century.[1,2] Ivar was believed to be short in stature with very fragile bones. He was so disabled that his troops were reported to have carried him into battle on their shields. Unfortunately, it was never possible to study his bones because they were destroyed by William the Conqueror.[2] In terms of actual identification of the syndrome, a study of the bones of an Egyptian mummy dating to approximately 1000 BC showed rather severe changes in the skull, teeth, and bones of the lower extremities—strongly suggestive of OI.[3] In 1788, O. J. Ekman[4] wrote a thesis in Latin to obtain a doctorate in Sweden; he described a case of "osteomalacia congenita" that ex-

tended for three generations in one family. In 1831, Edmund Axmann[5] of Germany described his own personal affliction with OI and detailed the status of his two brothers, who had the same disease. He and his brothers not only had fragile bones, but also had blue sclerae. Several years later, Lobstein[6] reported on the adult form of the disease. In 1849, Vrolik[7,8] described the disease in a newborn infant who died shortly after birth.

In 1859, Ormerod[9] described a woman who at 68 years of age was very short in stature; she had passed the disease to two children. He introduced the term "mollities ossium" to describe the syndrome.[2,9] Shortly thereafter, Ernest Gurlt[10] introduced the term "fragilitus osseum," and in 1889, Stilling[11] of Strasburg demonstrated the striking histologic alterations seen in the bones. At the turn of the 20th century, Eddowes[12] described the blue sclerae and tried to correlate this finding with bone and particularly skull disorders. This was confirmed by Adair-Dighton,[13] who in 1912 reported on four generations of patients with blue sclerae. Several authors introduced the terms "wormian bones" and "caput membranaceum" for the skull abnormalities.[7] They described "beading" of the ribs, translucent or brownish discoloration of the teeth (now known as "dentogenesis imperfecta"), and the "china blue" sclerae, known also as robin's egg blue, slate blue, or Wedgwood blue.[2,7,14-16] Hearing loss was described first by Buchanan[2,17] in 1903, and is frequently present in all forms of the disease.

Since the earliest identification of the syndrome, terminology has been a major issue. OI has been known as mollities ossium, fragilitus ossium, osteopsathyrosis idiopathica, periosteal dysplasia, la Maladie de Lobstein, Eddowes syndrome, van der Hoeve syndrome, and Vrolik's disease.[1,2,7-9,14-16,18-22] It was Looser,[23] however, who in 1906 introduced the terms "osteogenesis imperfecta congenita" for the severe disease in newborn children and "osteogenesis imperfecta tarda" for the milder form in older persons. Until recently, these terms have remained in orthopaedic and pediatric language; however, in 1979, David Sillence and his colleagues[24] described the four syndromes and their identifying characteristics, resulting in the classification system in use today.

Classification and Staging System for Osteogenesis Imperfecta

According to Sillence's classification system, there are four types of osteogenesis imperfecta.[24]

OI type I: A relatively mild to moderate form of the disease, type I affects both children and adults and is transmitted as an autosomal dominant. The children show bone problems after a year or two and may have sometimes extensive fractures. The disease is relatively mild and not greatly deforming or disabling, although the children are short and often have abnormal head shape and teeth. Blue sclerae are present, and patients become deaf at an early age. There are two forms of type I OI: type IA has normal teeth, and IB has dentinogenesis imperfecta.[2,25] The frequency is approximately 1 in 30,000 live births in the US; life expectancy is approximately the same as in the general population.[25]

OI type II: Type II is a severe form of the disease that is often detectable in utero using ultrasound. The children have extreme osseous fragility described as "crumbled bones," a markedly thin calvarium described as "wormian," severe spinal scoliotic and kyphotic deformity, and beading and enlargement of the ribs.[19,25-28] The disorder is also transmitted as an autosomal dominant, although there are forms that are recessive. The frequency is 1 in 60,000 live births in the US; most patients die in utero or within a year of birth.[29-32]

OI type III: Type III disease also occurs in children, but is milder and the patients are more likely to survive. They have moderately severe to severe osseous fragility, variable but often marked bone deformity, stunted growth, and spinal curvature, but usually no blue sclerae.[2,19,25] Spinal and disk deformities, rib abnormalities associated with respiratory problems, and protrusio acetabulae are common.[31,33-35] Children generally survive, but function poorly.[2,31,32,35] The disorder is often transmitted as an autosomal recessive disorder. The frequency is 1 in

70,000 live births in the US; if a child survives past the age of 10 years, the overall prognosis improves.

OI type IV: Type IV is an uncommon, milder disease with osseous fragility.[2,25] The disease is similar to type I, but patients have normal sclerae. Patients have moderate deformity of bones of the extremities. Short stature, calvarial deformity, and "triangular face" are commonly present.[2,33,36] The disease is transmitted as an autosomal dominant and is very rare compared to the other three forms of the disorder.

In 2000, Glorieux and his colleagues[37] added a type V syndrome, in which patients have osteoporosis, interosseous membrane ossification, and hypertrophic calluses. In addition, several other rarely encountered disorders have been described. The Bruck syndrome is characterized by bone fragility and joint contractures; in patients with the osteoporosis-pseudoglioma syndrome, the bone fragility is associated with blindness.[2,25,33,38,39] Another entity described fairly recently is the Cole-Carpenter syndrome, which is characterized by bone fragility, craniosynostosis, ocular proptosis, hydrocephalus, and distinctive facial features.[40] All four disorders in this paragraph are believed to be autosomal recessive and are quite rare.

Genetic Causes of Osteogenesis Imperfecta

Almost all patients with OI types I to IV have a genetic error in the synthesis of type I collagen, which results in mutations that cause the bony problems. The affected genes have been flagged to the chromosomal location 17q21.31-q22.05, which is responsible for the synthesis of this material.[2,21,25,41] Normal bone is a compound structure, consisting mostly of large-sized bundles of type I collagen that are impregnated with calcium salts in the form of crystals of calcium hydroxyapatite. Attached to the collagen fibers are some small segments of noncollagenous protein and glycosaminoglycans, including chondroitin sulfate, decorin, biglycan, and heparin, which are in part responsible for the deposit and maintenance of the crystalline calcium salts. These functions are dependent on the quality of the collagen structure. Type I collagen is synthesized by two genes: COL1A1, encoding for Pro-α1(I); and

COL1A2, encoding for Pro-α2(I). The carboxy terminal propeptides 1 and 2 combine to form type I procollagen molecules.[42] The triple helix form starts at the carboxy terminal end and then propagates to the amino terminal end of the molecule. Mutations of the type I collagen genes produce abnormal collagen, which results in OI and Ehlers-Danlos syndrome.[25,42-44]

A very large number of errors can occur in this system; over 250 mutations in both genes have been reported in patients with OI.[2,24,25,38,39,41,42,44-51] The majority of these are missence residues in the triple helical domains of the two chains. In one form, the mutant genetic COL1A1 makes an RNA that would ordinarily severely damage the Pro-α1(I) collagen segment, but the body is able to detect and destroy the erroneous RNA.[2] Thus the affected patient's collagen contains only the Pro-α2(I) chain. Similarly, some of the patients with forms of the disease have the error in the COL1A2 gene and thus lose that component. Other forms include errors that lead to a loss of 85 or more amino acids in the collagen I structure.[25,42] Another form is multiexon skipping and exon deletions, which seriously reduce the competence of the collagen structure.[42] Substitution of a cysteine molecule for glycine in the collagen fiber is sometimes present along with other forms of point mutations. All of these detected abnormalities cause an inadequate collagen structure that has a reduced capacity to form bone, hold crystals of calcium apatite, form teeth, or create a competent scleral component in the eye.

Alterations in Body Structure

Patients with OI have a number of significant problems that occur in almost all forms of the disease. For patients with type II disease, the disorders are much more severe and almost always present at birth. For patients with type I and type IV diseases, the problems may be delayed in onset and are sometimes relatively mild.[2,19,25,32,33] The problems include:

- **Size and stature:** If patients with OI survive, most are short in stature. They may be only 3.5 to 5 feet tall as adults.[1,2,19-21,25-27,52,53]
- **Intelligence.** Type II children are usually severely retarded. Type I, III, and IV patients usually have normal intelligence.[1,2,19,21,24,25,54]
- **Fractures.** All bones are subject to fracture. Fractures are much more severe in type II disease, in which the children may develop fractures in utero. Fractures are less of a problem for patients with type I or type IV disease. The fractures show a considerable amount of bony callus but do not really heal well and are subject to repeated fractures through the same sites.[1,2,19,21,26,33,35,40,55]
- **Extremity deformity**. Many patients experience easy bruising, and all patients with the disease are at risk for extremity deformity. The limbs are short and bowed; consequently, the adjacent joints are distorted and at times excessively mobile and poorly functional. Hips can dislocate, and elbows and knees may be unstable.[2,12,20,21,26,33,35,55,56] The changes are most severe in patients with type II and type III disease.
- **Rib and chest problems**. Patients with type II disease at birth show a deformity of the ribs characterized by beading; the sometimes enlarged and poorly ossified ribs may create a syndrome of pectus excavatum and progressive respiratory impairment, and sometimes result in death.[2,19,21,26,28-32] Rib problems may be present in the other forms of the disease, but are less severe or noticeable.
- **Skull deformities**. Children with type II disease almost always show a mosaic pattern of wormian bones and caput membranaceum (very thin cortices on skull radiographs). In addition, the skull is markedly deformed for nearly all patients.[2,26,36,40] Bulging of the most cephalic part of the calvarium and craniofacial defect lead to specific alterations known as a triangular face or overhanging occiput. The pattern is sometimes called "tam o'shanter skull."[2] Children with type I OI have micrognathia (small jaw) but less severe deformity of the skull.[2,21]
- **Blue sclerae**. The cause of the blue discoloration in the sclerae that is present in type I and II disease is probably related to marked thinning of the scleral structures so that the venous

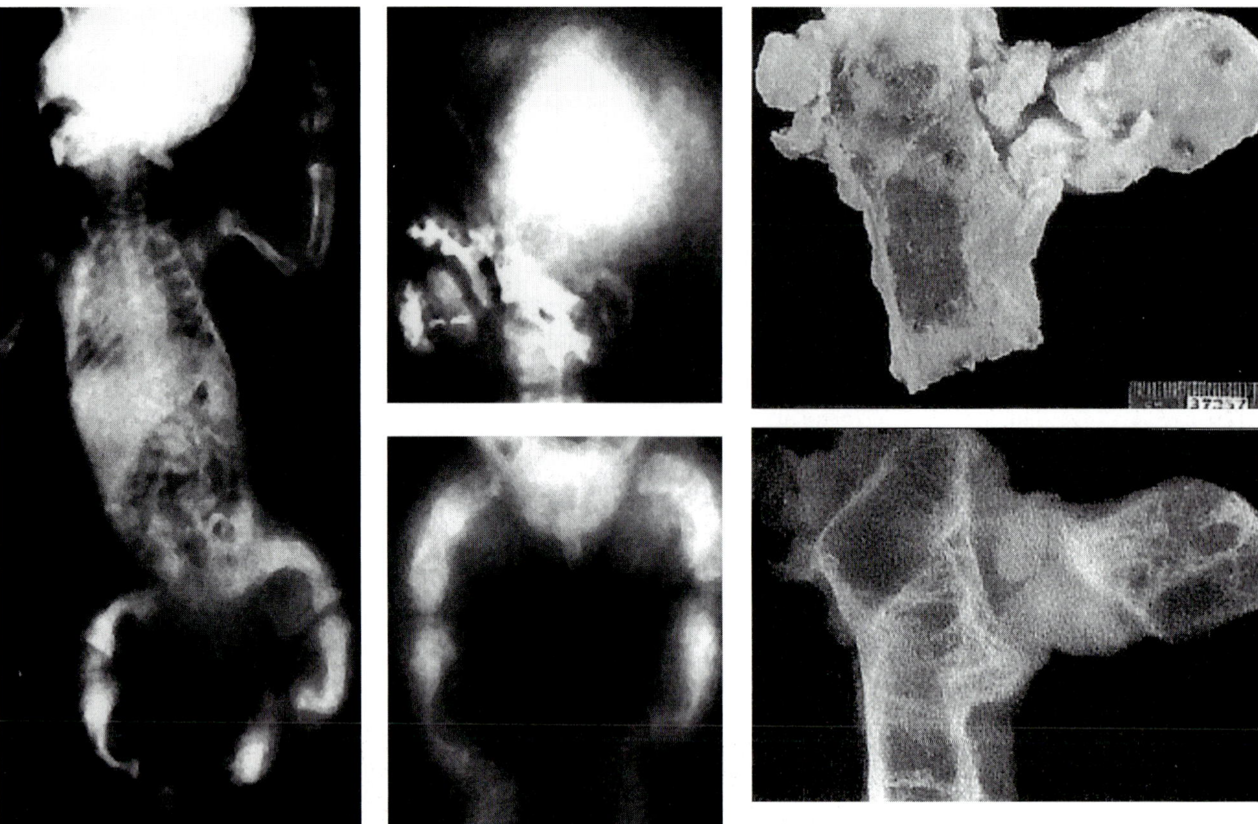

Figure 1
Radiographic studies of a newborn child with type II osteogenesis imperfecta showing the bone deformities. The bones are small and show deformity in part related to multiple fractures. The calvarium is distorted in shape and structure.

Figure 2
Gross specimen and radiograph of the proximal femur of a child with type II osteogenesis imperfecta obtained at autopsy. A fracture has occurred in the neck of the femur and the bones are grossly distorted and osteopenic.

blood system immediately behind the cornea projects through as a sometimes bright blue color.[2,7,14,17,21,36] Eye function is usually not impaired by the scleral abnormality, but some patients develop glaucoma.[2] Retinal hemorrhages after trauma are seen occasionally in patients with type I disease.[57]

- **Dental problems**. Almost all patients with OI have bluish or brownishly discolored and sometimes translucent teeth that are often small in size, loose, and irregularly placed in the mandible or maxilla.[58] The condition is known as dentinogenesis imperfecta, and also as "hereditary opalescent dentin."[1,3,36,58] It is caused by a disordered arrangement of tubulin and poor calcification of dentin, and is characterized by variable obliteration of the pulp chambers and root canals along with crumbling and loss of enamel.[2] The changes are

present in over half of the patients with type III disease, and are considerably less common in type IA or type IV disease.[2]

- **Spinal deformities**. Most patients with type II OI have severe alterations in the spinal structure with both scoliosis and kyphosis, at times leading to disk herniation and damage to the adjacent neural structures.[27,28,34,54,59,60] Type I problems are less marked, but type III disease may have severe changes known as "codfish" or "hourglass" biconcave configuration.[2,28,34]

- **Neural problems**. Neurologic complications include bilateral and progressive cerebellar disturbances and spinal cord compression.[2,27,54,60,61] Low pressure hydrocephalus may occur in patients with type III disease. Vertigo may be present and at times is disabling.[54] Seizure disorders have been

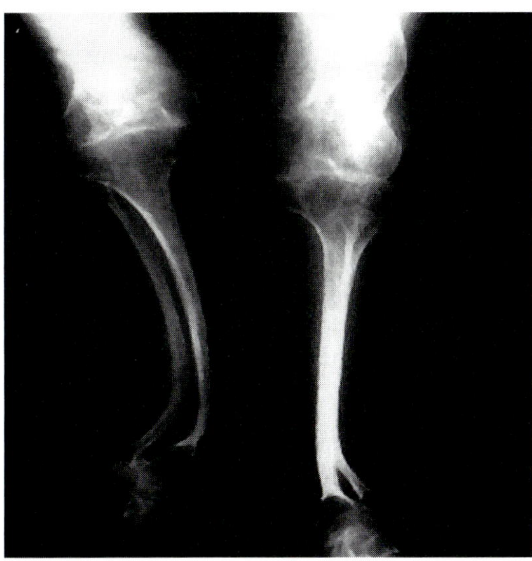

Figure 3
Tibial shaft deformities in an adult patient with type I osteogenesis imperfecta. There is marked deformity of the bones with enlargement of the metaphyseal area and marked thinning of the shafts. The joint is at best poorly functional.

reported and are sometimes difficult to treat.[21,30,54] Except for the type II patients, the intelligence of the patients is normal.[2]

- **Deafness:** Over half of the patients with types I, III, or IV OI develop tinnitus and become deaf by early or middle adult life.[2] The usual cause is otosclerosis, consisting of damage to the osseous structures around the eighth nerve cavity and canal structure.[1,2,14,17,21,36] The problem is most noticeable in the high sound range.

Patients with type I or type IV OI may have a relatively normal health status and life style that is only occasionally associated with fractures or deformities. Some of these patients may not even know they have the disease.

Imaging and Laboratory Studies

Radiographic studies of patients with the various forms of OI vary widely depending on the site, the class of disease, the severity of the syndrome, the age of the patient, the number of fractures that have occurred, and the alignment and quality of the adjacent joints.[1,2,14,16,19-21,25,26,28,33-35,37,42,56,60] Some patients with type I or type IV disease have virtually no changes in bone structure except a reduction in bone mass and possibly

the changes associated with fractures. In general, however, the bones are more radiolucent than normal and the cortices are thin and somewhat irregular in structure. The bones, particularly for patients with type II or type III disease, are short and deformed with bowing and torsional abnormalities (Figure 1). The presence of fracture and fracture callus is frequently evident. Although bone production occurs in response to the injury, union is slow and sometimes does not occur (Figure 2). The metaphyseal portions of the bones adjacent to the joints are often enlarged and show irregular trabecular structural alterations (Figure 3). The spine, particularly for type II or type III disease, often shows kyphoscoliotic deformities, which are quite severe and are associated with multiple fractures of the vertebral segments leading to hourglass configuration of the segments, often described as codfish vertebrae.[2,21,27,28,34,54,59,60] The skull shows the classic wormian bone and overhanging occiput pattern, with alterations in structure as defined in the discussion above.

Bone scans are often positive, particularly over fracture sites. Densitometry studies are difficult to perform, but when sites that are not deformed or have not had fractures are studied, the values are generally reduced compared to controls.[62] A recent study by Braga and associates[63] demonstrated that bone markers including alkaline phosphatase, serum osteocalcin, urinary free deoxypyridinoline, and urinary cross-linked n-telopeptides of type I collagen were higher than in controls, particularly for patients with type III and type IV disease.

Histologic Findings

The epiphyseal plates of immature patients with OI are relatively normal in structure and cell type.[20,26] The bone laid down in the zone of primary spongiosa has quite primitive features and is poorly formed[2,11,20,21,26,33,37,64] (Figure 4). "Woven bone" is characteristic, and the segments are small and seemingly purposeless. The hydroxyapatite crystals are smaller than normal.[65] The adjacent cortex is also woven, identified by some as fiber bone, and primitive in character (Figure 5). The periosteum is well delineated, but is clearly limited in function related to the relatively few osteoblasts present. The entire cortical structure is markedly thinned unless a fracture has occurred. Fractures often show extensive amounts of callus but the bone formed is of poor quality. Although present in large amounts, the callus does not really seem to strengthen the bone structure. The teeth show poor structure with irregular dentinal tubules and limited numbers of odontoblasts; this pattern is known as dentinogenesis imperfecta.[1-3,36,58]

Treatment of Osteogenesis Imperfecta

Just as the severity of the disease may vary considerably with age of the patient and the extent and type of disease, the treatment likewise may differ. Until recently, there seemed to be no plausible medical treatment for patients with these sometimes terribly disabling diseases; however, in the past decade, a number of new approaches have been introduced.[25,35,66] The principal addition is the use of bisphosphonates, which has resulted in a marked reduction in fracture frequency and improved bone densitometry.[2,35,43,53,67-73] The drug most frequently used is pamidronate, given every 4 to 6 months. Treated patients have a reduction in the rate of fractures, less bone pain, and improved psychological responses to an otherwise very depressing entity. The drug may be given to infants with type II disease and results in thickening of the cortices and vertebrae, which return to a more normal configuration and shape. Growth hormone has been introduced in an attempt to increase the height and size of the patients, but as yet no conclusive results have been reported.[74,75]

The use of mesenchymal stromal or stem cells and introduction of systems for genetic alteration have been tried recently, but are still under experimental protocols. The results are promising but somewhat unpredictable, and there is some concern about the safety of the procedures.[76-79]

Surgical procedures have been used for many years to heal fractures, straighten deformed limbs, reduce the effect of spinal abnormalities, improve dental status, or even decrease the degree of hearing loss. In general, orthopaedic procedures such as using rods to straighten bones or adding bone substitutes or bone grafts to increase the rate of bone healing for fractures have yielded some good results.[2,19,27,58-60,66,80-83] Osteotomies are sometimes successful as well.[84-87] However, not only are the bones fragile, but in many cases of type II or type III disease the patients are at risk during surgery. Heart or lung disease, neurologic complications,

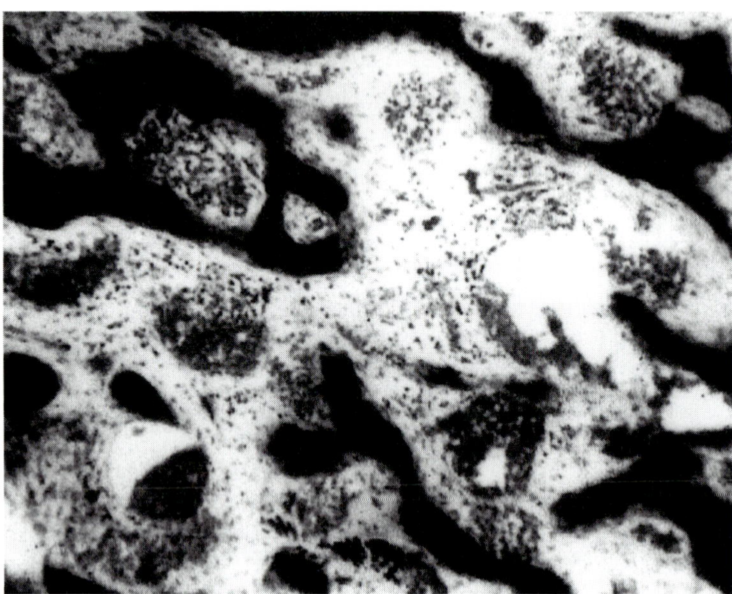

Figure 4

Histologic picture of the medullary bone from a child with osteogenesis imperfecta. The marrow space is wide and the bones are thin, poorly contoured, and purposeless. Hematoxylin and eosin × 60.

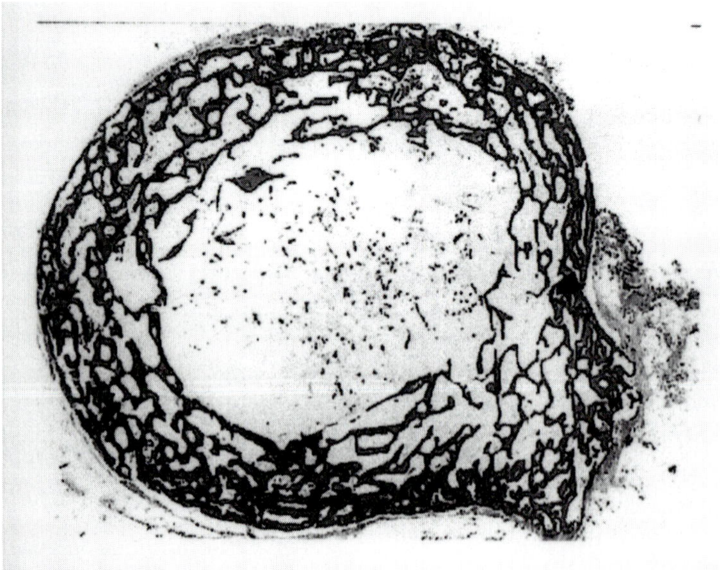

Figure 5

Cross-sectional anatomy of the femoral shaft of a newborn child with osteogenesis imperfecta shows a wide cortex with very poor structure and marked disorganization. Hematoxylin and eosin × 10.

110

and bleeding diatheses complicate the decision to do surgery.

Conclusions

In earlier times, dealing with OI was unfortunately fairly straightforward. The patients with OI congenita were always very ill and died quickly after birth, and those with OI tarda had some fractures and problems with disability but survived. Today we are faced with a much broader spectrum of disease types than these two, and even more entities are now appearing as we learn about the genetics of the syndromes. The disability level has not materially changed for many patients, but the use of bisphosphonates has greatly altered their bone strength, reduced their fracture rate, and made corrective surgery much more viable. Gene treatment may play a role; if given to patients (particularly those with type II OI) either at birth or in the uterus, it may radically alter their outcome. Many problems still exist with this type of treatment, however, given the fragility of the patients.

Despite all these issues, the diseases that comprise the array of OI syndromes have become even more fascinating. They are historically remarkable (who could forget Ivar the Boneless?), highly variable, and sometimes very puzzling and challenging in presentation. Of greatest importance, however, we now have an opportunity to medically, surgically, and soon perhaps genetically provide effective treatment of one of the true curses of the human race.

References

1. Seedorff KS: *Osteogenesis Imperfecta: A study of clinical features and heredity based on 55 Danish families comprising 189 affected persons.* Copenhagen, Denmark, Ejnar Munksgaard, 1949.

2. Tsipouras P: Osteogenesis imperfecta, in Beighton P (ed): *McKusick's Heritable Disorders of Connective Tissue,* ed 5. St. Louis, MO, Mosby, 1993, pp 281-314.

3. Gray PHK: A case of osteogenesis imperfecta associated with dentinogenesis imperfecta, dating from antiquity. *Clin Radiol* 1970;21:106-108.

4. Ekman OJ: *Dissetatio medica descriptionem et casus aliquot osteomalacia sistens.* Uppsala, Sweden, 1788.

5. Axmann E: Merkurdige fragilitat der knochen ohne dyskraische ursache als krankhafte eigenthumlichkeit dreir geschwister. *Ann Ges Heilk (Karlsruhe)* 1831;4:58-63.

6. Lobstein JG: *Lehrbuch der Pathologischen Anatomie.* Stuttgart, Germany, 1835, pp 179-190.

7. Baijet B: Aspects of the history of osteogenesis imperfecta (Vrolik's syndrome). *Ann Anat* 2002;184:1-7.

8. Vrolik W: *Tabulae ad illustrandam embrygenesim hominis et mammalium, tam naturalem quam abnormem.* Amsterdam, The Netherlands, J Muller, 1849.

9. Ormerod EL: An account of a case of mollities ossium. *BMJ* 1859;2:735-739.

10. Gurlt E: Handbuch der Lehre von den Knocheruchen. Berlin, Germany, 1862, pp 147-184.

11. Stilling H: Osteogenesis imperfecta. *Virchows Arch* 1889;115:357-364.

12. Eddowes A: Dark sclerotics and fragilitas ossium. *BMJ* 1900;2:222-227.

13. Adair-Dighton CA: Four generations of blue sclerotics. *Ophthalmoscope* 1912;10:188-189.

14. Bronson E: On fragilitas ossium and its association with blue sclerotics and otosclerosis. *Edinburgh Med J* 1917;18:240-281.

15. Conlon FA: Five generations of blue sclerotics and associated osteoporosis. *Boston Med Surg J* 1913;169:16-18.

16. Holcomb DY: A fragile-boned family: Hereditary fragilitas ossium. *J Hered* 1931;22:105-115.

17. Buchanan L: Case of congenital maldevelopment of the cornea and otosclerosis. *Trans Ophthal Soc U K* 1903;23:267-273.

18. Apert E: Les homes de verre. *Presse Med* 1928;36:805-808.

19. Hanscom DA, Winter RB, Lutter L, Lonstein JE, Bloom BA, Bradford DS: Osteogenesis imperfecta: Radiographic classification, natural history, and treatment of spinal deformities. *J Bone Joint Surg Am* 1992;74:598-616.

20. Jaffe HL: *Metabolic, Degenerative and Inflammatory Diseases of Bone and Joints.* Philadelphia, PA, Lea and Febiger, 1972.

21. Spranger JW, Langer LO Jr, Wiedemann HR: *Bone Dysplasias: An Atlas of Constitutional Disorders of Skeletal Development.* Philadelphia, PA, WB Saunders Company, 1974, pp 269-280.

22. van der Hoeve J, deKleyn A: Blaue sclerae, knochenbruchigkeit und schwerhorigkeit. *Arch Ophthalmol* 1918;95:81-88.

23. Looser E: Zur kenntniss der osteogenesis imperfecta congenita et tarda. *Mitt Grenzgeb Med Chir* 1906;15:161-207.

24. Sillence DO, Senn A, Danks DM: Genetic heterogeneity in osteogenesis imperfecta. *J Med Genet* 1979;16:101-116.

25. Cole WG: Advances in osteogenesis imperfecta. *Clin Orthop Relat Res* 2002;401:6-16.

26. Bullough PG, Davidson DD, Lorenzo JC: The morbid anatomy of the skeleton in osteogenesis imperfecta. *Clin Orthop Relat Res* 1981;159:42-57.

27. Engelbert RH, Gerver WJ, Breslau-Siderius LJ, et al: Spinal complications in osteogenesis imperfecta: 47 patients 1-16 years of age. *Acta Orthop Scand* 1998;69:283-286.

28. Versfeld GA, Beighton PH, Katz K, Solomon A: Costovertebral anomalies in osteogenesis imperfecta. *J Bone Joint Surg Br* 1985;67:602-604.

29. Cole WG, Dalgleish R: Perinatal lethal osteogenesis imperfecta. *J Med Genet* 1995;32:284-289.

30. McAllion SJ, Paterson CR: Causes of death in

osteogenesis imperfecta. *J Clin Pathol* 1996;49:627-630.

31. Paterson CR, Ogston SA, Henry RM: Life expectancy in osteogenesis imperfecta. *BMJ* 1996;312:351.

32. Singer RB, Ogston SA, Paterson CR: Mortality in various types of osteogenesis imperfecta. *J Insur Med* 2001;33:216-220.

33. Plotkin H: Syndromes with congenital brittle bones. *BMC Pediatr* 2004;4:16.

34. Renshaw TS, Cook RS, Albright JA: Scoliosis in osteogenesis imperfecta. *Clin Orthop Relat Res* 1979;145:163-167.

35. Sillence DO, Morley K, Ault JE: Clinical management of osteogenesis imperfecta. *Connect Tissue Res* 1995;31:S15-S21.

36. Waltimo-Siren J, Kolkka M, Pynnonen S, Kuurila K, Kaitila I, Kovero O: Craniofacial features in osteogenesis imperfecta: A cephalometric study. *Am J Med Genet A* 2005;133:142-150.

37. Glorieux FH, Rauch F, Plotkin H, et al: Type V osteogenesis imperfecta: A new form of brittle bone disease. *J Bone Miner Res* 2000;15:1650-1658.

38. Bank RA, Robins SP, Wijmenga C, et al: Defective collagen crosslinking in bone but not in ligament or cartilage in Bruck syndrome: Indications for homospecific telopeptide lysyl hydroxylase on chromosome 17. *Proc Natl Acad Sci USA* 1999;96:1054-1058.

39. Ha-Vinh R, Alanay Y, Bank RA, et al: Phenotypic and molecular characterization of Bruck syndrome (osteogenesis imperfecta with contractures of the large joints) caused by a recessive mutation in PLOD2. *Am J Med Genet A* 2004;131:115-120.

40. Cole DE, Carpenter TO: Bone fragility, craniosynostosis, ocular proptosis, hydrocephalus and distinctive facial features: A newly recognized type of osteogenesis imperfecta. *J Pediatr* 1987;110:76-80.

41. Byers PH, Tsipouras P, Bonadio JF, Starman BJ, Schwartz RD: Perinatal lethal osteogenesis imperfecta (OI Type II): A biochemically heterogeneous disorder usually due to new mutations in the gene for type I collagen. *Am J Hum Genet* 1988;42:237-248.

42. Cole WG: The Nicholas Andry Award 1996: The molecular pathology of osteogenesis imperfecta. *Clin Orthop Relat Res* 1997;343:235-248.

43. Dimeglio LA, Ford L, McClintock C, Peacock M: Intravenous pamidronate treatment of children under 36 months of age with osteogenesis imperfecta. *Bone* 2004;35:1038-1045.

44. Raff ML, Craigen WJ, Smith LT, Keene DR, Byers PH: Partial COL1A duplication produces features of osteogenesis imperfecta and Ehlers-Danlos syndrome type VII. *Hum Genet* 2000;106:19-28.

45. Barsh GS, Byers PH: Reduced secretion of structurally abnormal Type I procollagen in a form of osteogenesis imperfecta. *Proc Natl Acad Sci USA* 1981;78:5142-5146.

46. Schwarze U, Hata R, McKusick VA, et al: Rare autosomal recessive cardiac valvular form of Ehlers-Danlos syndrome results from mutations in the COL1A2 gene that activate the nonsense-mediated RNA decay pathway. *Am J Hum Genet* 2004;74:917-930.

47. Sillence DO, Barlow KK, Garber AP, Hall JG, Rimoin DL: Osteogenesis imperfecta type II delineation of the phenotype with reference to genetic heterogeneity. *Am J Med Genet* 1984;17:407-423.

48. Steinmann B, Superti-Furga A, Royce PM: Imperfect collagenesis in osteogenesis imperfecta: The consequences of cysteine-glycine substitutions upon collagen structure and metabolism. *Ann N Y Acad Sci* 1988;543:47-61.

49. Ward LM, Lalic L, Roughley PJ, Glorieux FH: Thirty-three novel COL1A and COL2A mutations in patients with osteogenesis imperfecta types I-IV. *Hum Mutat* 2001;17:434.

50. Wenstrup RJ, Hunter AG, Byers PH: Osteogenesis imperfecta type IV: Evidence of abnormal triple helical structure of type I collagen. *Hum Genet* 1986;74:47-53.

51. Willing MC, Deschenes SP, Scott DA, et al: Osteogenesis imperfecta type I: Molecular heterogeneity for COLI1A null alleles of type I collagen. *Am J Hum Genet* 1994;55:638-647.

52. Marini JC, Bordenick S, Chrousos GP: Endocrine aspects of growth deficiency in OI. *Connect Tissue Res* 1995;31:S55-S57.

53. Rauch F, Plotkin H, Zeitlin L, Glorieux FH: Bone mass, size and density in children and adolescents with osteogenesis imperfecta: Effect of intravenous pamidronate therapy. *J Bone Miner Res* 2003;18:610-614.

54. Charnas LR, Marini JC: Neurologic profile in osteogenesis imperfecta. *Connect Tissue Res* 1995;31:S23-S26.

55. Amako M, Fassier F, Hamdy RC, Aarabi M, Montpetit K, Glorieux FH: Functional analysis of upper limb deformities in osteogenesis imperfecta. *J Pediatr Orthop* 2004;24:689-694.

56. Violas P, Fassier F, Hamdy R, Duhaime M, Glorieux FH: Acetabular protrusion in osteogenesis imperfecta. *J Pediatr Orthop* 2002;22:622-625.

57. Ganesh A, Jenny C, Geyer J, Shouldice M, Levin AV: Retinal hemorrhages in type I osteogenesis imperfecta after minor trauma. *Ophthalmology* 2004;111:1428-1431.

58. Malmgren B, Norgren S: Dental aberrations in children and adolescents with osteogenesis imperfecta. *Acta Odontol Scand* 2002;60:65-71.

59. Janus GJ, Finidori G, Engelbert RH, Pouliquen M, Pruijs JF: Operative treatment of severe scoliosis in osteogenesis imperfecta: Results of 20 patients after halo traction and posterior spondylodesis with instrumentation. *Eur Spine J* 2000;9:486-491.

60. Oppenheim WL: The spine in osteogenesis imperfecta: A review of treatment. *Connect Tissue Res* 1995;31:S59-S63.

61. Groninger A, Schaper J, Messing-Juenger M, Mayatepek F, Rosenbaum T: Subdural hematoma as a clinical presentation of osteogenesis imperfecta. *Pediatr Neurol* 2005;32:140-142.

62. Boyde A, Travers R, Glorieux FH, Jones SJ: The mineralization density of iliac crest bone from children with osteogenesis imperfecta. *Calcif Tissue Int* 1999;64:185-190.

63. Braga V, Gatti D, Rossini M, et al: Bone turnover markers in patients with osteogenesis imperfecta. *Bone* 2004;34:1013-1016.

64. Stenvers HW: Radiological studies on the patients by J. Van der Hoeve and A. de Kleyn. *Arch Ophthalm (Leipzig)* 1918;95:94-96.

65. Vetter U, Eanes ED, Kopp JB, Termine JD, Robey PG: Changes in apatite crystal size in bones of patients with osteogenesis imperfecta. *Calcif Tissue Int* 1991;49:248-250.

66. Albright JA: Systemic treatment of osteogenesis imperfecta. *Clin Orthop Relat Res* 1981;159:88-96.

67. Arikoski P, Silverwood B, Tillmann V, Bishop NJ:

Intravenous pamidronate treatment in children with moderate to severe osteogenesis imperfecta: Assessment of indices of dual-energy X-ray absorptiometry and bone metabolic markers during the first year of therapy. *Bone* 2004;34:539-546.

68. Astrom E, Soderhall S: Beneficial effect of bisphosphonate during five years of treatment of severe osteogenesis imperfecta. *Acta Paediatr* 1998;87:64-68.

69. Bembi B, Parma A, Botte M, et al: Intravenous pamidronate treatment of osteogenesis imperfecta. *J Pediatr* 1997;131:622-625.

70. Glorieux FH: Bisphosphonate therapy for severe osteogenesis imperfecta. *J Pediatr Endocrinol Metab* 2000;13(suppl 2):989-992.

71. Glorieux FH, Bishop NJ, Plotkin H, Chabot G, Lanoue G, Travers R: Cyclic administration of pamidronate in children with severe osteogenesis imperfecta. *N Engl J Med* 1998;339:947-952.

72. Pizones J, Plotkin H, Parra-Garcia JI, et al: Bone healing in children with osteogenesis imperfecta treated with bisphosphonates. *J Pediatr Orthop* 2005;25:332-335.

73. Plotkin H, Rauch F, Bishop NJ, et al: Pamidronate treatment of severe osteogenesis imperfecta in children under 3 years of age. *J Clin Endocrinol Metab* 2000;85:1846-1850.

74. Antoniazzi F, Bertoldo F, Mottes M, et al: Growth hormone treatment in osteogenesis imperfecta with quantitative defect of type I collagen synthesis. *J Pediatr* 1996;129:432-439.

75. Vieira NE, Goans RE, Weiss GH, Hopkins E, Marini JC, Yergey AL: Calcium kinetics in children with osteogenesis imperfecta type III and IV: Pre- and post-growth hormone therapy. *Calcif Tissue Int* 2000;67:97-100.

76. Horwitz EM, Prockop DJ, Fitzpatrick LA, et al: Transplantability and therapeutic effects of bone marrow-derived mesenchymal cells in children with osteogenesis imperfecta. *Nat Med* 1999;5:309-313.

77. Marini JC, Gerber NL: Osteogenesis imperfecta: Rehabilitation and prospects for gene therapy. *JAMA* 1997;277:746-750.

78. Niyibizi C, Smith P, Mi Z, Robbins P, Evans C: Potential of gene therapy for treating osteogenesis imperfecta. *Clin Orthop Relat Res* 2000;379(suppl):S126-S133.

79. Prockop DJ, Azizi SA, Colter D, Digirolamo C, Kopen G, Phinney DG: Potential use of stem cells from bone marrow to repair the extracellular matrix and the central nerous system. *Biochem Soc Trans* 2000;28:341-345.

80. Karbowski A, Schwitalle M, Brenner R, Lehmann H, Pontz B, Worsdorfer O: Experience with Bailey-Dubow rodding in children with osteogenesis imperfecta. *Eur J Pediatr Surg* 2000;10:119-124.

81. Li YH, Chow W, Leong JC: The Sofield-Millar operation in osteogenesis imperfecta: A modified technique. *J Bone Joint Surg Br* 2000;82:11-16.

82. Mulpuri K, Joseph B: Intramedullary rodding in osteogenesis imperfecta. *J Pediatr Orthop* 2000;20:267-273.

83. Wilkinson JM, Scott BWS, Clarke AM, Bell MJ: Surgical stabilization of the lower limb in osteogenesis imperfecta using the Sheffield Telescopic Intramedullary Rod System. *J Bone Joint Surg Br* 1998;80:999-1004.

84. Niemann KMW: Surgical treatment of the tibia in osteogenesis imperfecta. *Clin Orthop Relat Res* 1981;159:134-140.

85. Porat S, Hellar E, Seidman DS, Meyer S: Functional results of operation in osteogenesis imperfecta: Elongating and non-elongating rods. *J Pediatr Orthop* 1991;11:200-203.

86. Sofield HA, Millar EA: Fragmentation, realignment and intramedullary rod fixation of deformities of the long bones in children: A ten year appraisal. *J Bone Joint Surg Am* 1959;41:1371-1391.

87. Williams PF: Fragmentation and rodding in osteogenesis imperfecta. *J Bone Joint Surg Br* 1965;47:23-31.

Chapter 16

Gaucher Disease: A Model for the Diagnosis and Management of Genetic Diseases

Genetic disorders remain serious problems in medical science and orthopaedic practice. In the past, many afflictions were determined to be familial and indeed defined not only in terms of the clinical characteristics of the problem but by the name of the physicians who described them. Hence "gargoylism" became known as Hurler's disease, "nail-patella syndrome" as Fong's disease, "fibrous dysplasia with precocious puberty" as Albright-Butler syndrome, and so forth. However, very limited information was available as to the genetic error that caused the disease or even the biologic abnormality that produced the symptoms and signs. Of even greater importance, no rational method of therapy based on the biochemistry or the gene abnormality could be defined for these disorders.

The situation changed dramatically with scientific advances and especially biologic studies of some rare disorders such as Gaucher disease. It became possible not only to define the characteristics of the clinical entities and describe the causes of the findings, but to discover the gene errors and introduce treatment protocols that could markedly improve the life of the patient. Such a systematic and indeed spectacular series of discoveries were made for Gaucher disease in the 12 decades since it was first described. This research has not only helped patients with Gaucher disease, but has now opened the gates for similar approaches to many other genetic diseases.

History of Gaucher Disease

The syndrome now known as Gaucher disease was first described in 1882 by Phillipe Charles Ernest Gaucher,[1] a French dermatologist who postulated that a patient who survived despite massive hepatosplenomegaly and a bleeding tendency had a benign form of leukemia. In 1924, Epstein[2] de-scribed a lipid material in the cells of the patients and defined the disease as a lipid storage disease. He also reported that the patients had bone lesions identifiable on radiograph. In 1948, Groen[3] defined the genetic transmission pattern of the disease and suggested that it was a classic autosomal recessive disease. Of critical importance was the work by Roscoe Brady and associates[4] in 1965; they not only defined the lipid-containing material within the abnormal Gaucher cells as glucosylceramide, but also identified the error that caused the disease as a genetic deficiency in the enzyme glucosylceramide hydrolase (also known as β-glucosidase). The absence of the enzyme allows the material glucosylceramide to accumulate in the lysosomal bodies of the cells of the reticuloendothelial system; this causes profound changes in the spleen, liver, and bone marrow, which create the clinical syndrome.[5-7] The enzyme could be introduced to the patient, but could not cross the cell membrane barrier to correct the error until the seminal studies of Barton and associates were conducted; they used a system of mannose alteration of the enzyme to target the macrophage, kill the affected cells, and improve the patient's condition.[8-14] Since then, the genetic error has been identified and the gene introduced in an effort to change the disease pattern; however, only limited success has been achieved.[14-18]

The Biologic Cause of Gaucher Disease and the Resultant Clinical Syndrome

Every 25 to 28 days, a red cell or a white cell breaks down and releases a material that consists of a sphingosine and a fatty acid (together known as ceramide), to which are attached three sugars—a galactose, a second galactose, and a glucose.[4,5,7,13,19] The ceramide and the sugar attachments are known

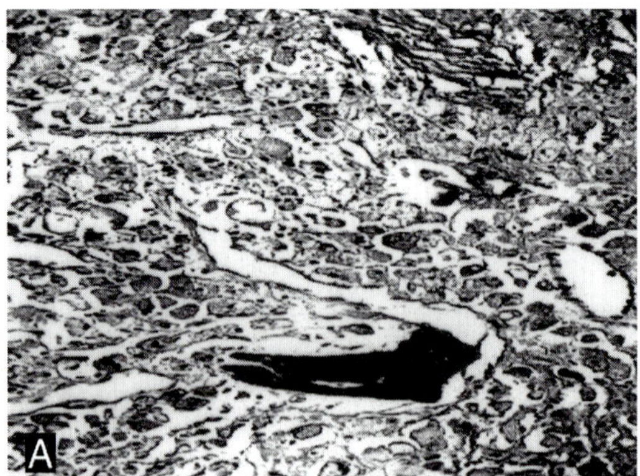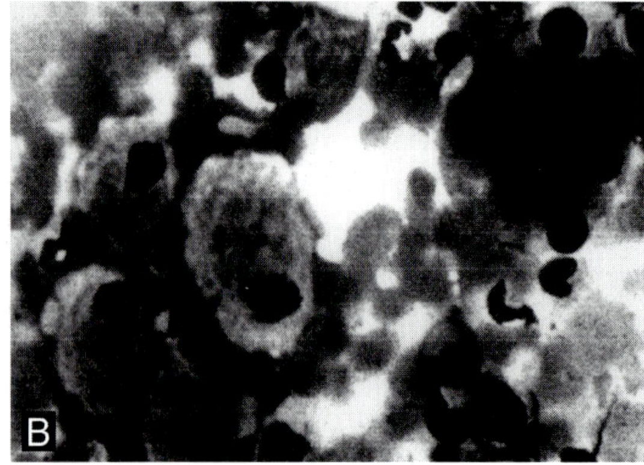

Figure 1

A, Low-power photograph of the bone marrow of a patient with Gaucher disease. Note the presence of a small spicule of bone, indicating the sometimes severe degree of osteoporosis seen in these patients. The majority of the cells in the section are Gaucher cells. Hematoxylin and eosin × 40. **B,** Close-up of the Gaucher cell in the marrow of an affected bone. Toludine blue stain × 400.

as ceramide trihexoside, which is in the serum and cannot be reutilized or excreted until the three sugars are removed. These actions require three enzymes: a ceramide trihexosidase (a galactosidase), a lactosylceramide hydrolase (also a galactosidase), and a glucosylceramide hydrolase (also known as a β-glucosidase). If the patient has a genetic error resulting in a deficiency of β-glucosidase, they have Gaucher disease.[7,14]

The classic appearance of the Gaucher cell is virtually diagnostic. The cell is large and the nucleus is small and eccentrically placed. The cytoplasm of the cell is filled with a grayish material that is irregular in texture, stains poorly, and has been said to resemble "wrinkled cigarette paper"[14,20-22] (Figure 1). This material represents a sometimes enormous volume of glucosylceramide, which exists as helical microtubular structures in the lysosomal bodies of the reticuloendothelial cells.[14,21,22] The presence of the glucosylceramide is believed to interfere with apoptotic activity, possibly rendering the cell "immortal;" this results in almost uncontrollable enlargement of the organs in which the Gaucher cells are sequestered. The spleen gets larger and larger as does the liver; between the hypersplenism and the damage to the marrow elements by the Gaucher cells, the patients develop a series of hematologic problems characterized by reduced hemoglobin, leucopenia, and thrombocytopenia.[14,19,23-25] The patients not only become anemic and bleed, but they also often have a macrophage incompetence for staphylococci and hence are at risk for infection.[26-28]

Clinical Types of Gaucher Disease

Type 1 Gaucher disease is most common in the US, Europe, and Israel. The disease is classified as mild to moderately severe, becomes evident in childhood or early adulthood, and is slowly progressive and non-neuronopathic. It is most common in Ashkenazi Jews and is characterized by hematologic complications, hepatosplenomegaly, and fairly marked skeletal deterioration that in some cases may dominate the picture.[14,23,29] Type 2 Gaucher disease is pan-ethnic and appears at infancy. The children often have very severe neurologic problems that may result in death by 2 years of age. Skeletal disease is uncommon.[5,14,19] Type 3 Gaucher disease occurs principally in children from the Norrbottnian region of Sweden who develop skeletal disease but also have neurologic problems, although much less severe than in type 2.[5,19,23] The patients may die earlier than the type 1 patients who often live for long periods, based in part on a diminished cholesterol level as a result of the lipid disorder in which the fatty acids are locked into the "immortal" cells of the reticuloendothelial system.[14,19,23,25] For this reason, heart disease also appears to be less common in patients with type 1 disease.[5,19,25]

The cause of Gaucher disease is an autosomal recessive inheritance of a gene error mapped to Iq21-q22.[18,19,23,30] For type 1 disease, there are five commonly identified abnormal alleles. The most frequent is N370S, which appears to result in milder disease and occurs with highest frequency in Ashkenazi Jews (approximately 70%). The other forms are 84GG, L444P, IVS2, and R463C, as well as several rarely seen alleles including G202R and E326K.[12,14,18,19,25,30-32] The severity of the disease is in part related to the type of abnormal allele.[18,25]

Type 1 Gaucher Disease
Clinical Syndrome

Patients with type 1 Gaucher disease usually develop symptoms and findings in childhood or adolescence.[23,25] They have hematologic disorders characterized by a low hematocrit, thrombocytopenia, and leucopenia; the principal finding is excessive hemorrhaging and collections of blood in soft tissues, organs, or bowels.[5,14,19,22,23,25,33] Splenomegaly is the first visceral abnormality encountered; the spleen can grow to enormous size and develop infarcts. The liver enlarges less rapidly until the patient has a splenectomy, as many did in the past, and then the liver may become enormous and develop infarcts, fibrosis, and clinical and chemical hepatic disease.[14,32,34] Pulmonary disease is less frequently encountered but may be severe and can cause death in susceptible patients.[35-39]

As indicated, patients with extensive disease have a high risk of infection, particularly for staphylococcus[28] as well as for virus disorders such as Epstein-Barr and influenza.[40] One of the recent findings in patients with Gaucher disease, even those who receive enzyme treatment, is what seems to be an increased incidence of Parkinson's disease, which is often progressive, severe, and not easily treated.[41-43] Amyloidosis has been reported in patients with Gaucher disease as well, and can lead to their demise.[44] Corrective or emergency surgery is sometimes associated with increased operative bleeding, which can be life-threatening.[45] Pregnant women with Gaucher disease as well as their fetuses may have hematologic difficulties, leading to decreased infant survival.[46]

Laboratory data are an important part of the patient's assessment. The hemoglobin is usually low, as are the number of thrombocytes and leukocytes in the absence of infection.[26,33] Patients with Gaucher disease almost always have an increased serum acid phosphatase.[5,14,19,25,47,48] Many of the patients have increased angiotensin-converting enzyme,[49] and in the face of liver disease they may have increased serum glutamic-oxaloacetic transaminase and serum glutamic- pyruvic transaminase.[34] Over 30% of patients have increased serum immunoglobulin IgG and IgA concentrations on immunoelectrophoresis, possibly related to the fact that the most frequent neoplasm in patients with Gaucher disease is myeloma; consequently, this must be carefully followed.[50-53] Two special tests recently discovered to be helpful in determining the success of treatment are the serum chitotriosidase,[54,55] which is markedly increased, and the serum and white blood cell glucosylceramide hydrolase, which are markedly diminished.[6,7,19,22]

Bone Disease in Patients With Gaucher Disease

The degree of bone disease in patients with Gaucher disease varies considerably with age, anatomic site studied, severity of the process, history of splenectomy, and the duration and amount of any enzyme therapy.[12,56-62] Some patients with type 1 Gaucher disease have few complaints and on imaging studies have few or no bone problems.[57,58] Others with the same abnormal allele have severe symptoms and extensive damage to the osseous system that requires them to be in wheelchairs or even bedbound.[14,57] Some of the factors that influence this variation include the general health of the patient, the history of splenectomy,[62,63] the extent of liver disease,[34] and the amount of enzyme that the patient receives.[57,60,61] However, there are still no clear guidelines as to why some patients have more severe bone changes than others. Those patients with bone disease need some special studies to define the degree of disease. These include radiographs, bone scan, bone densitometry, magnetic resonance imaging (MRI) of both lower extremities for a "Rosenthal score," and analysis of cortical thickness, usually on computed tomography of the femur.[14,25,58,60,64-69]

The bone changes seen include the following:
- *Failure in remodeling of the distal femora and proximal tibiae.* Patients with Gaucher disease appear to have a very lim-

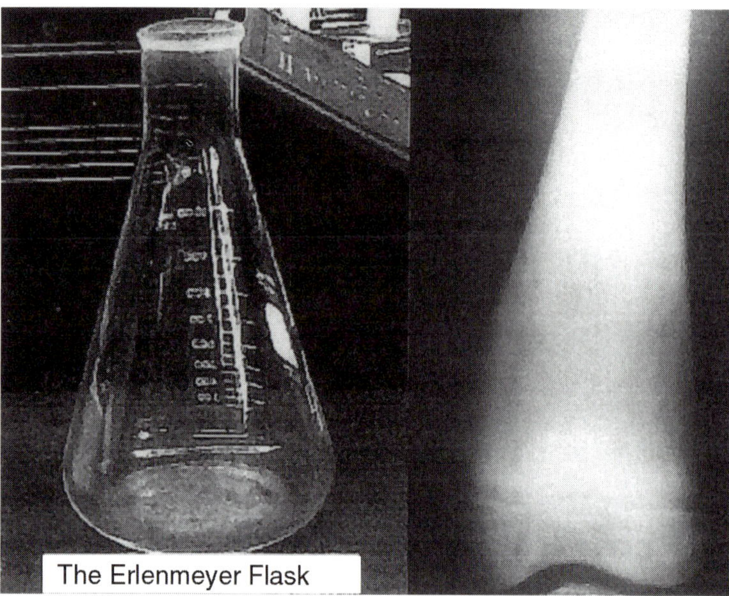

Figure 2
Classic appearance of the Erlenmeyer flask in the femur of a patient with type 1 Gaucher disease.

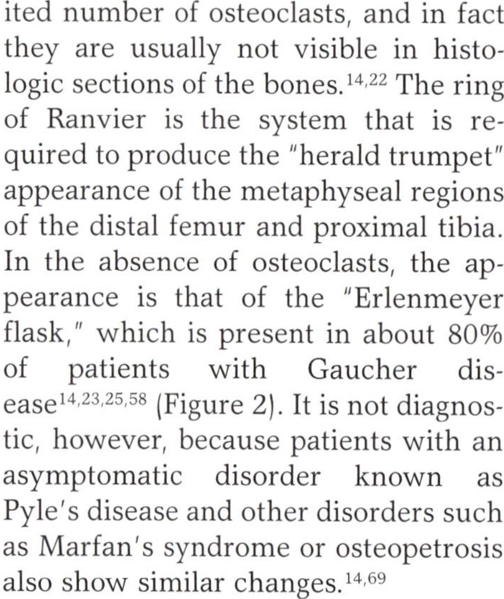

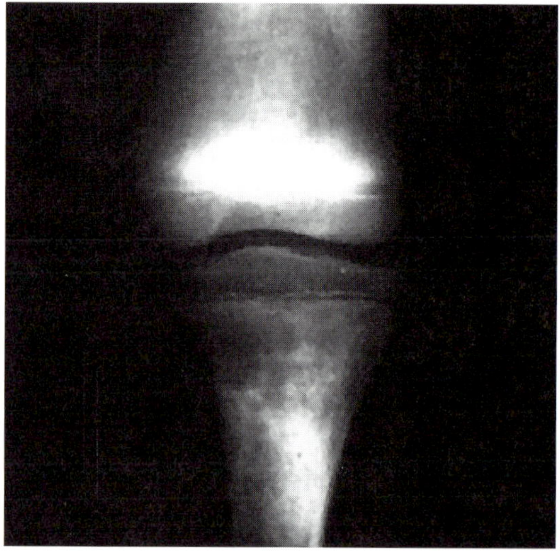

Figure 3
Radiograph showing the distal femur and proximal tibia of a child with type 1 Gaucher disease. In addition to the Erlenmeyer flask, an area of markedly increased density is evident, which is characteristic of osteonecrosis of the medullary cavity.

ited number of osteoclasts, and in fact they are usually not visible in histologic sections of the bones.[14,22] The ring of Ranvier is the system that is required to produce the "herald trumpet" appearance of the metaphyseal regions of the distal femur and proximal tibia. In the absence of osteoclasts, the appearance is that of the "Erlenmeyer flask," which is present in about 80% of patients with Gaucher disease[14,23,25,58] (Figure 2). It is not diagnostic, however, because patients with an asymptomatic disorder known as Pyle's disease and other disorders such as Marfan's syndrome or osteopetrosis also show similar changes.[14,69]

- *Medullary osteonecrosis and sometimes a related Gaucher crisis.* Loss of the blood supply to the medullary cavity, which in most patients with Gaucher disease is filled with Gaucher cells, results in the death of the large macrophages full of glucosylceramide. When the cells die, high concentrations of fatty acid are released; these seek a counterion, which in bone is logically calcium.[70] This produces a "calcium soap," which is insoluble in body fluids and remains lodged in the medullary cavity of the bone for years; the radiographic appearance is one of irregular dense cal-

cification, described as "smoke goes up the chimney"[14,58,64,70] (Figure 3). Although this medullary necrosis is ordinarily asymptomatic, if a sufficient amount of bone is damaged in this way, at the time of bone death it may result in a "Gaucher crisis," during which the patient develops severe pain in the affected limb, a high white blood cell count, and fever; on examination and imaging studies, they appear to have a large osteomyelitic focus.[31,58,65,70] The difference between the Gaucher crisis and osteomyelitis is often best assessed by a bone scan, which will be "cold" in the crisis and "hot" in infection.[27,28,31,65,70,71]

- *Corticocancellous osteonecrosis involving the proximal femur or proximal humerus.* These problems are much more pernicious and damaging to patients, and result in large osteonecrotic foci just subjacent to the joint. The damage to the subchondral cortices and the often uncontrolled healing process result in collapse of the articular surface and damage to the joint. Such a process is very disabling, particularly because many patients are also osteoporotic. The bones not only collapse, but in the face of poor blood supply and inadequate osteoblastic activity they fail to heal.

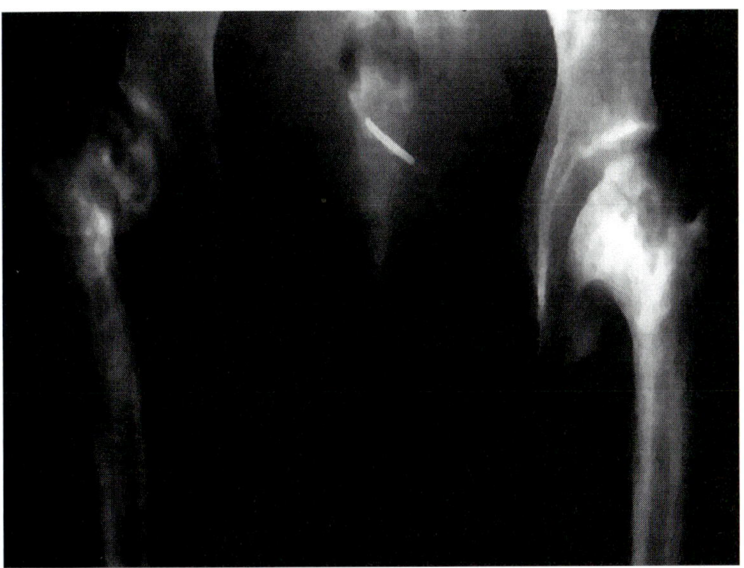

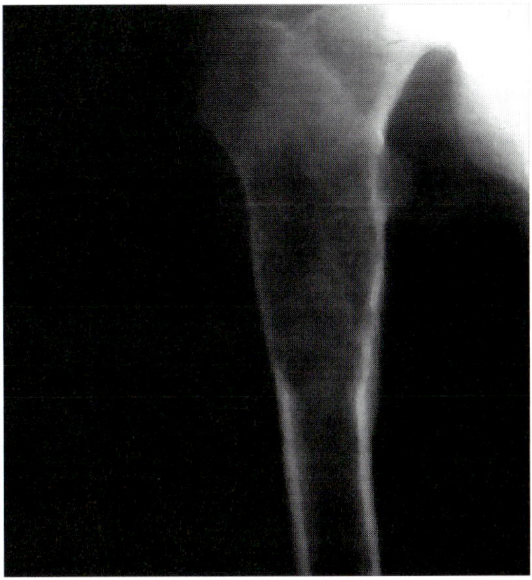

Figure 4
Radiograph demonstrating severe osteonecrosis of the proximal femora with marked joint deformity and structural change. The patient is a 33-year-old female with type 1 Gaucher disease.

Figure 5
Radiograph indicating severe osteoporosis in a 48-year-old female patient with type 1 Gaucher disease. In addition to the osteopenia, the site shows expansion and marked thinning of the cortex.

The process is often bilateral and frequently necessitates the use of crutches or even a wheelchair[14,58,63,70,72] (Figure 4).

- *Osteoporosis, lytic lesions, and fractures*: Patients with Gaucher disease have few cells that can be converted to osteoblasts, thus frequently develop sometimes very severe osteoporosis.[14,25,58] This is particularly true for females who at the time of menopause have a bone loss superimposed on their osteopenic state and frequently develop stress fractures, sometimes shattered extremities, and/or major collapsed spinal segments. Some of the sites show osteoporotic defects and enlargement of the bone, which presumably represents local collections of Gaucher cells that prevent bone healing or osteoblastic restoration[14,25,58] (Figure 5).

- *"Gaucheromas."* One occasionally sees enlargement of a bony site with marked cortical thinning resembling a bone tumor such as a giant cell tumor or an aneurysmal bone cyst. Biopsy of these lesional sites show only Gaucher cells with large amounts of poorly clotted blood.[14,73]

Treatment of Patients with Gaucher Disease

Aside from splenic enlargement and bleeding problems, the major issues for untreated patients with Gaucher disease are bony lesions, fractures, and Gaucher crises. In the past, splenectomy was the major approach for many patients. This eliminated the abdominal enlargement, but introduced a greater risk of liver disease and bone problems. The remarkable efforts of Roscoe Brady and his colleagues[4] at the National Institutes of Health led to the discovery of the enzyme deficit in the 1960s. When administration of the enzyme systemically was found to be ineffective, the finding in the early 1990s that a mannose-substituted enzyme could cross the cell membrane and destroy the otherwise immortal Gaucher cell markedly improved patient status.[8-14,57,59-61,74,75] Initially, Ceredase (alglucerase) (Genzyme Corp, Cambridge, MA), obtained from placental tissue, was found to be effective. It has since been replaced by Cerezyme (imiglucerase) (Genzyme Corp), which is produced in the laboratory by recombinant DNA technology. Now many of the patients with Gaucher disease receive enzyme treatment at a rate of 15 to 60 units/Kg every 2 to 3 weeks with remarkable changes. The spleen and liver reduce in size; the hemoglobin, white blood cell count, and platelets rise; the crises become far less frequent; and the acid phosphatase, angiotensin-converting enzyme, and chitotriosidase diminish. With all of these changes, the patient who was once quite ill now feels restored.[8-14,57,59-61,74,75] The problem that remains is that the bones do not respond at the same rate as the other organs; unless patients receive higher doses of enzyme, their bones remain osteopenic and their bone densitometry is abnormal.[14,56,60,66] Osteonecrosis appears to be less common but is still a problem for many patients who may require crutches or canes, wheelchairs, or surgical procedures such as osteotomies or total joint replacement surgery.[14,58]

Recently bisphosphonates have been added to the protocol for patients, which has resulted in improved densitometric studies and Rosenthal scores on MRI of the lower extremities.[76,77] The patients are still at some risk for fractures and sometimes bone crises. They are also at greater risk for myeloma and lymphoma,[50-53,78] as well as Parkinson's disease.[41-43] The oral drug miglustat was recently introduced for treatment of the disease; it may help with the visceral disease, but has not been demonstrated to improve bone status.[79-81] A number of attempts have been made to introduce materials to patients that might alter the gene error. Al-though some suggest that the systems are promising and will likely at some point be applicable, no long-term success has yet been demonstrated and experimental studies still continue.[14-18]

Gaucher Disease as a Model for Other Genetic Disorders

There are some 30,000 patients with Gaucher disease in the US, and the number of patients seen by orthopaedists and other clinicians is very limited. The wonderful lesson in the Gaucher story is that the system by which the disease was identified, described, and genetically and chemically defined represents a significant approach to the definition of other genetic disorders. Of even greater importance was the discovery and development of a system of administration of an enzyme that could ameliorate and to some extent eliminate the clinical aspects of the syndrome. With genetic studies underway, it is possible that Gaucher disease will become a disease of the past.

Similar studies are also now underway on a variety of diseases, some of them orthopaedic in nature. These include Fabry's disease, the mucopolysaccharidoses, Pompe's disease, Niemann-Pick disease, Tay-Sachs disease, neurofibromatosis, and others. Our hope is that the research will ultimately make the world a better place for patients whose only fault is a gene error. What a joy that will be!

References

1. Gaucher PCE: *De l'epithelloma primitif de la rate liypertropie idiopathique del la rate sans leucemie.* (MD thesis) Paris, France, 1882.

2. Epstein E: Beitrag zur chemie der Gaucherschen krankheit. *Biochem Z* 1924;145:398-414.

3. Groen JF: The hereditary mechanism of Gaucher's disease. *Blood* 1948;3:1238-1249.

4. Brady RO, Kanfer JN, Shapiro D: Metabolism of glucocerebrocides: II. Evidence of an enzymatic deficiency in Gaucher's disease. *Biochem Biophys Res Commun* 1965;18:221-225.

5. Beutler E: Gaucher's disease. *N Engl J Med* 1991;325:1354-1360.

6. Beutler E, Kuhl W: The diagnosis of the adult type of Gaucher's disease and its carrier state by demonstration of deficency of beta-glucosidase activity in peripheral blood leukocytes. *J Lab Clin Med* 1970;76:747-755.

7. Brady RO, Barranger JA: Glucosylceramide lipidosis: Gaucher disease, in Stanbury JB, Wyngaarden Fredrickson DS, Goldstein JL, Brown MS (eds): *The Metabolic Basis of Inherited Disease,* ed 5. New York, NY, McGraw-Hill 1983, pp 842-856.

8. Barton NW, Brady RO, Dambrosia JM: Enzyme replacement therapy for Gaucher's disease. *N Engl J Med* 1993;328:1564-1568.

9. Barton NW, Brady RO, Dambrosia JM, et al: Replacement therapy for inherited enzyme deficiency: Macrophage-targeted glucocerebrosidase for Gaucher's disease. *N Engl J Med* 1991;342:1464-1470.

10. Barton NW, Brady RO, Dambrosia JM, et al: Dose-dependent responses to mannose-terminated glucocerebrosidase in a child with Gaucher's disease. *J Pediatr* 1992;120:277-280.

11. Barton NW, Furbish FS, Murray GJ: Therapeutic response to intravenous infusions of glucocerebrosidase in a patient with Gaucher's disease. *Proc Natl Acad Sci USA* 1990;87:1913-1916.

12. Grabowski GA, Leslie N, Wenstrup R: Enzyme therapy for Gaucher disease: The first 5 years. *Blood Rev* 1998;12:115-133.

13. Mankin HJ: Gaucher's disease: A novel treatment

and an important breakthrough. *J Bone Joint Surg Br* 1993;75:2-3.

14. Mankin HJ, Rosenthal DI, Xavier R: Gaucher disease: New approaches to an ancient disease. *J Bone Joint Surg Am* 2001;83:748-762.

15. Barranger JA, Rice EO, Swaney WP: Gene transfer approaches to the lysosomal storage disorders. *Neurochem Res* 1999;24:601-615.

16. Havenga M, Fisher R, Hoogerbrugge P, Roberts B, Valerio D, van Es HH: Development of safe and efficient retroviral vectors for Gaucher disease. *Gene Ther* 1997;4:1393-1400.

17. Hong YB, Kim EY, Yoo JW, Jung SC: Feasibility of gene therapy in Gaucher disease using an adeno-associated virus vector. *J Hum Genet* 2004;49:536-543.

18. Rice EO, Mifflin TE, Sakallah S, Lee RE, Sansieri CA, Barranger JA: Gaucher disease: Studies of phenotype, molecular diagnosis and treatment. *Clin Genet* 1996;49:111-118.

19. Beutler E, Grabowski GA: Glycosylceramide lipidoses: Gaucher disease, in Scriver CL, Beaudet AL, Sly WS, Valle D (eds): *The Metabolic Basis of Inherited Diseases*, ed 7. New York, NY, McGraw-Hill, 1993, pp 730-759.

20. Lee RE: Pathology of Gaucher disease, in Desnick RJ, Gatt S, Grabowski GA (eds): *Gaucher Disease: A Century of Delineation and Research. Proceedings of the First International Symposium on Gaucher Disease.* New York, NY, Alan R. Liss Inc, 1982, pp 151-176.

21. Parkin JL, Brunning RD: Pathology of the Gaucher cell. *Prog Clin Biol Res* 1982;95:151-175.

22. Pastores GM: Gaucher's disease: Pathological features. *Baillieres Clin Haematol* 1997;10:739-749.

23. Cox TM, Schofield JP: Gaucher's disease: Clinical features and natural history. *Baillieres Clin Haematol* 1997;10:657-689.

24. Medoff AS, Boyd ED: Gaucher's disease in 29 patients: Hematologic complications and the effect of splenectomy. *Ann Intern Med* 1954;40:481-492.

25. Zimran A, Kay A, Gelbart T, et al: Gaucher disease: Clinical, laboratory, radiologic, and genetic features of 53 patients. *Medicine* 1992;71:337-353.

26. Aker M, Zimran A, Abrahamov A, Horowitz M, Matzner Y: Abnormal neutrophil chemotaxis in Gaucher disease. *Br J Haematol* 1993;83:187-191.

27. Bell RS, Mankin HJ, Doppelt SH: Osteomyelitis in Gaucher disease. *J Bone Joint Surg Am* 1986;68:1380-1388.

28. Finkelstein R, Nachum Z, Reissman P, et al: Anaerobic osteomyelitis in patients with Gaucher's disease. *Clin Infect Dis* 1992;15:771-773.

29. Kolodny EH, Ulman MD, Mankin HJ, et al: Phenotypic manifestations of Gaucher disease: Clinical features in 48 biochemically verified Type 1 patients and comment on Type 2 patients, in Desnick RJ, Gatt S, Grabowski GA (eds): *Gaucher Disease: A Century of Delineation and Research. Proceedings of the First International Symposium on Gaucher Disease.* New York, NY, Alan R. Liss Inc, 1982, pp 33-66.

30. Sidransky E, Tsuji S, Martin BM, Stubblefield B, Ginns EI: DNA mutation analysis of Gaucher patients. *Am J Med Genet* 1992;42:331-336.

31. Yosipovitch Z, Katz K: Bone crisis in Gaucher disease: An update. *Isr J Med Sci* 1990;26:593-595.

32. Zimran A, Gelbart T, Westwood B, Grabowski GA, Beutler E: High frequency of the Gaucher disease mutation at nucleotide 1226 among Ashkenazi Jews. *Am J Hum Genet* 1991;49:855-859.

33. Billett HH, Rizvis S, Sawitsky A: Coagulation abnormalities in patients with Gaucher disease: Effect of therapy. *Am J Hematol* 1996;51:234-236.

34. James SP, Stromeyer FW, Stowens DW, Barranger JA: Gaucher disease: Hepatic abnormalities in 25 patients, in Desnick RJ, Gatt S, Grabowski GA (eds): *Gaucher Disease: A Century of Delineation and Research. Proceedings of the First International Symposium on Gaucher Disease.* New York, NY, Alan R. Liss Inc, 1982, pp 131-142.

35. Amir G, Ron N: Pulmonary pathology in Gaucher's disease. *Hum Pathol* 1999;30:666-670.

36. Aydin K, Karabulut N, Demirkazlk F, Arat A: Pulmonary involvement in adult Gaucher's disease: High resolution CT appearance. *Br J Radiol* 1997;70:93-95.

37. Miller A, Brown LK, Pastores GM, Desnick RJ: Pulmonary involvement in type 1 Gaucher disease: Functional and exercise findings in patients with and without clinical interstitial lung disease. *Clin Genet* 2003;63:368-376.

38. Mistry PK, Sirrs S, Chan A, et al: Pulmonary hypertension in type 1 Gaucher's disease: Genetic and epigenetic determinants of phenotype and response to therapy. *Mol Genet Metab* 2002;77:91-98.

39. Theise ND, Ursell PC: Pulmonary hypertension and Gaucher's disease: Logical association or mere coincidence? *Am J Pediatr Hematol Oncol* 1990;12:74-76.

40. Eapen M, Hostetter M, Neglia JP: Massive splenomegaly and Epstein-Barr virus-associated infectious mononucleosis in a patient with Gaucher disease. *J Pediatr Hematol Oncol* 1999;21:47-49.

41. Bembi B, Zambito Marsala S, Sidransky E, et al: Gaucher's disease with Parkinson's disease: Clinical and pathological aspects. *Neurology* 2003;61:99-101.

42. Tayebi N, Walker J, Stubblefield B, et al: Gaucher disease with parkinsonian manifestations: Does glucocerebrosidase deficiency contribute to a vulnerability to parkinsonism? *Mol Genet Metab* 2003;79:104-109.

43. Varkonyi J, Rosenbaum H, Baumann N, et al: Gaucher disease associated with parkinsonism: Four futher case reports. *Am J Med Genet A* 2003;116:348-351.

44. Kaloterakis A, Filiotou A, Koskinas J, et al: Systemic AL amyloidosis in Gaucher disease: A case report and review of the literature. *J Intern Med* 1999;246:587-590.

45. Katz K, Tamary H, Lahav J, Soudry M, Cohen IJ: Increased operative bleeding during orthoapedic surgery in patients with type I Gaucher disease and bone involvement. *Bull Hosp Jt Dis* 1999;58:188-190.

46. Elstein Y, Eisenberg V, Granovsky-Grisaru S, et al: Pregnancies in Gaucher disease: A 5-year study. *Am J Obstet Gynecol* 2004;190:435-441.

47. Bull H, Murray PG, Thomas D, Fraser AN, Nelson PM: Acid phosphatases. *Mol Pathol* 2002;55:65-72.

48. Robinson DB, Glew RH: Acid phosphatase in Gaucher's disease. *Clin Chem* 1980;26:371-382.

49. Lieberman J, Beutler E: Evaluation of serum angiotensin-converting enzyme in Gaucher disease. *N Engl J Med* 1976;294:1442-1444.

50. Brady K, Corash L, Bhargava V: Multiple myeloma arising from monoclonal gammopathy of undetermined significance in a patient with Gaucher's disease. *Arch Pathol Lab Med* 1997;121:1108-1111.

51. Brautbar A, Elstein D, Pines G, Abrahamov A, Zimran A: Effect of enzyme replacement therapy on gammopathies in Gaucher disease. *Blood Cells Mol Dis* 2004;32:214-217.

52. Kaloterakis A, Cholongitas E, Pantelis E, Papadimitriou C, Durakis S, Filiotou A: Type 1 Gaucher disease with severe skeletal destruction, extraosseous extension, and monoclonal gammopathy. *Am J Hematol* 2004;77:377-380.

53. Turesson I, Rausing A: Gaucher's disease and benign monoclonal gammopathy. *Acta Med Scand* 1975;197:507-512.

54. Giraldo P, Cenarro A, Alfonso P, et al: Chitotriosidase genotype and plasma activity in patients type 1 Gaucher's disease and their relatives (carriers and non carriers). *Haematologica* 2001;86:977-984.

55. Wajner A, Micelin K, Burin MG, et al: Biochemical characterization of chitotriosidase enzyme: Comparison between normal individuals and patients with Gaucher and with Niemann-Pick diseases. *Clin Biochem* 2004;37:893-897.

56. Ciana G, Martini C, Leopaldi A, et al: Bone marker alteration in patients with type 1 Gaucher disease. *Calcif Tissue Int* 2003;72:185-189.

57. Damiano AM, Pastores GM, Ware JE: The health-related quality of life of adults with Gaucher's disease receiving enzyme replacement therapy: Results from a retrospective study. *Qual Life Res* 1998;7:373-386.

58. Elstein D, Itzchaki M, Mankin HJ: Skeletal involvement in Gaucher's disease. *Baillieres Clin Haematol* 1997;10:793-816.

59. Hermann G, Pastores GM, Abdelwahab IF, Lorberboym AM: Gaucher disease: Assessment of skeletal involvement and therapeutic responses to enzyme replacement. *Skeletal Radiol* 1997;26:687-697.

60. Lebel E, Dweck A, Foldes AJ, et al: Bone density changes with enzyme therapy for Gaucher disease. *J Bone Miner Metab* 2004;22:597-601.

61. Pastores GM, Hermann G, Norton KI, Lorberboym M, Desnick RJ: Regression of skeletal changes in type 1 Gaucher disease with enzyme replacement therapy. *Skeletal Radiol* 1996;25:485-488.

62. Rose JS, Grabowski GA, Barnett SH, Desnick RJ: Accelerated skeletal deterioration after splenectomy in Gaucher type 1 disease. *AJR Am J Roentgenol* 1982;139:1202-1204.

63. Rodrigue SW, Rosenthal DI, Barton NW, Zurakowski D, Mankin HJ: Risk factors for osteonecrosis in patients with type 1 Gaucher disease. *Clin Orthop Relat Res* 1999;362:201-207.

64. Cremin BJ, Davey H, Goldblatt J: Skeletal complications of type I Gaucher disease: The magnetic resonance features. *Clin Radiol* 1990;41:244-247.

65. Katz K, Mechlis-Frish S, Cohen IJ, Horev G, Azizov R, Lubin E: Bone scans in the diagnosis of bone crisis in patients who have Gaucher disease. *J Bone Joint Surg Am* 1991;73:513-517.

66. Pastores GM, Wallenstein S, Desnick RJ, Luckey MM: Bone density in type 1 Gaucher disease. *J Bone Miner Res* 1996;11:1801-1807.

67. Rosenthal DI, Barton NW, McKusick KA, et al: Quantitative imaging of Gaucher disease. *Radiology* 1992;185:841-845.

68. Rosenthal DI, Scott JA, Barranger JA, et al: Evaluation of Gaucher disease using magnetic resonance imaging. *J Bone Joint Surg Am* 1986;68:802-808.

69. Vanhoenacker FM, De Schepper AM, Gielen JL, Parizel PM: MR imaging in the diagnosis and management of inheritable musculoskeletal disorders. *Clin Radiol* 2005;60:160-170.

70. Mankin HJ: Nontraumatic necrosis of bone (osteonecrosis). *N Engl J Med* 1992;326:1473-1479.

71. Bilchik TR, Heyman S: Skeletal scintigraphy of pseudo-osteomyelitis in Gaucher's disease: Two case reports and a review of the literature. *Clin Nucl Med* 1992;17:279-282.

72. Katz K, Horev G, Rivlin E, et al: Upper limb involvement in patients with Gaucher's disease. *J Hand Surg [Am]* 1993;18:871-875.

73. Springfield DS, Landried M, Mankin HJ: Gaucher hemorrhagic cyst of bone: A case report. *J Bone Joint Surg Am* 1989;71:141-144.

74. Parker RI, Barton NW, Read EJ, Brady RO: Hematologic improvement in a patient with Gaucher's disease on long-term enzyme replacement therapy: Evidence for decreased splenic sequestration and improved red blood cell survival. *Am J Hematol* 1991;38:130-137.

75. Weinreb NJ, Charrow J, Andersson HC, et al: Effectiveness of enzyme replacement therapy in 1028 patients with type 1 Gaucher disease after 2-5 years of treatment: A report from the Gaucher Registry. *Am J Med* 2002;113:112-119.

76. Ostlere L, Warner T, Meunier PJ, et al: Treatment of type 1 Gaucher's disease affecting bone with aminohydroxypropylidene bisphosphonate (pamidronate). *Q J Med* 1991;79:503-515.

77. Wenstrup RJ, Bailey L, Grabowski GA, et al: Gaucher disease: Alendronate disodium improves bone mineral density in adults receiving enzyme therapy. *Blood* 2004;104:1253-1257.

78. Shiran A, Brenner B, Laor A, Tatarsky I: Increased risk of cancer in patients with Gaucher disease. *Cancer* 1993;72:219-224.

79. Elstein D, Hollak C, Aerts JM, et al: Sustained therapeutic effects of oral miglustat (Zavesca, N-butyldeoxynojirimycin, OGT 918) in type 1 Gaucher disease. *J Inherit Metab Dis* 2004;27:757-766.

80. Mistry PK: Treatment of Gaucher's disease with OGT918. *Lancet* 2000;356:676-677.

81. Samuel R, Katz K, Papapoulos SE, Yosipovitch Z, Aziaov R, Liberman UA: Aminohydroxy propylidene bisphosphonate (APD) treatment improves the clinical skeletal manifestations of Gaucher's disease. *Pediatrics* 1994;94:385-389.

Chapter 17

Osteopetrosis

Osteopetrosis, also known as "marble bone disease," is a genetic abnormality principally affecting the skeleton that is caused by a failure of the osteoclasts to destroy bone. Because osteoblastic synthesis continues, the bones become dense and marrow space is significantly reduced, decreasing the ability to produce blood elements. There are two major forms of osteopetrosis. An autosomal recessive form occurs in newborn infants and almost always results in devastating illness and early death; a second form is autosomal dominant and far less life-threatening, although it causes deformity and strange bone structure.

The diseases are very rare, possibly occurring in fewer than 1 in 300,000 live births in the US. The recessive form is quite devastating, however, because untreated children have marked deformity, visual and hearing loss, mandibular and maxillary problems, fractures, hemorrhages, and extensive uncontrollable infections. These patients generally die by 2 years of age. The autosomal dominant form is far less aggressive in presentation; some patients and their physicians may not be aware of the extent of the disease even late in life.

History of Osteopetrosis

In 1904, Albers-Schönberg[1] described a patient whose bones appeared to be "marmorized" on radiograph and named the disorder "Marmorknochen," which has been translated to the commonly used term marble bone disease. The bones were believed to be stronger than normal,[2] and the patients were said to have bones with the "hardness of ivory."[2,3] Several reports, however, noted that osteopetrotic bones cut like chalk and suggested that they should be called "chalky bones" rather than marble bones.[2] In 1931, Windholz[3] noted marked periostitis, suggesting an inflammatory characteristic to the lesion. The malignant childhood disease pattern was described by numerous authors and included such characteristics as ocular, facial, and neurologic problems; the autosomal recessive transmission of the disease; and the relationship of the genetic and clinical characteristic of the disease to mouse, rabbit, and avian models.[3-21] In 1977, Loria-Cortes and associates[22] described the increased frequency of the disease in patients from Costa Rica, which seems to be the only country with greater frequency of the genetic error.

Differentiation and Resorbing Activities of Normal Osteoclasts and the Gene Errors

Over the past 30 years, considerable research has been conducted to define the genetic errors and the relationship of the disease to aspects of osteoclast development and function.

Osteoblasts have a monocytic lineage, and cultures of peripheral blood monocytes can differentiate into osteoclasts. The formation of the osteoclasts from monocytes results from the action of an array of cytokines including PU.1, a myeloid-specific transcription factor, and macrophage colony-stimulating factor.[23-27] These materials stimulate the production of the preosteoclast from the monocyte. A material known as receptor activator of nuclear factor κB (RANK) is produced by osteoblasts and binds to the monocytic osteoclast precursor cells.[28] A ligand of this material (RANKL), also produced by osteoblasts, binds to the RANK and induces osteoclast differentiation.[27,29] Signaling following the RANK-RANKL action is mediated by tumor necrosis factor receptor-associated factor 6 (TRAF6), nuclear factor κB, and c-fos.[27,30]

After differentiation, the osteoclasts require further activation to perform bone destruction. They come under the influence of vitronectin and $\alpha_v\beta$ integrin, and develop podosomes (tiny footlike processes) that serve as attachments to bone.[15,27,31] The materials achieve this attachment by close association with the osteopontin on the bone surface. Resorption of the bone occurs as a result of acidification; this causes dissolution of the crystalline bone mineral calcium hydroxyapatite, which produces soluble calcium and acid phosphate. In addition, the osteoclasts secrete enzymes (especially cathepsin K, ATPase, and carbonic anhydrase) that digest the collagen and proteoglycan of the bone, leaving a space that is histologically described as a Howship's lacuna.[23,27,32-35]

The most frequent genetic error that causes the autosomal recessive malignant osteopetrotic syndrome is believed to be in the ATP6i gene, which mediates the acidification of the bone osteoclast interface.[27,36-38] Another is the CLCN-7, which appears to act through interference with the osteoclast-specific chloride channel;[27,36,39] yet another is a defect in the TCIRG1 subunit of the vacuolar proton pump.[27,40] A fourth rare form may be related to carbonic anhydrase II dysfunction.[27,35,37,41] Regardless of genetic error, any alteration in the production of PU.1, RANKL, ATPase, TRAF6, or carbonic anhydrase can cause osteoclast failure and lead to marble bones. Other less frequently found errors for the milder autosomal dominant form of the disease include alteration in chromosome 16p13.3.[42] Even less common is an error in the LPR5 gene, which seems to function by increasing osteoblastic activity.[27,43]

The Clinical Syndromes of the Two Major Forms of Osteopetrosis

As noted above, the etiology of the problem is the failure of osteoclast resorbtion of bone, which results in a marked increase in the density of the bone and striking abnormalities of osseous structure[11,21,22,27,36,44-51] (Figure 1). A major additional problem caused by the marble bones is the marked decrease in marrow space, which leads to diminution in blood elements (namely platelets, red cells, and white cells).[12,27,48,49,52] Damages to neural elements as a result of cranial and spinal osteopetrosis may cause blindness, hearing loss, and neurologic abnormalities.[7,13,19,22,48,53-55]

The "malignant" autosomal recessive osteosclerotic syndrome occurs principally in newborn children and is often recognizable at birth or at the latest by 3 months of age.[22,27,45,48,49,51] Males and females are equally involved and although generally very rare throughout the world, the disease occurs more frequently in children in Costa Rica.[22] The earliest findings include failure

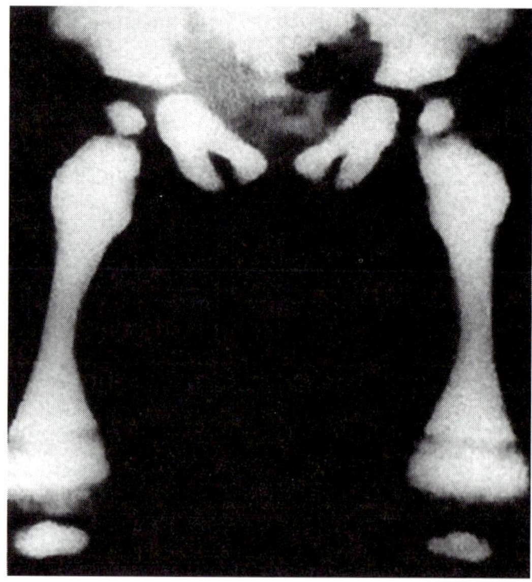

Figure 1
Classic radiographic image of a very young child with osteopetrosis, or "marble bone disease." The shafts show very dense bone and the metaphyses show Erlenmeyer flasking.

to achieve normal visual milestones, roving eye movements, and a peculiar craniofacial appearance consisting of macrocephaly and frontal bossing.[6,7,10,27,48,53,54] Within a relatively short time, the patients may develop anemia and excessive bleeding. Depression of the white blood cell count can lead to infection, which may be nasal, oral, pulmonary, osseous, or otologic and can be life-threatening.[5,12,27,48,52,55] Splenomegaly and at times hepatomegaly result from extraosseous hematopoiesis in response to the diminished blood elements and platelets from the marrow cavity.[12,27,48,50] Blindness, failure to thrive, and mental impairment supervene fairly quickly in many of the severely affected patients.[6,13,27] Convulsive disorders are frequent, as is damage to peripheral nerves as a result of bony encroachment in the calvarium and spinal canal.[7,10,13] If children live long enough, abnormal dentogenesis leads to unusual structure of the oral cavity and teeth.[19,22,51,54,56] Bone abnormalities are the major finding in all children with the disorder, and the classic radiographic appearance of marble bones in children under 2 years of age is virtually diagnostic.[5,12,44,48-50] Despite the appearance of increased density on imaging studies, the bones of many patients are fragile and fractures are quite common. Limb distortion, growth failure, and joint derangements lead to marked anatomic and structural change.[9,12,44,48-50] Parathyroid hormone is often elevated and acid phosphatase and creatinine kinase are increased, related to increased release of the materials from defective osteoclasts.[12,27,49,50] Some patients develop rickets, and a small number also show signs of scurvy.[56-58] For most patients who are not treated, death as a result of infection, bleeding, or cardiac abnormalities occurs within 2 years. The diagnosis may sometimes be made by imaging studies while the child is in the uterus.[59,60]

Albers-Schönberg disease, first described by him in 1904,[1] is also known as autosomal dominant osteopetrosis, type II (ADOII). The disease is more common than the malignant recessive form but is also caused by an increased skeletal mass due to impaired osteoclast function.[45,61-63] Seven different gene abnormalities have been described; the exact mechanism of interference with osteoclastic resorption may vary for different patients.[25,27,36,38,42,43,61,63,64] The patients develop symptoms much later than in the malignant recessive form, and may have only limited findings and disabilities.[49,61,63,65] Roughly half the patients are asymptomatic, and the diagnosis is made by radiography that discloses marble bone disease.[63] Patients may have bone pain; develop fractures (in about 40%); and present with cranial nerve entrapment syndromes, carpal tunnel syndrome, osteoarthritis, or mandibular abnormalities.[65] Serum acid phosphatase is usually increased, as well as the bone-specific alkaline phosphatase.[65] Imaging studies show increased osseous density, which is more marked in the base of the skull. The spine may show deformity and the classic "rugger jersey" appearance.[8,9,12,48,49,61,65] Sclerosis is common in the pelvis and may show "bone within a bone," also known as endobone.[9,12,27,48,49,58,65] Another feature is transverse banding of the metaphysis, which may be noted in this disorder and not in the malignant autosomal recessive variant.[12,49,58,65] Because the bone marrow is usually not compromised in this form of the disease, patients are at less risk for appearance of splenomegaly or the development of infections and bleeding.[61,65]

Another extremely rare form of the autosomal dominant form of the disease is type I (ADOI).[8,61,63] The disease is extremely mild

with very limited bone changes, far fewer fractures, no marrow abnormality, and a low alkaline phosphatase.[27,58,61] Histologic findings do not show the characteristic pattern seen in either the malignant autosomal recessive form or ADOII.[49,58,63] Another very rarely encountered variant of the disease is a mild autosomal recessive form in which patients survive far longer and have far fewer problems than in the malignant recessive form.[66]

Structural, Imaging, and Histologic Findings

For malignant autosomal recessive neonatal patients, the bones on gross examination are excessively heavy. Examination of the internal structure of the bones shows excessive amounts of compacted osseous tissue; the normal reddish color of marrow is no longer present, and the bones have a grayish coloration.[5,12,47,48] Ribs show beading at the osteochondral junctions and the vertebrae may be entirely dense without any marrow cavity in the structure. Epiphyseal areas are poorly structured and do not seem to be actively causing increased bone length.[12,48] The changes seen in patients with autosomal dominant disease are similar, but more marrow is present and the amount of dense bone is less than that seen in children with the severe form of the disease.[61,63]

Radiographs show very dense white bone, with almost no marrow cavity (Figure 1). The bones are wider than normal and almost always show Erlenmeyer flasking of the distal femora and proximal tibiae (Figure 2). The base of the skull is frequently very dense and the calvaria is enlarged and deformed[10,47,48,50,53,55,62] (Figure 3). The spine may show scoliosis, bowing, and the classic rugger jersey appearance.[9,47,48,50] Sclerosis is common in the pelvis and may show endobone. Another feature is transverse banding of the metaphysis, which may be noted in the autosomal dominant milder disorder but not in the malignant autosomal recessive variant.[48,50,62,65] Fractures are common in both types of disease but are more frequent and often show greater displacement in patients with the malignant autosomal recessive disease.[44,47-49,51,61]

Histologic study shows that the bones have little marrow space; most of the tissue consists of dense bone with little structural

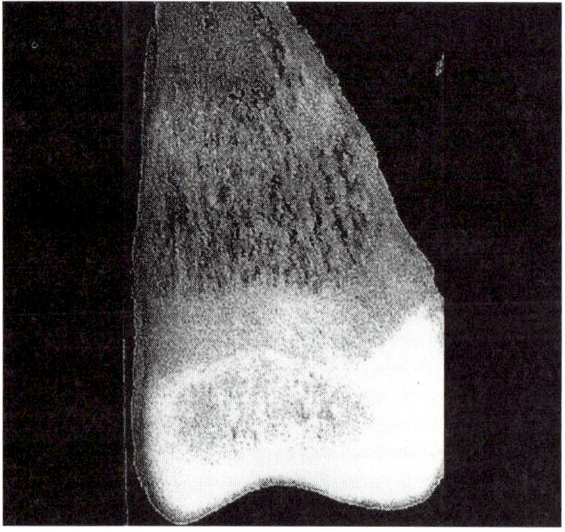

Figure 2

Cut section of the bone from a patient who died of osteopetrosis, showing the marked reduction in the marrow space and the enormous width of the metaphyseal region. The epiphyseal cartilage is relatively normal, but the epiphysis shows similar changes.

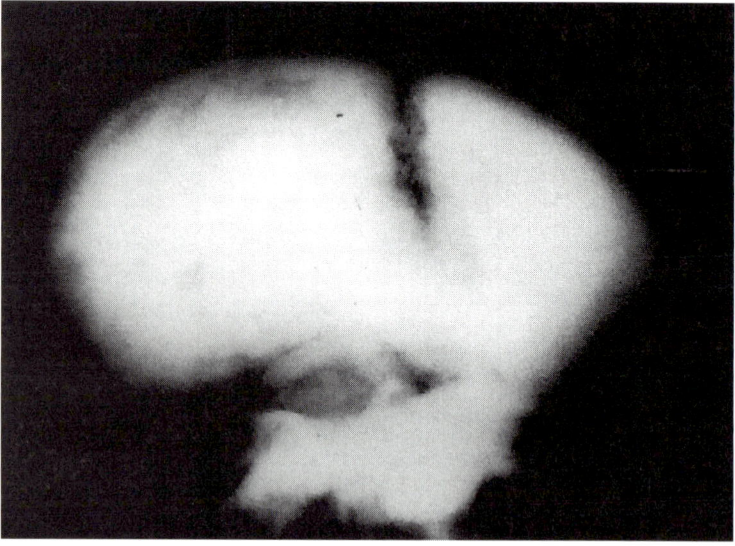

Figure 3

Radiograph of the calvarium of a child with severe osteopetrosis that shows the classic marble bone characteristics and the marked enlargement of the bony structure. Children with this kind of picture are usually blind, deaf, and may have difficulty swallowing.

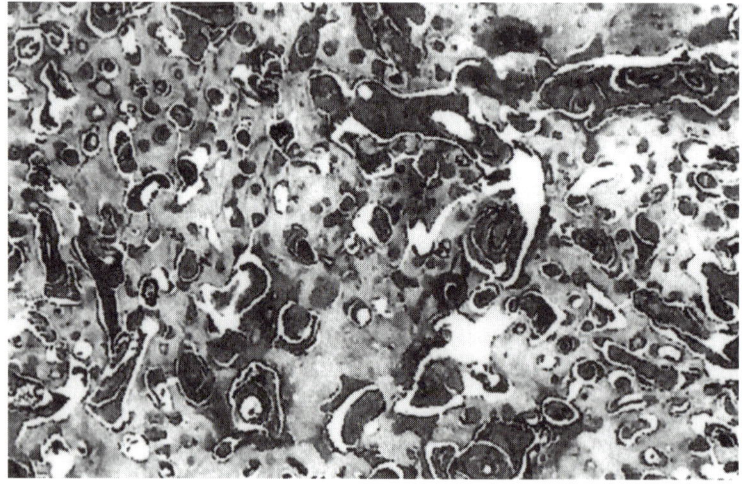

Figure 4

Histologic picture of the femur of a child with osteopetrosis. The bone is almost completely without marrow and consists of large segments of bone with no order or organization to the structure. Osteoclasts are absent. Hematoxylin and eosin × 40.

configuration, particularly in terms of definition of the cortex[12,48] (Figure 4). Within the irregular bone, trabecular collections of calcified cartilage are observed that presumably represent retained foci of endochondral ossification. The osseous tissue is relatively poor in numbers of cells. With advancing time, the segments get larger and larger. Osteoblasts are rarely seen and virtually no osteoclasts are encountered.[12,48] Vascularity is generally poor, and islands of osteonecrosis can be observed with advancing age.[48]

Outcome and Treatment of Osteopetrosis

As noted above, many of the patients with malignant autosomal recessive disease die by 2 years of age.[9,13,22,27,45,49] Some live beyond that age, but are greatly disabled with mental retardation, blindness, hearing loss, fractures, displaced joints, and spinal curvature. Of even greater concern, many patients develop severe marrow failure problems with bleeding, anemia, and leukopenia. Extraosseous hematopoiesis causes sometimes extraordinary enlargement of the liver and spleen. Infections including pulmonary disease and osteomyelitis may dominate the child's health status.[22,27,48,49,51,58]

The treatment options for such patients include calcitriol to stimulate dormant osteoclasts, and calcitonin or corticosteroids to increase osteoclastic resorption.[27,51,67-70] Erythropoietin can be used to improve the anemia, and antibiotics as necessary will protect against infectious disease.[27] Recently, gamma interferon has been found to produce some long-term benefits by improving white blood cell function.[71,72]

The approach that is currently advocated when all else fails is bone marrow transplant or introduction of stem cells, which may reverse the marrow failure and metabolic abnormalities.[27,44,49,73-77] The treatment is difficult, particularly in terms of febrile and respiratory complications and possible infections, all of which may be life-threatening.[78] Gene therapy coding for an osteoclast-specific vacuolar pump was recently introduced, and other genes are now being mapped and cloned.[27] These approaches may reduce the symptoms and risks for the child with very severe disease.

Patients with autosomal dominant osteopetrosis may not require treatment if they are relatively asymptomatic. Interferon and calcitonin can be helpful for them.[27,49]

Both groups of patients require orthopaedic management of fractures and deformities. The malignant form of the disease may require extensive rehabilitation protocols to improve function.[44,48,49,51] Surgical procedures for ocular disturbances are difficult and complex, as is spine surgery for neural compressive syndromes.[6,19]

Conclusion

Osteopetrosis is a rare disorder that has multiple presentations. The most distressing is the malignant autosomal recessive form, which for most of the children appears at birth and causes extensive neurologic, osseous, hematologic, and infectious problems; death generally occurs by 2 or 3 years of age. A fascinating aspect of the disease is the other forms that may occur—the milder autosomal recessive form, the relatively mild type II autosomal dominant adult form, and the even milder type I adult disease. Regardless of genetic cause (and there is considerable variation in this aspect), all of them have marble bones and therefore may present with abnormalities on imaging studies, fractures, structural abnormalities, dislocations, deformities, growth disturbances, and even a form of rickets. The disorders are bizarre but clearly are related to insufficient osteoclastic bone destruction. There is now some hope for these patients that calcitriol, corticosteroids, calcitonin, marrow or stem cell transplants, or gene therapy may ultimately cure or prevent the disease. Let us hope so!

References

1. Albers-Schönberg HE: Röntgenbilder einer seltenen Knockenerkrankung. *Munch Med Wochenschr* 1904;51:365-368.

2. Bick EM: *Source Book of Orthopaedics*. New York, NY, Hafner Publishing Company, 1968, pp 154-177.

3. Windholz F: Osteosclerosis fragilitis (marmorknochenkrankheit) mit periostaler Knochenneubildung. *Zeitschr F Kinderheil* 1931;51:708-728.

4. Biltz RM, Pellegrino ED: Avian osteopetrotic bone: A correlation of its chemical composition with its roentgenopraphic and histological appearance. *J Bone Joint Surg Am* 1965;47:1365-1377.

5. Cohen J: Osteopetrosis: Case report, autopsy findings and pathologic interpretation: Failure of treatment with vitamin A. *J Bone Joint Surg Am* 1951;33:923-938.

6. Cummings TJ, Proia AD: Optic nerve compression in infantile malignant recessive osteopetrosis. *J Pediatr Ophthalmol Strabismus* 2004;41:241-244.

7. Dort JC, Pollak A, Fisch U: Facial nerve dysfunction in osteopetrosis. *Laryngoscope* 1994;104:517-522.

8. Engfeldt B, Fajers CM, Lodin H, Pehrson M: Studies on osteopetrosis: III. Roentgenological and pathologic-anatomical investigations on some of the bone changes. *Acta Paediatr* 1960;49:391-408.

9. Fairbank HAT: Osteopetrosis, osteopetrosis generalisata, marble bones, Albers-Schönberg disease, osteosclerosis fragilities generalisata. *J Bone Joint Surg Br* 1948;30:339-356.

10. Giaccai L, Salaam M, Zellweger H: Cleidocranial dysostosis with osteopetrosis. *Acta Radiol* 1954;41:417-424.

11. Hasenhuttl K: Osteopetrosis: Review of the literature and comparative studies on a case with twenty-four year followup. *J Bone Joint Surg Am* 1962;44:359-370.

12. Jaffe HL: *Metabolic, Degenerative and Inflammatory Diseases of Bone and Joints*. Philadelphia, PA, Lea and Febiger, 1972, pp 178-192.

13. Lehman RAW, Reeves JD, Wilson WB, Wesenberg RI: Neurological complications of infantile osteopetrosis. *Ann Neurol* 1977;2:378-384.

14. Nussey AM: Osteopetrosis. *Arch Dis Child* 1938;13:161-172.

15. McHugh KP, Hodivala-Dilke K, Zheng MH, et al: Mice lacking β3 integrins are osteosclerotic because of dysfunctional osteoclasts. *J Clin Invest* 2000;105:433-440.

16. Pincus JB, Gittleman IF, Kramer B: Juvenile osteopetrosis: Metabolic studies in two cases and further observations on the composition of the bones in this disease. *Am J Dis Child* 1947;73:458-472.

17. Pines B, Lederer M: Osteopetrosis (Albers-Schönberg disease: Marble bone disease): Report of a case and morphologic study. *Am J Pathol* 1947;213:755-781.

18. Seifert MF, Popoff SN, Jackson ME, MacKay CA, Cielinski M, Marks SC Jr: Experimental studies of osteopetrosis in laboratory animals. *Clin Orthop Relat Res* 1993;294:23-33.

19. Stocks RM, Wang WC, Thompson JW, Stocks MC II, Horwitz EM: Malignant infantile osteopetrosis:

Otolaryngological complications and management. *Arch Otolaryngol Head Neck Surg* 1998;124:689-694.

20. Tondravi MM, McKercher SR, Anderson K, et al: Osteopetrosis in mice lacking haematopoietic factor PU.1. *Nature* 1997;386:81-84.

21. Zawisch C: Marble bone disease: A study of osteogenesis. *Arch Pathol* 1947;43:55-75.

22. Loria-Cortes R, Quesada-Calvo E, Codero-Chaverri C: Osteopetrosis in children: A report of 26 cases. *J Pediatr* 1977;91:43-47.

23. Blair HC, Schlesinger PH, Ross FP, Teitelbaum SL: Recent advances toward understanding osteoclast physiology. *Clin Orthop Relat Res* 1993;294:7-22.

24. Holtrop ME, Kig GJ: The ultrastructure of the osteoclast and its functional implications. *Clin Orthop Relat Res* 1977;123:177-196.

25. Marks SC Jr: Osteopetrosis: Multiple pathways for the interception of osteoclast function. *Appl Pathol* 1987;5:172-183.

26. Teitelbaum SL, Ross FP: Genetic regulation of osteoclast development and function. *Nat Rev Genet* 2003;4:638-649.

27. Tolar J, Teitelbaum, Orchard PJ: Osteopetrosis. *N Engl J Med* 2004;351:2839-2849.

28. Dougall WC, Glaccum M, Charrier K, et al: RANK is essential for osteoclast and lymph node development. *Genes Dev* 1999;13:2412-2424.

29. Sankar U, Patel K, Rosol TJ, Ostrowski MC: RANKL coordinates cell cycle withdrawal and diffentiation in osteoclasts through the cyclin-dependent kinase inhibitors p27KIP1 and p21CIP1. *J Bone Miner Res* 2004;19:1339-1348.

30. Lomaga MA, Yeh WC, Sarosi I, et al: TRAF6 deficiency results in osteopetrosis and defective interleukin-1, CD40, and LPS signaling. *Genes Dev* 1999;13:1015-1024.

31. Teti A, Migiaccio S, Taranta A, et al: Mechanisms of osteoclast dysfunction in human osteopetrosis: Abnormal osteoclastogeneisis and lacking osteoclast-specific adhesion structures. *J Bone Miner Res* 1999;14:2107-2117.

32. Blair HC: How the osteoclast degrades bone. *Bioessays* 1998;20:837-846.

33. Blair HC, Teitelbaum SL, Ghiselli R, Gluck S: Osteoclastic bone resorption by a polarized vacuolar proton pump. *Science* 1989;245:855-857.

34. Cotter M, Connell T, Colhoun E, Smith OP, McMahon C: Carbonic anhydrase II deficiency: A rare autosomal recessive disorder of osteopetrosis, renal tubular acidosis, and cerebral cacification. *J Pediatr Hematol Oncol* 2005;27:115-117.

35. Whyte MP: Carbonic anhydrase II deficiency. *Clin Orthop Relat Res* 1993;294:52-63.

36. de Vernejoul MC, Benichou O: Human osteopetrosis and other sclerosing disorders: Recent genetic developments. *Calcif Tissue Int* 2001;69:1-6.

37. Kornak U, Schulz A, Friedrich W, et al: Mutations in the a3 subunit of the vacuolar H(+)-ATPase cause infantile osteopetrosis. *Hum Mol Genet* 2000;9:2059-2063.

38. Van Hul W, Bollerslev J, Gram J, et al: Localization of a gene for autosomal dominant osteopeotrosis (Albers-Schonberg disease) to chromosome 1p21. *Am J Hum Genet* 1997;61:363-369.

39. Frattini A, Pangrazio A, Susani L, et al: Chloride channel ClCN-7 mutations are responsible for severe recessive dominant and intermediate osteopetrosis. *J Bone Miner Res* 2003;18:1740-1747.

40. Frattini A, Orchard PJ, Sobacchi C, et al: Defects in the TCIRG1 subunit of the vacuolar proton pump are responsible for a subset of human autosomal recessive osteopetrosis. *Nat Genet* 2000;25:343-346.

41. Sly WS: The carbonic anhydrase II deficiency syndrome: Osteopetrosis with renal tubular acidosis and cerebral calcification, in Scriver CR, et al (eds): *The Metabolic Basis of Inherited Disease*. New York, NY, McGraw Hill, 1989, pp 2857-2868.

42. Benichou O, Cleiren E, Gram J, Bollersley J, de Vernejoul MC, Van Hul W: Mapping of autosomal dominant osteopetrosis type II (Albers-Schonberg disease) to chromosome 16p13.3. *Am J Hum Genet* 2001;69:647-654.

43. Alatalo SL, Ivaska SG, Waguespack MJ, Econs MJ, Vaananen HK, Halleen JM: Osteoclast-derived serum tartrate-resistant acid phosphatase 5B in Albers-Schonberg disease (Type II autosomal dominant osteopetrosis). *Clin Chem* 2004;50:883-890.

44. Armstrong DG, Newfield JJ, Gillespie R: Orthopaedic management of osteopetrosis: Results of a survey and a review of the literature. *J Pediatr Orthop* 1999;19:122-132.

45. Felix R, Hofstetter W, Cecchini MG: Recent developments in the understanding of osteopetrosis. *Eur J Endocrinol* 1996;134:143-156.

46. Gerritsen EJA, Vossen JM, van Loo IH, et al: Autosomal recessive osteopetrosis: Variability of findings at diagnosis and during the natural course. *Pediatrics* 1994;93:247-253.

47. Helfrich MH, Aronson DC, Everts V, et al: Morphologic features of bone in human osteopetrosis. *Bone* 1991;12:411-419.

48. Milgram JW, Jasty M: Osteopetrosis: A morphological study of twenty-one cases. *J Bone Joint Surg Am* 1982;64:912-929.

49. Shapiro F: Osteopetrosis: Current clinical considerations. *Clin Orthop Relat Res* 1993;294:34-44.

50. Shapiro F, Glimcher MJ, Holtrop ME, Tashjian AH Jr, Brickley-Parsons D, Kenzora JE: Human osteopetrosis: A histological, ultrastructural, and biochemical study. *J Bone Joint Surg Am* 1980;62:384-389.

51. Wilson CJ, Vellodi A: Autosomal recessive osteopetrosis: Diagnosis, management and outcome. *Arch Dis Child* 2000;83:449-452.

52. Beard CJ, Key L, Newburger PE, et al: Neutrophil defect associated with malignant infantile osteopetrosis. *J Lab Clin Med* 1986;108:498-505.

53. Elster AD, Theros EG, Key LL, Chen MY: Cranial imaging in osteopetrosis: Part I. Facial bones and calvarium. *Radiology* 1992;183:129-135.

54. Elster AD, Theros EG, Key LL, Chen MY: Cranial imaging in osteopetrosis: Part II. Skull base and brain. *Radiology* 1992;183:137-144.

55. Osborn R, Boland T, DeLuchi S, Beirne OR: Osteomyelitis of the mandible in a patient with malignant osteopetrosis. *J Oral Med* 1985;40:76-80.

56. Kaplan FS, August CS, Fallon MD, Gannon F, Haddad JG: Osteopetrorickets: The paradox of plenty. Pathophysiology and treatment. *Clin Orthop Relat Res* 1993;294:64-78.

57. Oliveira G, Boechat MI, Amaral SM, Young LW: Osteopetrosis and rickets: An intriguing association. *Am J Dis Child* 1986;140:377-378.

58. Whyte MP: Osteopetrosis and the heritable forms of rickets, in Steinmann B, Royce PM (eds): *Connective Tissue and Its Heritable Disorders: Medical, Genetic and Molecular Aspects*. New York, NY, Wiley Liss, 1993, pp 563-589.

59. Jenkinson EL, Phisterer WH, Latterier KK, Martin M: A prenatal diagnosis of osteosclerosis. *Am J Radiol* 1943;49:455-462.

60. Ogur G, Ogur E, Celasun B, et al: Prenatal diagnosis of autosomal recessive osteopetrosis, infantile type, by X-ray evaluation. *Prenat Diagn* 1995;15:477-481.

61. Bollerslev J, Mosekilde L: Autosomal dominant osteopetrosis. *Clin Orthop Relat Res* 1993;294:45-51.

62. Hinkel CL, Beiler DD: Osteopetrosis in adults. *AJR Am J Roentgenol* 1955;74:46-64.

63. Johnston CC, Lavy N, Lord T, Vellios F, Merritt AD, Deiss WP Jr: Osteopetrosis: A clinical, genetic, metabolic, and morphologic study of the dominantly inherited, benign form. *Medicine* 1968;47:149-167.

64. Iglesias A, Iglesias S, Levis BA, et al: Autosomal dominant hyperostosis osteosclerosis with high serum alkaline phosphatase activity. *J Clin Endocrinol Metab* 2003;88:2650-2655.

65. Benichou OD, Laredo JD, de Vernejoul MC: Type II autosomal dominant osteopetrosis: Clinical and radiological manifestations in 42 patients. *Bone* 2000;26:87-93.

66. Kahler SG, Burns JA, Aylsworth AS: A mild autosomal recessive form of osteopetrosis. *Am J Med Genet* 1984;17:451-464.

67. Key L, Carnes D, Cole S, et al: Treatment of congenital osteopetrosis with high-dose calcitriol. *N Engl J Med* 1984;310:409-415.

68. Key LL, Ries WL: Osteopetrosis: The pharmacophysiologic basis for treatment. *Clin Orthop Relat Res* 1993;294:85-89.

69. Reeves JD, Huffer WE, August CS, et al: The hematopoietic effects of prednisone therapy in four infants with osteopetrosis. *J Pediatr* 1979;94:210-214.

70. van Lie Peters EM, Aronson DC, Everts V, Dooren LJ: Megadose methylprednisolone treatment for malignant osteopetrosis. *Eur J Pediatr* 1994;154:779-780.

71. Key LL, Ries WL, Rodriguiz RM, Hatcher HC: Recombinant human interferon gamma therapy for osteopetrosis. *J Pediatr* 1992;121:119-124.

72. Key LL, Rodriguiz RM, Willi SM, et al: Long term treatment of osteopetrosis with recombinant human interferon. *N Engl J Med* 1995;332:1594-1599.

73. Driessen GJ, Gerritsen EJ, Fischer A, et al: Long-term outcome of haematopoietic stem cell transplantation in autosomal recessive osteopetrosis: An EBMT report. *Bone Marrow Transplant* 2003;32:657-663.

74. Frattini A, Blair HC, Sacco MG, et al: Rescue of ATPa3-deficient murine malignant osteopetrosis by hematopoietic stem cell transplantation in utero. *Proc Natl Acad Sci USA* 2005;102:14629-14634.

75. Gerritsen EJA, Vossen JM, Fasth A, et al: Bone marrow transplantation for autosomal recessive osteopetrosis: A report from the Working Party on Inborn Errors of the European Bone Marrow Transplantation Group. *J Pediatr* 1994;125:896-902.

76. McMahon C, Will A, Hu P, Shah GN, Sly WS, Smith OP: Bone marrow transplantation corrects osteopetrosis in the carbonic anhydrase II deficiency syndrome. *Blood* 2001;97:1947-1950.

77. Schulz AS, Classen CF, Mihatsch WA, et al: HLA-haploidentical blood progenitor cell transplantation in osteopetrosis. *Blood* 2002;99:3458-3460.

78. Steward CG, Pellier I, Mahajan A, et al: Severe pulmonary hypertension: A frequent complication of stem cell transplantation for malignant infantile osteopetrosis. *Br J Haematol* 2004;124:63-71.

Chapter 18

Neurofibromatosis and Neural Tumors

Tumors of neurologic origin are common, and frequently affect the body's soft tissues and bone. The principal disorder associated with bone and soft-tissue lesions that may appear in an orthopaedic setting is neurofibromatosis type 1 (NF1), also known as von Recklinghausen's disease. This is a common autosomal dominant genetic disturbance believed to occur in 1 of every 3,000 live births, in the world. The disease, equally distributed by gender, causes an array of findings that include skin and soft-tissue lesions, ophthalmic abnormalities, gross soft-tissue tumors, and sometimes bizarre deformities of limbs. Bone changes include osseous cortical thinning, scoliosis, and pathologic fractures of bones. Malignant soft-tissue tumors occur with considerable frequency and have a high rate of local recurrence and metastasis.

Neural Disease Terminology

Many abnormalities arise from the nervous system, and it is important to recognize the differences among them. NF1 affects the entire body, while neurofibromatosis type 2 (NF2) principally affects the nerves within the calvarium and most frequently the acoustic nerves.[1-3] The tumors that arise in NF1 are known as neurofibromas; usually not encapsulated, they have a localized diffuse and sometimes plexiform pattern.[1-6] The other major form of nerve tumor is a schwannoma, which arises from the sheath of Schwann and has a distinctive histology.[2,3,7,8] Schwannomas stain heavily with S100 and generally occur sporadically as individual tumors or occasionally with NF2.[2,3,8] Further confusion arises with the use of terms such as neurilemmoma, neuroblastoma, malignant peripheral nerve sheath tumors, and malignant schwannoma.[2,3,8]

History of Neurofibromatosis Type 1

Although based on study of the Ebers papyrus, the disease may have existed in ancient Egypt,[9] the earliest definition of the disorder was by Friedrich D. von Recklinghausen (1833-1910), an eminent German pathologist at the turn of the century who was appointed assistant to Professor Rudolf Virchow and subsequently served as Professor at the University of Strasbourg.[2] Although the first description of the disease was by Professor Robert Smith in 1849,[10] it was von Recklinghausen's[11] clear description and definition of the disease published in 1882 that resulted in the eponym for the entity. In 1889, Chaffaurd[12] described pseudoxanthoma elasticum and the café au lait spots. The hereditary nature of the disease was recognized by Thomson in 1900,[13] and numerous authors subsequently described other aspects of the disease. These features include ophthalmic lesions (Lisch granules and optic glioma), café au lait spots resembling the "coast of California," axillary freckling, fibroma molluscum nodules, plexiform neurofibromas, elephantiasis, bone deformities, and pathologic fractures.[14-30] In the past 20 years the genetic character of the disease has been defined,[31-37] as well as the psychological and cardiac problems,[38] the degree of disability,[20,36,39,40] and the frequency of malignancy.[4,41-45] Although the authors of two different texts[2,3] have gone to great lengths to distinguish the lesions of NF1 from schwannoma, the two disorders are still sometimes confused in the literature and by pathologists.[5,8]

Biologic and Histologic Characteristics of Neurofibromatosis Type 1

Neurofibromatosis is an autosomal dominant disorder with high penetrance, but over half of the cases occur as a sporadic mutation, resulting from deletions, insertions, or mutations in the NF1 gene.[3,35,36,46] The gene, located in chromosome 17, is mapped at 17q11.2 and spans 350 kb genomic DNA; it comprises 60 exons encoding

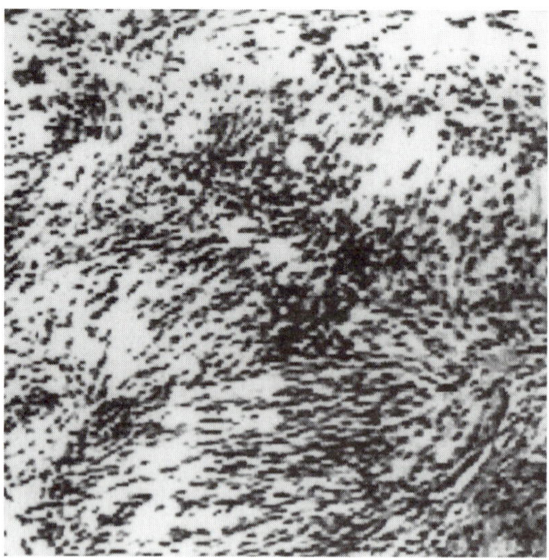

Figure 1

Histologic features of the schwannoma, showing elongated cells in clusters and groups. There is no evidence of atypism, giant cells, or synthetic activity. Hematoxylin and eosin × 100.

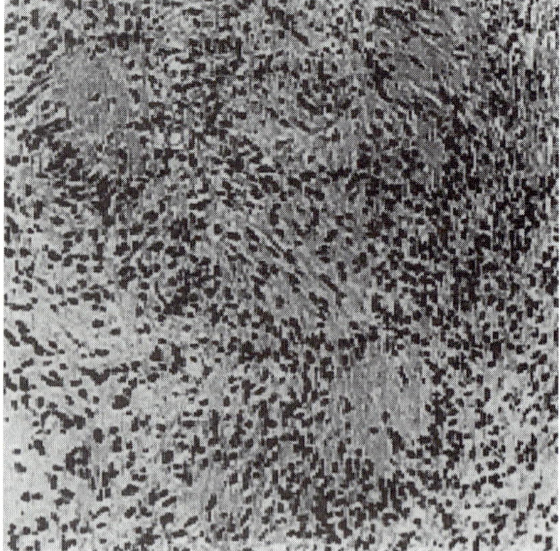

Figure 2

Histology of the neurofibroma showing Antoni B cells clustered around focal regions of myxoid and myomyxoid material. Hematoxylin and eosin × 100.

an 11-13 kb transcript.[31,32,45,47] Exons 21-27a of NF1 encode a 360 amino acid domain in a protein called neurofibromin, which shows homology with a family of proteins known as guanosine triphosphatase-activating proteins.[33,35,36,47,48] Because there are several isoforms of neurofibromin, this results in a marked variability in the presentation of the disease, and even more so a variation in the degree of development of malignant components in various sites.[36] In addition, because of the size and the variability in structure of the NF1 gene, it is difficult to assess the nature of the disease by genetic studies in an adult, and virtually impossible prenatally.[35,36]

The histologic characteristics of neurofibromatosis are quite variable, particularly if the findings seen in schwannomas are included. The latter lesions, sometimes known as neurilemmomas, arise from the sheath of Schwann surrounding neural elements. Schwannomas are ordinarily not related to NF1 and are more common in relation to NF2.[2,3,5,8] They have some distinctive features, notably the Antoni A and Antoni B patterns, and a peculiar characteristic known as Verocay bodies[3,7,8] (Figure 1). Neurofibromas show a much more "fibrous" pattern and less uniformity of structure[3,5,6,8] (Figure 2). They may show some Schwann cells but also show Wagner-Meissner bodies, which are rounded acellular structures sur-

rounded by fibroblast-like cells.[3,6] Almost all schwannomas stain intensely with S100; this is far less common for neurofibromas.[3,8] To add to the confusion, there are also special forms of schwannomas (including ancient schwannomas, cellular schwannomas, epitheliod schwannomas, and plexiform schwannomas) that all have somewhat different cellular patterns and a modest difference in clinical behavior.[3,6] Malignant schwannomas are uncommon, particularly in patients with NF1; most patients who develop malignancies have neurofibrosarcomas.[3,49]

Clinical Findings in Patients With Neurofibromatosis Type 1

Because genetic identification is so difficult, in 1988 the National Institutes of Health established criteria for clinical diagnosis of NF1.[41,50] A patient with any two of the following findings is considered to have the disease: (1) six or more café au lait spots > 5 mm in diameter; (2) two neurofibromas or one plexiform neurofibroma; (3) optic glioma; (4) two or more Lisch nodules in the iris; (5) freckles in the axilla or inguinal region; (6) distinctive osseous changes that include cortical lesions with external scallops, pseudarthrosis, or dystrophic scoliosis; and (7) a first-degree relative with clinical neurofibromatosis according to criteria 1 through 6.

As noted above, the physical findings for

patients with neurofibromatosis vary considerably. In very young children, there may be no findings other than the café au lait spots and perhaps axillary freckling. As patients get older, additional findings may develop; with very severe disease, patients may show extensive and disabling changes.

The features of the disease that are most evident include:

- *Café au lait spots.*[2,23,25,26] Patients with NF1 may have many café au lait spots; some are quite large. Unlike those seen in patients with fibrous dysplasia with irregular borders (coast of Maine), these have smooth borders (coast of California) (Figure 3).
- *Axillary or inguinal freckling.*[2,23,25,26] Multiple brown spots in the axilla or inguinal region is virtually diagnostic of NF1. Some patients, particularly young ones, may have fewer or no freckles.
- *Lisch granules in the iris.*[3,24,26] These granules are quite distinctive and show as multiple tiny brown spots along the periphery of the iris. They do not cause visual disturbances as a rule, but optic glioma—the other ocular abnormality and a cause of unilateral exophthalmos and blindness—is fortunately rare.
- *Fibroma molluscum bodies.*[2,3,16,29] These small nodular neurofibroma bodies are located subcutaneously and project out as tiny, most often painless, lumps. Some patients have thousands of them throughout the chest, abdomen, extremities, face, and skull. They are sometimes very deforming (Figure 4).
- *Pachydermatocele.*[1-3,23,25-27] These large masses of skin and soft tissues extend like a cape over a shoulder, hip, thigh, or sometimes even the face. They may be discolored and can contain blood vessels sufficient to make them bleed excessively if surgery is attempted.
- *Plexiform neurofibromas.*[1-3,6,23] These large collections of many neurofibromas in a thigh, chest wall, or arm result in enormous enlargement. The lesions sometimes feel like a collection of worms or small nodules. Vascular malformations may be present in these lesions as well (Figure 5).
- *Hemihypertrophy.*[1,2,18,36] Hemihypertrophy usually affects one limb, and leads to gigantism of a body part. Patients

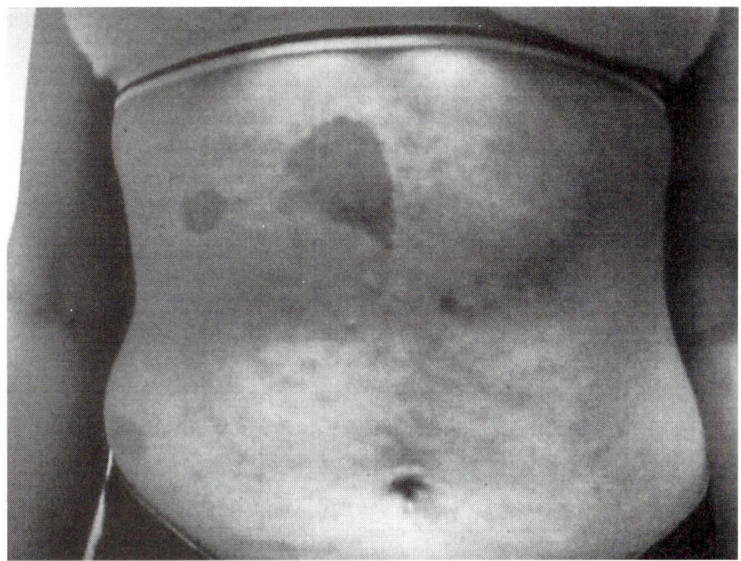

Figure 3
Café au lait skin lesions in a patient with neurofibromatosis type 1, showing the characteristic rounded features of the coast of California.

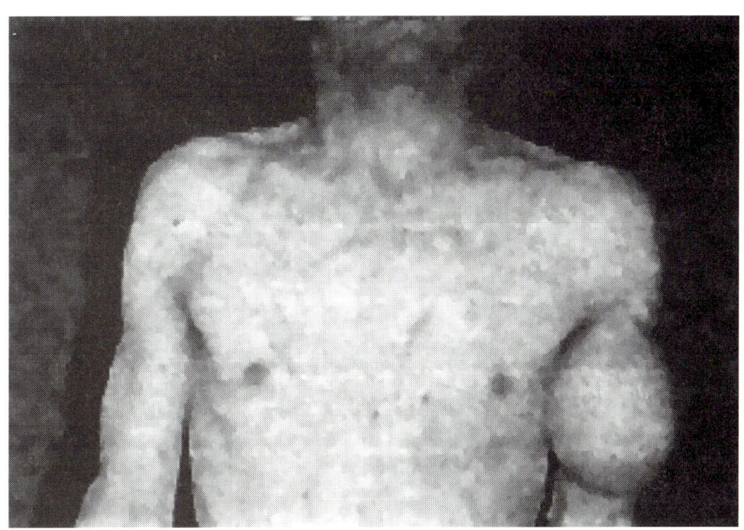

Figure 4
A patient with a severe form of neurofibromatosis type 1 showing a mass on his left arm and multiple fibroma molluscum bodies in his skin.

with this problem sometimes have enormous lower or upper extremities with skin and soft-tissue thickening; the condition has been mistaken for elephantiasis.

- *Neurofibromas.*[2,3,5,25,27] Patients with neurofibromatosis frequently present with masses that are closely attached to nerves. The nerves may be large ones, such as the sciatic, or small, eg, a motor nerve within a muscle. The masses are usually firm, nontender, and often movable. If they cause com-

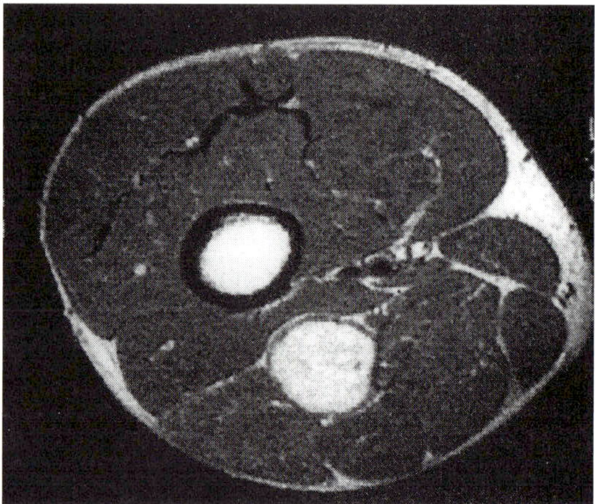

Figure 6
Magnetic resonance image of a solitary lesion of the thigh showing the classic finding of bright color on T1. The lesion is round and presumably is a schwannoma arising from a nerve in the thigh.

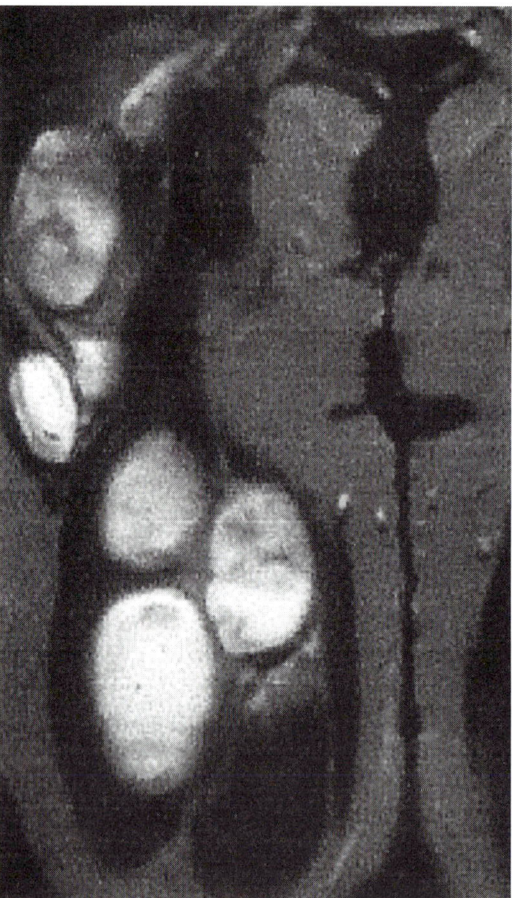

Figure 5
Magnetic resonance image of a plexiform neurofibroma of the thigh, showing numerous rounded nodules that are bright on T2.

pression on the nerve, the patient may experience weakness or numbness in the part distally. Histologically, the masses show all the characteristics of neurofibromas and occasionally may show a pattern consistent with a schwannoma. The lesions are best seen on magnetic resonance imaging (MRI), where they are most frequently light on T2 due to the amount of fluid contained within the tumors (Figure 6).

- *Relationship to fibrous dysplasia and osteomalacia.*[51-53] One of the unusual features of neurofibromatosis is its seeming relationship to disseminated fibrous dysplasia. Both diseases have café au lait spots (coast of Maine for fibrous dysplasia versus coast of California for NF1) and bone deformities (scallops from within in fibrous dysplasia, and scallops from without in NF1). Both disorders also may present with a form of vitamin D-resistant rickets and osteomalacia, which can be quite severe.

- *Mental impairment and psychological problems.*[36,38] Over 30% of the patients with extensive NF1 have modest to moderate diminution in mental capacity, which is not severe enough to require internment but often interferes with school and subsequent work activities. Patients also have psychological problems in part related to their deformities, skin alterations, and limitations of function. They are often reluctant to be involved in social situations.

- *Malignancy.*[2-4,42-45,49] Patients with NF1 have a 10% to 15% chance of developing a neurofibrosarcoma; this not only causes pain and further limitation of function but can metastasize and result in death. The tumors are best seen on MRI and are almost always bright on T2. Most of the lesions are high-grade and one occasionally encounters a malignant schwannoma. Despite the aggressive appearance of both the neurofibrosarcomas and malignant schwannomas, the death rate for both types of tumor is relatively low. In one series of over 100 patients that included both those in whom the tumors arose spontaneously and those with NF1, the survival rate was 81% at 10 ± 5 years; this is considerably better than some other forms of soft-tissue sarcoma.[54]

Bone Disease in Patients With Neurofibromatosis Type 1

Bone disease in patients with NF1 can exhibit the following features:

- *Spinal deformities.*[19,21,36,39,55,56] Approximately 20% of the pediatric patients with NF1 have scoliosis. The majority of them are quite distinctively identified as presenting a "dystrophic" pattern,[36] which shows a sharply angulated curve over several adjacent vertebrae and scalloping of the posterior margins of the segments. The foramina are often enlarged, the canal is widened, the pedicles are defective, and ribs show ribbon-like deformities. These changes are thought to be related to intraspinal neurofibromata and pseudomeningoceles that erode the adjacent bones. The destruction not only leads to sometimes severe scoliosis but also a kyphotic lesion and bony destruction, destabilization, and deformity. Combined kyphosis and scoliosis can result in marked shortening, and sometimes severe pulmonary limitation as well. Surgical treatment of these types of curves is not only difficult, but fraught with danger of excessive bleeding, osseous destabilization and neural injury leading to paraplegia.

- *Nonunion of one or several long bones.*[14,15,19,20,22,36,40,51,55,57-59] Well over 15% of the patients with neurofibromatosis develop nonunion of one or several long bones, often at an early age. The earliest finding is one of bowing—usually of the tibia, but occasionally the ulna, fibula, or femur. The bones may contain cystic lesions and show striking "scalloping from without" cortical erosions that can be quite destructive (Figure 7). The nonunions, which occur often by age 10 years, are sometimes very difficult to treat. Braces can be helpful, but surgical treatment with bone grafts and metallic devices are sometimes more successful. Despite the use of such devices, amputation is sometimes required for tibial or fibular lesions or for problems with the ulna and radius.

- *Other bone and joint problems.*[36,60-62] Deformities of hands, feet, and extremi-

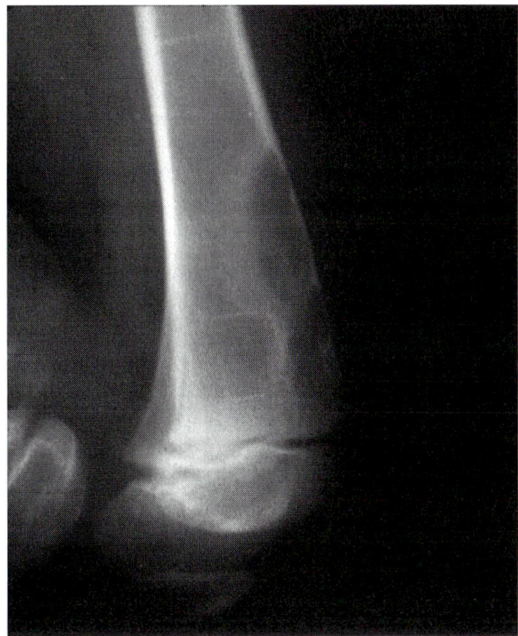

Figure 7
Radiograph of the distal femur of a teenager with a lesion affecting the distal femur. The characteristic pattern observed is a "scallop from without."

ties may be the cause of severe functional impairment and disturbing appearance. Massive enlargement of a limb may be associated with joint destruction or dislocation of the hip, knee, elbow, or shoulder. Macrodactyly can result in hands and feet that function poorly and may require surgical corrections, including partial amputations.

- *Malignancy.*[6,36,43,45,62] As noted above, patients with NF1 are likely to develop neurofibrosarcoma and occasionally malignant schwannoma; however, other types of tumors may occur in the extremities as well. Osteosarcomas, malignant fibrous histiocytomas, and other sarcomas have been reported to occur within a bone of a patient with NF1 and have a high rate of metastasis and patient demise.

The Future for Patients With Neurofibromatosis Type 1

von Recklinghausen's disease probably remains the most common congenital disease today. Many of the patients have a series of deforming afflictions that cause pain, disability, psychological distress, and in some cases early demise. One can treat the individual problems in the extremities, namely the fractures, pseudarthroses, the solitary and even the plexiform neurofibromas, and sometimes the scoliosis. However, the gigantism, hemihypertrophy, blindness, macrodactyly, and especially the skin problems and pachydermatoceles become major problems for many of the patients. We have limited ability to help these individuals. The best hope at this point might be some form of genetic therapy. Regrettably, there are so many deviations and abnormalities in the gene structure that until this point none of the usual approaches seem likely to have any effect. For the sake of the patients, families, and physicians who deal with this frequently occurring disease, we hope that some reasonable approach will be forthcoming in the near future.

References

1. Crowe FW, Schull JW, Neel JV: *A Clinical, Pathological and Genetic Study of Multiple Neurofibromatosis.* Springfield, IL, Charles C. Thomas, 1956.

2. Hajdu SI: *Pathology of Soft Tissue Tumors.* Philadelphia, PA, Lea and Febiger, 1979, pp 427-482.

3. Weiss S, Goldblum JR: *Enzinger and Weiss Soft Tissue Tumors,* ed 4. St. Louis, MO, Mosby Inc, 2001, pp 1111-1263.

4. Doorn PF, Molenaar WM, Buter J, Hoekstra NJ: Malignant peripheral nerve sheath tumors in patients with and without neurofibromatosis. *Eur J Surg Oncol* 1995;21:78-82.

5. Ferner RE, O'Doherty MJ: Neurofibroma and schwannoma. *Curr Opin Neurol* 2002;15:679-684.

6. Korf BR: Clinical features and pathobiology of neurofibromatosis 1. *J Child Neurol* 2002;17:573-577.

7. Antoni NRE: *Ueber Ruckenmarkstumoren und Neurofibrome.* Munich, Germany, JF Bergman, 1920.

8. Reith JD, Goldblum JR: Multiple cutaneous plexiform schwannomas: Report of a case and review of the literature with particular reference to the association with types 1 and 2 neurofibromatosis and schwannomatosis. *Arch Pathol Lab Med* 1996;120:399-401.

9. Sanchez GM, Siuda T: Ebers papyrus case #873: A probable case of neurofibromatosis type 1. *S D J Med* 2002;55:529-535.

10. Smith RW: *Treatise on the Pathology, Diagnosis and Treatment of Neuroma.* Dublin, Ireland, Hodges and Smith, 1849.

11. von Recklinghausen FD: *Über die Multiplen Fibromen der Haut und Ihre Beziehung zu den Multplen Neuromen.* Berlin, Germany, A Hirschwald, 1882.

12. Chaffaurd AME: Xanthelasma dissemine et symmetrique, sans insuffisance hepatique. *Bull Mem Soc Med Hosp* 1889;6:412-423.

13. Thomson R: *On Neuroma and Neurofibromatosis.* Edinburgh, Scotland, Turnbull and Spears, 1900.

14. Ali MS, Hooper G: Congenital pseudarthrosis of the ulna due to neurofibromatosis. *J Bone Joint Surg Br* 1982;64:600-602.

15. Barber CG: Congenital bowing and pseudarthrosis of the lower leg: Manifestations of von Recklinghausen's neurofibromatosis. *Surg Gynecol Obstet* 1939;69:618-626.

16. Brasfield RD, Das Gupta TK: Von Recklinghausen's disease: A clinicopathological study. *Ann Surg* 1972;175:86-104.

17. Findlay M, Denny MBM: Radiological features of neurofibromatosis. *Afr J Med Med Sci* 1955;29:375-381.

18. Floyd A, Percy-Lancaster R: The elephant woman: Neurofibromatosis associated with psuedoarthrosis of the humerus. *J Bone Joint Surg Br* 1987;69:121-123.

19. Friedman MM: Neurofibromatosis of bone. *AJR Am J Roentgenol* 1944;51:623-630.

20. Green WT, Rudo N: Pseudarthrosis and neurofibromatosis. *Arch Surg* 1943;46:639-651.

21. Holt JF, Wright EM: The radiologic features of neurofibromatosis. *Radiology* 1948;51:647-664.

22. Hunt JC, Pugh DG: Skeletal lesions in neurofibromatosis. *Radiology* 1961;76:1-20.

23. Karnes PS: Neurofibromatosis: A common neurocutaneous disorder. *Mayo Clin Proc* 1998;73:1071-1076.

24. Lubs ML, Bauer MS, Formas ME, Djokic B: Lisch nodule in neurofibromatosis type 1. *N Engl J Med* 1991;324:1264-1266.

25. Morse RP: Neurofibromatosis type 1. *Arch Neurol* 1999;56:364-365.

26. Otsuka F, Kawashima T, Iamakado S, Usuki Y, Hon-Mura S: Lisch nodules and skin manifestations in neurofibromatosis type 1. *Arch Dermatol* 2001;137:232-233.

27. Reynolds RM, Browning GG, Nawroz I, Campbell IW: Von Recklinghausen's neurofibromatosis: Neurofibromatosis type 1. *Lancet* 2003;361:1552-1554.

28. Riccardi VM: Von Recklinghausen neurofibromatosis. *N Engl J Med* 1981;305:1617-1627.

29. Kaplan P, Rosenblatt B: A distinctive facial appearance in neurofibromatosis von Recklinghausen. *Am J Med Genet* 1985;21:463-470.

30. Uhlmann E, Grossman A: Von Recklinghausen's neurofibromatosis with bone manifestations. *Ann Intern Med* 1940;14:225-241.

31. Barker D, Wright E, Nguyen L: Gene for von Recklinghausen neurofibromatosis is in the pericentromeric region of chromosome 17. *Science* 1987;236:1100-1102.

32. Chong JA, Moran MM, Teichmann M, Kaczmarek JS, Roeder R, Clapham DE: TATA-binding protein (TBP)-like factor (TLF) is a functional regulator of transcription: Reciprocal regulation of the neurofibromatosis type 1 and c-fos genes by TLF/TRF2 and TBP. *Mol Cell Biol* 2005;25:2632-2643.

33. Horan MP, Osborn M, Cooper DN, Upadhyaya M: Functional analysis of polymorphic variation within the promoter and 5' untranslated region of neurofibromatosis type 1 (NF1) gene. *Am J Med Genet A* 2004;131:227-231.

34. Stephens K: Genetics of neurofibromatosis 1-associated peripheral nerve sheath tumors. *Cancer Invest* 2003;21:897-914.

35. Viskochil D: Genetics of neurofibromatosis 1 and the NF1 gene. *J Child Neurol* 2002;17:562-570.

36. Vitale MG, Guha A, Skaggs DL: Orthopaedic manifestations of neurofibromatosis in children: An update. *Clin Orthop Relat Res* 2002;401:107-118.

37. Ward K, O'Connell P, Carey JC, et al: Diagnosis of neurofibromatosis I by using tightly linked, flanking DNA markers. *Am J Hum Genet* 1990;46:943-949.

38. Johnson NS, Saal HM, Lovell AM, Schorry EK: Social and emotional problems in children with neurofibromatosis type 1: Evidence and proposed interventions. *J Pediatr* 1999;134:767-772.

39. Funasaki H, Winter RB, Lonstein JB, Denis F: Pathophysiology of spinal deformities in neurofibromatosis: An analysis of seventy-one patients who had curves associated with dystrophic changes. *J Bone Joint Surg Am* 1994;76:692-700.

40. Jacobs JE, Kimmelsteil P, Thompson KR Jr: Neurofibromatosis and pseudarthrosis: Report of a case. *Arch Surg* 1949;59:232-239.

41. DeBella K, Szudek J, Friedman JM: Use of the National Institutes of Health criteria for diagnosis of neurofibromatosis 1 in children. *Pediatrics* 2000;105:608-614.

42. Korf BR: Malignancy in neurofibromatosis type 1. *Oncologist* 2000;5:477-485.

43. Poyhonen M, Niemela S, Herva R: Risk of malignancy and death in neurofibromatosis. *Arch Pathol Lab Med* 1997;121:139-143.

44. Shearer P, Parham D, Kovnar E: Neurofibromatosis type 1 and malignancy: Review of 32 pediatric cases treated in a single institution. *Med Pediatr Oncol* 1994;22:78-83.

45. Sorensen SA, Mulvihill JJ, Nielsen A: Long-term follow-up of von Recklinghausen neurofibromatosis: Survival and malignant neoplasms. *N Engl J Med* 1986;314:1010-1015.

46. Arun D, Gutmann DH: Recent advances in neurofibromatosis type 1. *Curr Opin Neurol* 2004;17:101-105.

47. Garavelli L, Donadio A, Sigorini M, Grassi L, Banchini G: Genetics of type 1 neurofibromatosis. *Acta Biomed Ateneo Parmense.* 2000;71:89-95.

48. Gutmann DH: Recent insights into neurofibromatosis type 1: Clear genetic progress. *Arch Neurol* 1998;55:778-780.

49. Cashen DV, Parisien RC, Raskin K, Hornicek FJ, Gebhardt MC, Mankin H: Survival data for patients with malignant schwannoma. *Clin Orthop Relat Res* 2004;426:69-73.

50. Conference of the National Institutes of Health Consensus Development: Neurofibromatosis. Conference statement. *Arch Neurol* 1988;45:575-578.

51. Aegerter EE: The possible relationship of neurofibromatosis, congenital pseudarthrosis and fibrous dysplasia. *J Bone Joint Surg Am* 1950;32:618-626.

52. Hogan DB, Anderson C, MacKenzie RA, Crilly RG: Hypophosphatemic osteomalacia complicating von Recklinghausen's neurofibromatosis: Increase in spinal density on treatment. *Bone* 1986;7:9-12.

53. Mundy GR: Osteomalacia and rickets, in *Bone Remodeling and Its Disorders,* ed 2. London, England, Martin Dunitz, 1999, pp 200-207.

54. Mankin HJ, Hornicek FJ: Diagnosis, classification and management of soft tissue sarcomas. *Cancer Control* 2005;12:5-21.

55. Brooks B, Lehman EP: The bone changes in Recklinghausen's neurofibromatosis. *Surg Gynecol Obstet* 1924;38:587-595.

56. Chaglassian JH, Riseborough EJ, Hall JE: Neurofibromatous scoliosis: Natural history and results of treatment of thirty-seven cases. *J Bone Joint Surg Am* 1976;58:695-702.

57. Boyd HB: Pathology and natural history of congenital pseudarthrosis of the tibia. *Clin Orthop Relat Res* 1982;166:5-13.

58. Hayashi S, Kobayashi D, Satsuma S, Yoshiya S, Kurosaka M: Acquired pseudarthrosis of the radius and ulna in a neurofibromatosis patient with radiographic normal bone: A case report. *J Hand Surg [Am]* 2005;30:168-171.

59. Stevenson DA, Birch PH, Friedman JM, et al: Descriptive analysis of pseudarthrosis of the tibia in patients with neurofibromatosis type 1. *Am J Med Genet* 1999;84:413-419.

60. Hensley CC Jr: The rapid development of a "subperiosteal bone cyst" in multiple neurofibromatosis. *J Bone Joint Surg Am* 1953;35:197-203.

61. Sane S, Yunis E, Greer R: Subperiosteal or cortical cyst and intramedullary neurofibromatosis: Uncommon manifestations of neurofibromatosis. *J Bone Joint Surg Am* 1971;53:1194-1201.

62. Weber FP: Periosteal neurofibromatosis with a short consideration of the whole subject of neurofibromatosis. *Q J Med* 1930;23:151-165.

Chapter 19

Scurvy

Scurvy is one of the oldest diseases of the human race. Studies have shown findings suggestive of the disorder in ancient Egyptians and the prehistoric people who lived in Peru and the southern US.[1-3] The disorder was very prevalent in seamen, who were confined to sailing vessels for long periods of time and were limited in their access to certain key foods.[4-8] They bled from their gums; lost teeth; and had sometimes severe extremity problems with bleeding, poor wound healing, and vascular disturbances.[4-14] Psychological issues were common, along with brain injury; many of the crew members on long excursions died from the disease.[4-7,15]

A second group of patients who developed a severe form of the disorder were children who received very limited dietary supplements of fresh citrus fruits. In addition to the bleeding, oral, and psychological disturbances similar to the adults, the children very frequently presented with bone and especially epiphyseal and periosteal disorders, as well as motor weakness and deformities.[16-22]

The disease in humans is a consequence of a genetic error in enzyme production, which appears to have originated as a mutation in a primitive primate precursor of man as long as 60 million years ago.[23-26] In order to avoid scurvy, glucose must be converted in the liver to produce l-ascorbate, an endogenous vitamin C that prevents the disease.[23,24] The conversion requires four enzymes. Most animals have all four and are successful in producing l-ascorbate; however, humans, guinea pigs, and a few other unfortunate creatures are incapable of synthesizing the fourth enzyme (l-gulonolactone oxidase) in the liver; this material is necessary for the last step in the synthetic process for the l-ascorbate.[25,26] Without the product of this enzyme production, collagen and proteoglycan synthesis is diminished and the patient develops a bizarre syndrome known as scurvy. If untreated, scurvy can lead to very serious physical and mental problems and can

cause death. With the addition of either citrus fruits in the diet or exogenous administration of ascorbate in the form of vitamin C, the disease can be eliminated and the patients restored to good health in a relatively short period of time.[11,25,27-30]

History of Scurvy

The history of scorbutic disorders is a remarkable saga—one that really has no parallel among other disease states. The earliest reported cases were in sailors who were at sea for prolonged periods.[5,6] In 1499, Vasco da Gamma lost two thirds of his crew when sailing from the Mediterranean to India; in 1520, Magellan lost more than 80% of his sailors on his vessel on his voyage across the Pacific.[5,6,8,11] In 1535, Jacques Cartier and his crew sailed up the St. Lawrence River in midwinter and his ships were frozen in ice for 5 months. Twenty-five of his 112 sailors died of a disease that was later identified as scurvy; the rest survived because they received some plant food that contained l-ascorbate from Indians.[7] The illness that affected all of these sailors was clearly described. It was characterized by generalized weakness, ecchymoses, joint pain, internal hemorrhages, "black legs," loss of teeth, gingival hemorrhages and enlargement, proptosis, foul breath, "corkscrew hair" on the extremities, draining wounds, and psychological disturbances.[5-7,15,31] Many of the patients became irritable and demented, and finally became unresponsive and died.[5-8,15,31-33] In "The Rime of the Ancient Mariner," written by Samuel Taylor Coleridge in 1798,[34] the sailor's problems were remarkably well described with two famous lines—"With throats unslaked, with black lips baked we could not laugh nor wail", and "Four times fifty living men (and I heard not a sigh nor a groan) with heavy thump, a lifeless lump, they dropped down one by one."

The sailors' world changed dramatically with a remarkable discovery by Scottish physician James Lind (1716-1794), who worked with the Royal Navy.[35] In 1747, Lind conducted a classic experiment aboard the

Salisbury.[8] He chose 12 patients with severe scorbutic findings and for a 6-day period gave each of the 6 pairs of men either cider, elixir of vitriol, vinegar, seawater, nutmeg paste, or oranges and lemons. The patients receiving the oranges and lemons made a remarkable recovery in 6 days, and it was apparent that the citrus fruits were the "cure" for the scorbutic changes.[6,8,15,35,36] Sailors in the Royal Navy became known as "limeys" for that reason, and to this date the protocol proposed by Lind and supported by many others provides a means of introducing ascorbic acid in the form of vitamin C, preventing the disease.[6,37]

A second form of the disease is known as "infantile scurvy" or Barlow's disease. Moller[38] described scorbutic children in his article on rickets published in 1859. In 1882, Cheadle[17] described a disease characterized by osteal and periosteal lesions associated with cachexia. A year later, Thomas Barlow[16] established infantile scurvy as a clinical entity based on the study of a group of children who were thought to have rickets but clearly had findings more characteristic of scurvy. The scurvy in children became known as Moller-Barlow disease. The children had swollen ecchymotic limbs with marked subperiosteal hemorrhages and often severe damage to the epiphyses, along with bleeding, dental, and gingival problems analogous to those seen in the 18th century sailors.[11,17-21,33,39-48] Some of the patients died of the disease before Barlow appropriately suggested that citrus fruits could effectively prevent or cure the disorder.[16]

Of considerable importance was the identification of vitamin C by Szent-Gyorgyi in 1929.[37] Since these basic discoveries, the disease has become far less common. With the use of vitamin C, along with increased popularity of fresh orange juice and lemons and limes, scurvy is rarely encountered today. Many of the patients with the disease are either in disadvantaged countries where child starvation is a problem, or have other disease states or bizarre eating habits that limit their access to ascorbic acid.[9,22,42,47,49-58]

Perhaps the most unusual cause of scurvy is the treatment of orange juice and milk with excessive heat by overconcerned parents in order to prevent infection. These procedures inactivate the ascorbic acid, and the children are unable to obtain vitamin C without additional sources.[21,42,49,59,60]

Orthopaedic Findings in Patients With Scurvy

Scurvy in adults is now quite rare; most of the manifestations of the adult form of the disease in sporadic reports are vascular or affect the skin, teeth, and gingival tissue.[13,14,39,43-45,47,52,61] Proptosis, partial blindness, and skull deformities may be present as well as irritability and mental confusion.[9,45,46,62] The childhood variant, however, is primarily nutritional and orthopaedic in nature and produces some very unusual findings both clinically and on imaging studies. The disease is rare in children under the age of 6 months.[18-20,41] After age 6 months, the scorbutic child becomes progressively smaller in height and weighs far less than normal.[18,21,41] Skin pallor is the rule; frequently ecchymotic spots are noted, along with wounds that heal slowly.[18,63] The limbs are noted to be markedly tender and swollen, and in older children may be covered with corkscrew hair.[18,21] The patients may show pseudoparalysis and contractures of the limbs, and are often irritable and anorexic with a poor attention span.[21,22] They occasionally are febrile and have respiratory difficulties.[18] Blood studies show anemia and sometimes a low white blood cell count.[21,52] The alkaline phosphatase is almost always low; the serum ascorbic acid and especially the white cell ascorbic acid are very low.[18,21]

Scurvy of the bones and epiphyses is another "eponymic playground." The terms "Wimberger epiphyses,"[64] "Pelkan's spurs,"[65] "white line of Fraenkel,"[66] and the scurvy line and scorbutic rosary[27] are all uniquely related to the clinical findings and especially to the radiographic imaging of children with the disease. In severe cases, the findings may be striking.[19,21,27,48] Because there is a failure of appropriate synthesis of collagen and proteoglycan, the bony and cartilaginous tissues do not grow normally. Children show slow epiphyseal growth and are frequently stunted in height.[19,21,27] Their deciduous teeth do not appear at the appropriate age and at times fall out; the gums are swollen and bleed excessively.[13,18,21] The bones have thin cortices and the marrow cavity has few trabeculae, thus the patients are prone to fracture[19,21,27,48] (Figure 1). Radiographs of the long bones show a finding described as ground glass medullary bone, as a

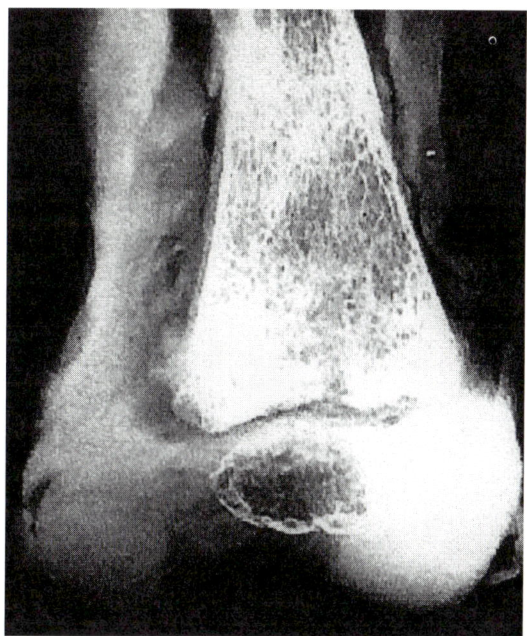

Figure 1

Photograph of a section of the distal femur showing the poorly developed bone, radiolucent epiphysis, and the hemorrhagic subperiosteal collection.

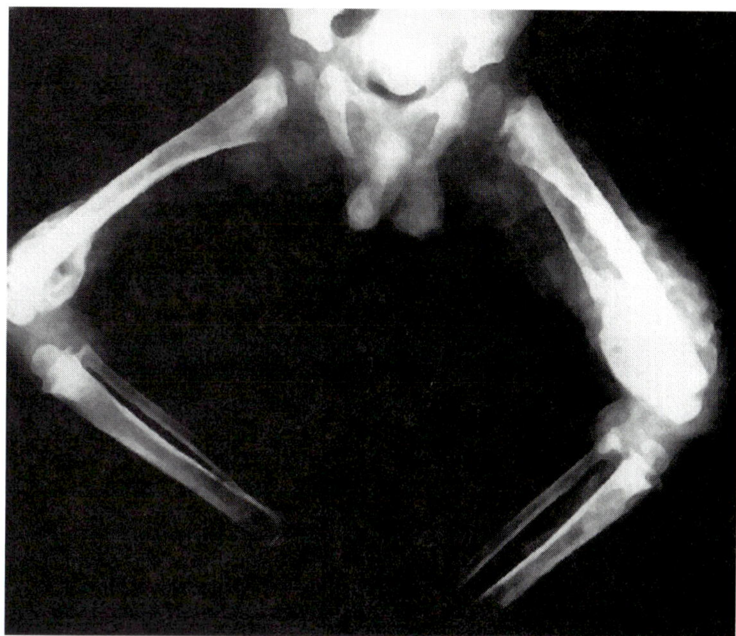

Figure 2

Radiograph of the lower extremities of a child with very severe scurvy shows the periosteal collections of blood that calcify and lead to marked pain and deformity.

result of the absence or limited size of trabecular segments.[18,27,65] One of the remarkable features is the subperiosteal hemorrhaging, which results in marked swelling and pain in the affected limb and severe limitation in movement and ambulation.[18,27] The femur, tibia, humerus, or radius may show enormously wide bony structures on radiographic examination; these often calcify (Figure 2).

The striking features on imaging of the long bones are the radiolucent central portion of the epiphysis known as Wimberger's epiphysis[64] (Figure 3), the dense white line adjacent to the metaphyseal region but apart from the zone of primary spongiosa that is known as the white line of Fraenkel,[66] and the spurring of the metaphyseal bone just adjacent to the epiphyseal plate that is known as Pelkan's spurs.[65] Frequently a radiolucent line is seen adjacent to the white line of Fraenkel; this anomaly is called scurvy line.[27]

The histologic pictures confirm these findings. The metaphyseal regions have large numbers of osteoblasts that do not form bone; usually little or no osteoid can be seen.[27] The marrow space is filled with poorly arranged, loose fibrous tissue; only a few red and white blood cells are evident.

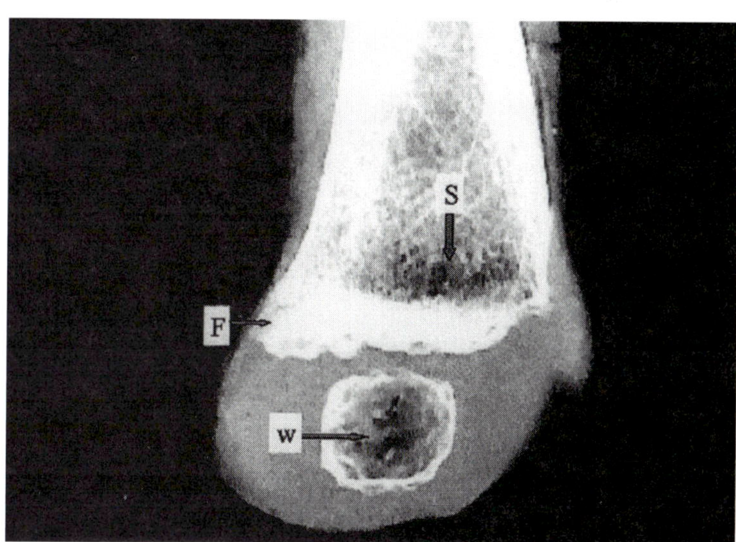

Figure 3

The distal femoral epiphysis and metaphysis of a child with severe scorbutic disease. Note the thin cortices and ground glass appearance of the medullary bone. W = Wimberger's epiphysis, F = white line of Fraenkel, S = scurvy line.

The white line of Fraenkel in the metaphysis is an irregular calcific dense line a short distance from the calcified zone and zone of primary spongiosa of the epiphyseal plate, and the scurvy line is a region of poor bone formation on the metaphyseal side of the white line[27] (Figure 4). Pelkan's spurs are prominent projections of the metaphyseal bone, more often on the medial than the lateral side and presumably caused by fractures or malformations. Wimberger's epiphyses are caused by the absence of bone in the central portion of the physis.

The ribs may show the changes described above, but frequently have another remarkable and very deforming abnormality. The cartilaginous portions of the ribs at the costochondral junctions subluxate because of malformation of cartilaginous tissue and poor bone formation at the site.[27] This results in a marked prominence of the bony end of the ribs known as the scorbutic rosary[27,48] (Figure 5). This change must be distinguished from the rachitic rosary, which consists of enlargements of the costochondral junctions as a result of excessive epiphyseal cartilage masses but without displacement of the tissues.[27]

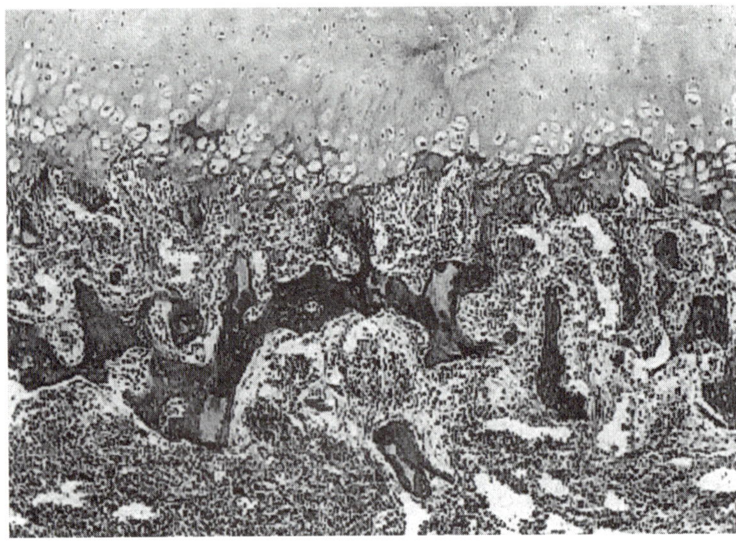

Figure 4
Histologic section of the distal femoral metaphysis of a child with scurvy showing the dense bone present in the white line of Fraenkel. Hematoxylin and eosin × 60.

Treatment of Scurvy

Scurvy clearly can be prevented or eliminated by administration of ascorbic acid in citrus fruits or other foodstuffs or in pill form as vitamin C. Clinical scurvy is rare in the US today except in the presence of some unusual entities such as anorexia,[51,56] Crohn's disease,[55] and some forms of cancer.[53] Some parts of the world have extraordinary frequency of the entity, particularly in children. Afghanistan and other countries with poor dietary supplements and lack of additional oral vitamin capsules may have large numbers of children with scorbutic lesions.[50] Even if citrus fruits are unavailable, vitamin C supplements are inexpensive and should be administered to all children.

The daily requirements for vitamin C vary with age.[59,60,67] For infants, 30 to 40 mg per day is adequate, while for children and adults the daily dose should be increased to 45 to 70 mg per day. Pregnant women and lactating mothers should have higher doses of 70 to 95 mg per day. Food sources of vitamin C include citrus fruits, berries, cantaloupe, broccoli, cauliflower, cabbage, spinach, potatoes, and tomatoes. Heating these foods, particularly the fruits and their juices, can destroy the ascorbate.

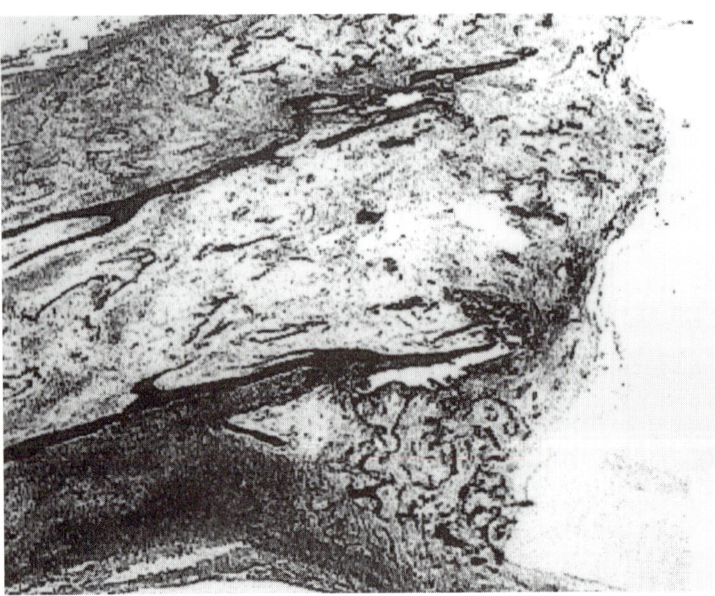

Figure 5
Histologic section of the rib at the costochondral junction showing the displacement and new bone formation characteristic of the scorbutic rosary. Hematoxylin and eosin × 40.

References

1. Nerlich AG, Rhorbach H, Zink A: Paleopathology of ancient Egyptian mummies and skeletons: Investigations on the occurrence and frequency of specific diseases during various time periods in the necropolis of Thebes-West. *Pathologe* 2002;23:379-385.

2. Ortner DJ, Butler W, Cafarella J, Milligan L: Evidence of probable scurvy in subadults from archeological sites in North America. *Am J Phys Anthropol* 2001;114:343-351.

3. Ortner DJ, Kimmrele EH, Diez M: Probable evidence of scurvy in subadults from archeological

sites in Peru. *Am J Phys Anthropol* 1999;108:321-331.

4. Bartholomew M: James Lind's Treatise of the Scurvy (1753). *Postgrad Med J* 2002;78:695-696.

5. Burnby J, Bierman A: The incidence of scurvy at sea and its treatment. *Rev Hist Pharm (Paris)* 1996;44:339-346.

6. Cook GC: Scurvy in the British Mercantile Marine in the 19th century and the contribution of the Seamen's Hospital Society. *Postgrad Med J* 2004;80:224-229.

7. Martini E: Jacques Cartier witnesses a treatment for scurvy. *Vesalius* 2002;8:2-6.

8. Sutton G: Putrid gums and 'dead men's cloaths': James Lind aboard the Salisbury. *J R Soc Med* 2003;96:605-608.

9. DeSantis J: Scurvy and psychiatric symptoms. *Perspect Psychiatr Care* 1993;29:18-22.

10. Hirschmann JV, Raugi GJ: Adult scurvy. *J Am Acad Dermatol* 1999;41:895-906.

11. Hodges RE, Hood J, Canham JE, Sauberlich HE, Baker EM: Clinical manifestations of ascorbic acid deficiency in man. *Am J Clin Nutr* 1971;24:432-443.

12. Reuler JB, Broudy VC, Cooney TG: Adult scurvy. *JAMA* 1985;253:805-807.

13. Touyz LZ: Oral scurvy and periodontal disease. *J Can Dent Assoc* 1997;63:837-845.

14. Warshauer DM, Hayes ME, Shumer SM: Scurvy: A clinical mimic of vasculitis. *Cutis* 1984;34:539-541.

15. Pimentel L: Scurvy: Historical review and current diagnostic approach. *Am J Emerg Med* 2003;21:328-332.

16. Barlow T: On cases described as "acute rickets" which are probably a combination of scurvy and rickets, the scurvy being an essential and thrice a variable element. *Med Surg Trans* 1883;66:159-219.

17. Cheadle WB: Osteal or periosteal cachexia and scurvy. *Lancet* 1882;2:48-49.

18. Clemetson CA: Barlow's disease. *Med Hypotheses* 2002;59:52-56.

19. Fairbank T: Infantile scurvy, in *An Atlas of General Affections of the Skeleton*. Edinburgh, Scotland, E & S Livingstone, Ltd, 1951, pp 231-240.

20. Griffith JPC, Jenning CG, Morse JL: The America Pediatric Society's collective investigation of infantile scurvy in North America. *Boston Med Surg J* 1898;138:605-609.

21. Rajakumar K: Infantile scurvy: A historical perspective. *Pediatrics* 2001;108:E76.

22. Tamura Y, Welch DC, Zie JA, Cooper WO, Stein SM, Hummell DS: Scurvy presenting as painful gait with bruising in a young boy. *Arch Pediatr Adolesc Med* 2000;154:732-735.

23. Burns JJ: Biosynthesis of l-ascorbic acid; basic defect in scurvy. *Am J Med* 1959;26:740-748.

24. Chatterjee IB: Evolution and the biosynthesis of ascorbic acid. *Science* 1973;182:1271-1272.

25. Inai T, Ohta Y, Nishikimi M: The whole structure of the human nonfunctional L-gulono-gamma-lactone oxidase gene: The gene responsible for scurvy and the evolution of repetitive sequences thereon. *J Nutr Sci Vitaminol (Tokyo)* 2003;49:315-319.

26. Padayatty SJ, Levine M: New insights in the physiology and pharmacology of vitamin C. *CMAJ* 2001;164:353-355.

27. Jaffe H: Scurvy and certain other vitamin-conditioned disorders, in *Metabolic, Degenerative and Inflammatory Diseases of Bones and Joints*. Philadelphia, PA, Lea and Febiger, 1973, pp 448-478.

28. Johnston CS, Solomon RE, Corte C: Vitamin C depletion is associated with alterations in blood histamine and plasma free carnitine in adults. *J Am Coll Nutr* 1996;15:586-591.

29. Parsons LG: Scurvy treated with ascorbic acid. *Proc R Soc Med* 1933;23:1533.

30. Wilson LG: The clinical definition of scurvy and the discovery of Vitamin C. *J Hist Med Allied Sci* 1975;30:40-60.

31. Oeffinger KC: Scurvy: More than historical relevance. *Am Fam Physician* 1993;48:609-613.

32. Sudbury S, Ford P: Femoral head destruction in scurvy. *J Rheumatol* 1990;17:1108-1110.

33. Yalcin A, Ural AU, Beyan C, Tastan B, Demiriz M, Cetin T: Scurvy presenting with cutaneous and articular signs and decrease in red and white blood cells. *Int J Dermatol* 1996;35:879-881.

34. Coleridge ST: The Rime of the Ancient Mariner: Part III. 1798.

35. Lind J: *A Treatise of the Scurvy*. Edinburgh, Scotland, Sands Murray and Cochrane, 1753.

36. Dunn PM: James Lind (1716-94) of Edinburgh and the treatment of scurvy. *Arch Dis Child Fetal Neonatal Ed* 1997;76:F64-F65.

37. Szent-Gyorgyi A: Observations on the function of peroxidase system and the chemistry of the adrenal cortex: Description of a new carbohydrate derivative. *Biochem J* 1929;22:137-140.

38. Moller JO: Uber acute rachitis. *Konigsberg Med J* 1859;1:377-379.

39. Adelman HM, Wallach PM, Gutierrez F, et al: Scurvy resembling cutaneous vasculitis. *Cutis* 1994;54:111-114.

40. Adetona N, Kramarenko W, McGavin CR: Retinal changes in scurvy. *Eye* 1994;8:709-710.

41. Akikusa JD, Garrick D, Nash MC: Scurvy: Forgotten but not gone. *J Paediatr Child Health* 2003;39:75-77.

42. Bingham AC, Kimura Y, Imundo L: A 16-year-old boy with purpura and leg pain. *J Pediatr* 2003;142:560-563.

43. Blankenhorn MA: Effect of vitamin deficiency on the heart and circulation. *Circulation* 1955;11:288-291.

44. Bloxham CA, Clough C, Beevers DG: Retinal infarcts and hemorrhages due to scurvy. *Postgrad Med J* 1990;66:687.

45. De Luna RH, Colley BJ III, Smith K, Divers SG, Rinehart J, Marques MB: Scurvy: An often forgotten cause of bleeding. *Am J Hematol* 2003;74:85-87.

46. Hood J, Hodges RE: Ocular lesion in scurvy. *Am J Clin Nutr* 1969;22:559-567.

47. Nguyen RT, Cowley DM, Muir JB: Scurvy: A cutaneous clinical diagnosis. *Australas J Dermatol* 2003;44:48-51.

48. Quiles M, Sanz TA: Epiphyseal separation in scurvy. *J Pediatr Orthop* 1988;8:223-225.

49. Barratt JA, Summers GD: Scurvy, osteoporosis and megaloblastic anaemia due to alleged food intolerance. *Br J Rheumatol* 1996;35:701-702.

50. Cheung E, Mutahar R, Assefa F, et al: An epidemic of scurvy in Afghanistan: Assessment and response. *Food Nutr Bull* 2003;24:247-255.

51. Christopher K, Tammaro D, Wing EJ: Early scurvy complicating anorexia nervosa. *South Med J* 2002;95:1065-1066.

52. Cohen SA, Paeglow RJ: Scurvy: An unusual cause of anemia. *J Am Board Fam Pract* 2001;14:314-316.

53. Fain O, Mathieu E, Thomas M: Scurvy in patients with cancer. *BMJ* 1998;316:1661-1662.

54. Hampl JS, Johnston CS, Mills RA: Scourge of black-leg (scurvy) on the Mormon trail. *Nutrition* 2001;17:416-418.

55. Linaker BD: Scurvy and vitamin C deficiency in Crohn's disease. *Postgrad Med J* 1979;55:26-29.

56. Mehta CL, Cripps D, Bridges AJ: Systemic pseudo-vasculitis from scurvy in anorexia nervosa. *Arthritis Rheum* 1996;39:532-533.

57. Shetty AK, Buckingham RB, Kilian PH, Girdany D, Meyerowitz R: Hemarthrosis and femoral head destruction in an adult diet faddist with scurvy. *J Rheumatol* 1988;15:1878-1880.

58. Walter JF: Scurvy resulting from a self-imposed diet. *West J Med* 1979;130:177-179.

59. Gerster H: Human vitamin C requirements. *Z Ernahrungswiss* 1987;26:125-137.

60. Levine M, Rumsey SC, Daruwala R, Park JB, Wang Y: Criteria and recommendations for vitamin C intake. *JAMA* 1999;281:1415-1423.

61. Pangan AL, Robinson D: Hemarthrosis as initial presentation of scurvy. *J Rheumatol* 2001;28:1923-1925.

62. Sloan B, Kulwin DR, Kersten RC: Scurvy causing bilateral orbital hemorrhage. *Arch Ophthalmol* 1999;117:842-843.

63. Shtasel DL, Krell H: Scurvy in schizophrenia. *Psychiatr Serv* 1995;46:293.

64. Wimberger H: Klinisch-radiologische diagnostik von rachitis, skorbut und lues congenita in kinde-salter. *Ergebn Inn Med U Kinderh* 1925;28:264-270.

65. Pelkan KF: Roentgenogram in early scurvy. *Am J Dis Child* 1925;30:174-188.

66. Fraenkel E: *De Moller-Barlowshe Krankheit*. Hamburg, Germany, L Grafe and Sillem, 1908.

67. Bartley W, Krebs HA, O'Brien JRP: *Vitamin C requirements in human adults*. Medical Council Research Report Series No 280. London, England, Her Majesty's Stationary Office, 1953, pp 1-179.

Chapter 20

Rickets, Osteomalacia, and Renal Osteodystrophy

Rickets and osteomalacia are disorders of bone mineral metabolism that occur as a result of insufficient amounts of available calcium, phosphorus, and/or vitamin D, all of which are required to maintain normal skeletal structure. Rickets occurs in childhood and affects not only the bone structure, but in a very unusual way the epiphyseal cartilage as well. The Latin term osteomalacia suggests weakened or softened adult bone. Rickets and osteomalacia have cursed the human race since ancient times, causing poor growth, skeletal deformities, mental disturbances, fractures, and sometimes severe disability. Despite the momentous discovery that vitamin D prevents or cures the disease, large geographic segments of the world still have children with rickets and adults with osteomalacia because of poor diet and inadequate health care systems. Renal osteodystrophy describes the bone lesions associated with chronic renal disease. The bones show changes of osteomalacia but are also associated with often quite severe hyperparathyroidism, another cause of structural loss of bone from the skeleton.

History of Rickets

Rickets (or "rachitis") is an ancient disease. The abnormalities seen in the skeleton were recorded centuries before the early medical literature citations. Some of the figures seen in early paintings of religious events suggest rachitic changes in the bones and skull, and there is little doubt that the changes associated with rickets occurred in children throughout the early days of human development. The structural alterations in the skeleton associated with rickets were first described by Daniel Whistler in 1645,[1] but the disease was not identified as an entity until Francis Glisson described the disorder in a group of patients in 1650.[2] According to Glisson and others, the name rickets probably derived from the old English terms "wrick" or "wrikken," meaning to twist an anatomic part, or possibly from the term "wrygates" meaning crooked gait.[2] Some authors have proposed that the term rachitis may come from the Greek word "rachis," meaning spine. Glisson's description was remarkably accurate. He described children 6 months of age or older with altered bony anatomy, bowing or knock-knee deformities of the lower extremities, prominence of the epiphyseal ends of the bones, frontal bossing of the calvarium, and prominent rib ends (now known as the rachitic rosary).[2] Because of the similarity of rachitic and scorbutic changes in the bone and soft tissues, rickets and scurvy were confused in early times. Thomas Barlow[3] successfully separated the findings of the two diseases and clearly established rickets as a clinical entity in 1883. Barlow was born in 1845 and lived to be 100 years old—thus he survived long enough to not only describe the disease but to identify sunlight and clean air as treatment protocols for rickets. McCollum[4,5] discovered that fresh milk and cod liver oil were a competent treatment system for animals made rachitic by diet. In 1903, Jakob Erdheim[6] described the increased size and activity of the parathyroid glands in patients with osteomalacia, suggesting that parathyroid hormone (PTH) may play an essential role in the rachitic syndromes. Acting on Erdheim's seminal discovery, Collip[7] later defined the major role of PTH in calcium absorption and function. Bourdillon and Askew and their associates[8,9] then identified and purified the fat-soluble material now known as vitamin D as the principal agent that effectively prevented or cured nutritional rickets and osteomalacia. In 1937, Fuller Albright and his colleagues[10] described a form of rickets that was resistant to normal or even high doses of vitamin D and introduced the term "refractory rickets." Eight years later, Edward Reifenstein, Fuller Albright, and another associate[11] defined the effects of vitamin D on the kidneys, intestinal tract, and bones.

Fuller Albright (1900-1969) was a gifted clinician-scientist at the Massachusetts General Hospital who performed much of the original research on the biology and biochemistry of the rachitic syndromes and was one of the great contributors to our understanding of the disease.[12] His studies also included discoveries relating to other metabolic bone diseases, including hyperparathyroidism,[13,14] fibrous dysplasia with precocious puberty,[15,16] osteoporosis,[17] Cushing's syndrome,[18] and pseudohypoparathyroidism.[19]

The Clinical Characteristics of Rickets and Osteomalacia

Although nutritional rickets and osteomalacia are the oldest and best known forms of the hypocalcemic disorders, there are a number of causes for the syndromes. Some are genetic, some are associated with other disorders, some are related to unusual dietary or drug-related syndromes, and some are of unknown cause. Most of them, however, share very similar histologic changes as well as clinical, laboratory, and radiographic characteristics.

Nutritional rickets was once the most common form of the disease and resulted from a diminished intake of vitamin D.[20-30] The majority of the cases occurred in relation to dietary restrictions, but other factors have been implicated as causes of the disease, including decreased stomach acidity, chelating agents such as phytate or oxalate in the diet, rapid transport through the gastrointestinal tract (the "dumping syndrome"), chronic liver disease, aluminum toxicity (leading to phosphate loss), and chronic bowel disorders.[5,22-24,31-42] If there is insufficient vitamin D in the diet, the synthesis of 1,25 dihydroxy vitamin D is decreased and this leads to a diminished intestinal absorption of calcium.[23,27,29,33,35,39,43-51] As a result, the patient develops hypocalcemia; this causes a secondary hyperparathyroidism,[43,52-54] which brings the calcium level relatively close to normal. The increased parathyroid activity causes the phosphate concentration to diminish as a result of the decreased tubular reabsorption of phosphate (TRP). This results in hyperphosphaturia and hypophosphatemia.[24,31,43,53,55-60] The bone changes are related to a decrease in the available calcium and phosphorus needed to synthesize calcium hydroxyapatite and a secondary hyperparathyroidism, which causes osteoclastic destruction of the existing bony structure.[24,29,33,43,48,56,61-65] The findings described above are characteristic for nutritional rickets or osteomalacia associated with an inadequate intake of vitamin D.

There are four forms of vitamin D-resistant rickets or osteomalacia; these result in changes similar to those noted above for the nutritional form of the disease. The first form, credited to Albright and associates,[10] is described as a sex-linked genetic error with homologies to endopeptidases that results in an error in phosphate reabsorbtion (increased TRP). This causes hyperphosphaturia and hypophosphatemia syndrome[10,57,66,67] and leads to a rachitic syndrome that can be severe and intractable, particularly if only vitamin D is used to treat them. The syndrome will respond best to administration of high concentrations of neutral phosphate; patients can be cured with this protocol even without administration of increased amounts of vitamin D.[24]

Two other forms of the resistant rickets, known as type 1 and type 2 dependent rickets, are associated with two forms of failure of production or function of 1,25 dihydroxy vitamin D.[49,68-74] Type 1 dependent rickets or osteomalacia is characterized by a failure of the kidney to synthesize 1,25 dihydroxy vitamin D in sufficient quantities to prevent rachitic disease. In type 2 dependent disease, a sufficient amount of 1,25 dihydroxy vitamin D is synthesized, but the intestinal absorptive cells seem to fail to recognize the material; as a result, the patients may become profoundly rachitic or osteomalacic. Both of these disorders are sometimes associated with alopecia.[68,73,74] Either type 1 or type 2 dependent disease can be effectively treated with exogenously administered 1,25 dihydroxy vitamin D.[30,74]

The fourth form of the disease is related to the syndrome of renal tubular acidosis, which is characterized by a hyperchloremic, hyponatremic, hypocalcemic acidosis with an alkaline urine. There are two forms of this disease: distal (classic), which represents a failure of production of hydrogen ion in the distal tubule; and proximal, which is related to a bicarbonate wastage.[24,31,33,42,47,57,58] Either of these syndromes can be effectively treated by systemic alka-

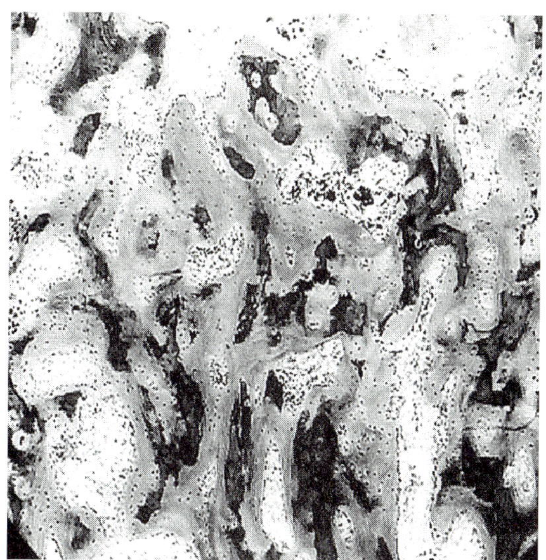

Figure 1

Low-power histologic view of the bone structure of a patient with rickets. The bone trabeculae are thin and irregular in outline. Of particular importance is the presence of osteoid seams surrounding the calcified bones. Hematoxylin and eosin × 60.

linization, using oral agents to reverse the acidic state and restore the calcium concentration to normal.

Additional causes of rickets and osteomalacia that are related to other conditions include two that are associated with genetic disorders. These are resistant rickets in patients with multiple sites of fibrous dysplasia associated with café au lait skin lesions (with irregular borders like the coast of Maine)[15,24,25,34,75]; and a second type of resistant rickets in patients with type 1 neurofibromatosis, who also have café au lait spots but with smooth borders, like the coast of California.[24,25] The causes of either of these rare syndromes are as yet unknown. A third form is an unusual disorder known as oncologic osteomalacia, in which some cytokines produced by benign or malignant bone or soft-tissue tumors seem to interfere with the renal production of 1,25 dihydroxy vitamin D. This results in intractable rickets or osteomalacia.[76,77] The syndrome has recently been found to be related to fibroblast growth factor-23.[78,79] When the tumor is completely removed, the rickets and osteomalacia disappear but return shortly after the tumor recurs; this is perhaps the best available marker for recurrent tumors.

Another unusual cause of the rachitic or osteomalacic syndrome is related to anticon-vulsant medication. Patients with convulsive disorders are given an array of anticonvulsant medications, most of which interfere with microsomal p450 enzymes in the liver.[24,25,50,80,81] This results in a decrease in synthesis of 25 hydroxy vitamin D, which leads to a reduction in the synthesis of 1,25 dihydroxy vitamin D and causes a slowly developing rachitic syndrome. Although this syndrome is mild, if the serum calcium diminishes then the muscular, peripheral, and central nervous systems become more easily stimulated; this increases the likelihood of increased convulsions and may lead to serious overuse of anticonvulsant agents.[26,45,82] The syndrome can be reversed by administration of sufficient amounts of vitamin D or, more importantly, 1,25 dihydroxy vitamin D.[29]

Histologic Changes in the Bony and Epiphyseal Structures in Rickets and Osteomalacia

The rachitic or osteomalacic disorders result in marked thinning of the cortices and diminished amounts of medullary bone[22,24,25,61-65,83,84] (Figure 1). The bony architecture is characterized by the presence of thinned segments, somewhat irregular in structure, and osteoid seams,[24,25,32,84,85] The osteoid seams are thin layers of poorly calcified or uncalcified bone surrounding the calcified segment; thus the staining characteristic with hematoxylin and eosin or other staining systems shows a striking alteration in the coloration. Although osteoid seams are not specifically diagnostic of rickets or ostemalacia and may be seen in other syndromes affecting the bony structure, they are usually so marked in extent and so uniformly present in rickets and osteomalacia as to be a major histologic feature of the disease.[24,63,64] The presence of markedly increased concentrations of osteoid may be seen in transverse linear defects in the cortex; these are notable not only on histologic study but also on radiographic imaging. These lytic areas are usually located in the concave sides of the long bones, the neck of the femur, pubic and ischial rami, the axillary border of the scapula, and the ribs. The lesions are known as Looser's lines, umbauzonen, or Milkman's pseudofractures[24,25] (Figure 2). With increased parathyroid activity, osteoclasts are increased in number and

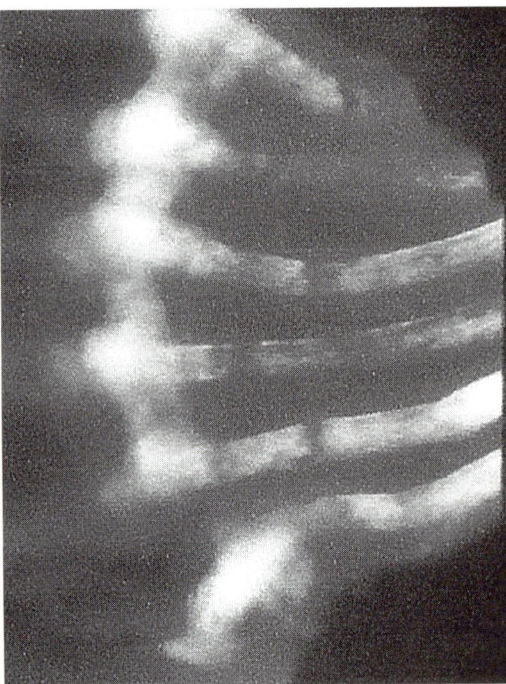

Figure 2
Radiograph of the ribs of a patient with severe rickets showing pseudofractures of the bones known as Looser's lines, umbauzonen, or Milkman's psuedofractures. Several of these appear to have resulted in fractures.

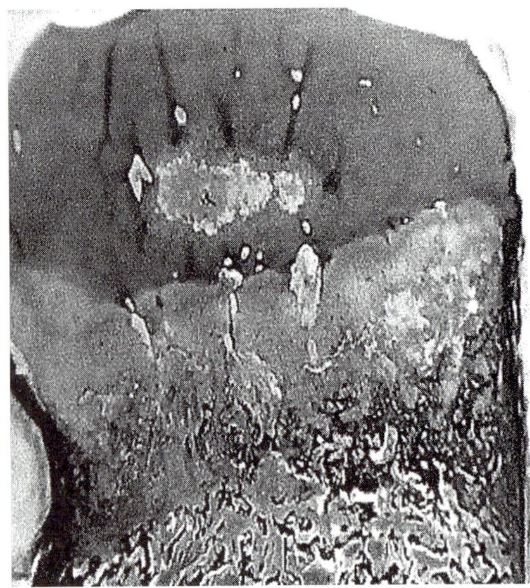

Figure 3
Histologic study of the epiphyseal plate from the proximal femur of a patient who died with rickets. The cartilaginous component of the physeal region is irregular in structure and enormously increased in axial height. The bone in the subchondral region is poorly organized and irregular in structure. Hematoxylin and eosin × 40.

bone destruction with some form of rickets and osteomalacia may dominate the histologic picture.[24-26,31,43,65]

Structural changes in the epiphyseal plates are quite remarkable and are virtually diagnostic for rickets in growing children.[22,24,25] The resting and proliferative zones are relatively normal in appearance, but there is a marked increase in the size and number of cells in the intermediate zone, with a profligate profusion of cell organization and structure (Figure 3). The zone of provisional calcification contains very little calcific material, and the zone of primary spongiosa has small irregular trabeculae with little bone and wide osteoid seams. The axial height of the epiphyseal cartilage is much greater than normal and may extend far into the metaphysis of the underlying bone. This is especially true for the anatomic sites of rapid growth, such as the distal femur, proximal tibia, and proximal radius, where the epiphyseal center is not only much longer than normal but also wider. When the changes occur in the ribs, they produce marked enlargement of the costochondral junction with extension of

the cartilage deep into the rib structure. This is the cause of marked prominence of the junctions of the bone with cartilage at the rib ends, described clinically as the rachitic rosary[24-26,64,65,84] (Figure 4).

Clinical Findings in Rickets and Osteomalacia

By definition, rickets is a disease of childhood; however, it is rarely seen before the age of 6 months.[22-25,28,29] It is more frequently seen in children from countries with cold climates or in children from impoverished families.[22,28,29] The children with nutritional rickets have a history of inadequate vitamin supplement administration and diets limited in foods containing vitamin D or ergosterol.[28,29] The children are usually small for their age, lethargic, apathetic, and irritable; they sometimes complain of severe bone pain associated with muscular hypertonia. Back pain and spinal deformity may be a prominent finding. Physical examination shows short stature, prominence of the frontal bones, abdominal protrusion, and tender bones and joints.[22,24,28,29] The most striking features in many of the patients 2 years of age or older are bowing or knock-knee deformities of the lower extremities (Figure 5)

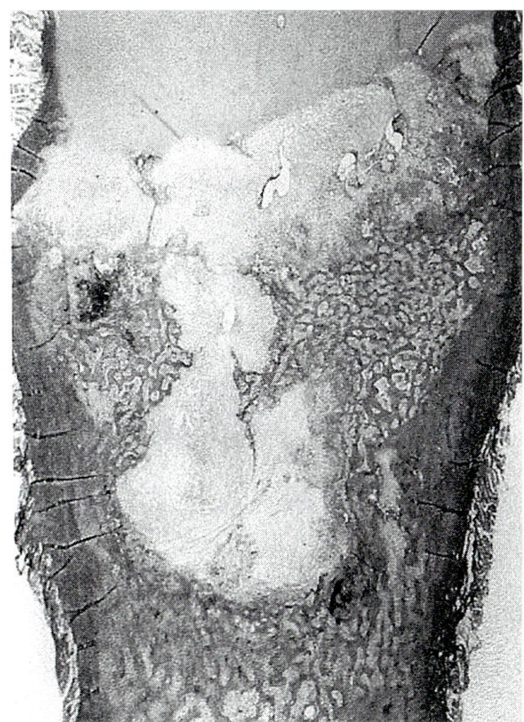

Figure 4
Histologic picture of the costochondral junction showing the degree of expansion of the cartilaginous portion, producing the rachitic rosary. Hematoxylin and eosin × 20.

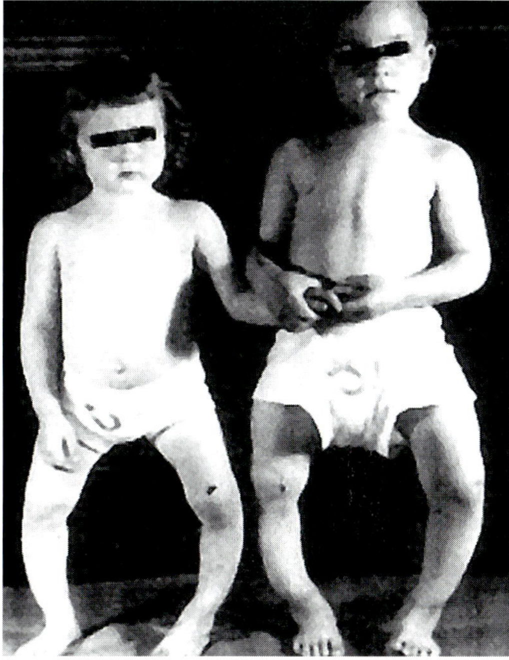

Figure 5
Two children with a severe familial rachitic syndrome showing an extraordinary degree of bowing.

and forearms; prominence and tenderness of the epiphyseal portions of the distal femur, proximal tibia, and distal radius; multiple costochondral enlargements (the rachitic rosary); and back deformities.[28,29] Fractures are common.

Laboratory studies usually show the calcium and phosphate to be low and the PTH concentration to be high. Vitamin D levels are low and the level of TRP is usually low.[24,28,29]

Most patients with adult osteomalacia are either elderly persons whose dietary intake of calcium, vitamin D, or phosphate is inadequate; those who have had complex abdominal surgery (eg, stomach procedures for ulcers or excessive weight); people with dumping syndrome, Crohn's disease, or chronic ulcerative colitis; or those who have had resections of large segments of bowel.[12,20,22,24-26,33-35,43,86,87] The patients usually present with a fracture and are found to be lethargic, irritable, and difficult to communicate with. They complain of bone pain and frequently have trouble with ambulation, particularly stairs. Back pain and deformity are common; scoliosis, lordosis, and kyphosis have all been described.[22,24,33-35,87] Laboratory studies of adults are similar to those of rachitic children.

Imaging Studies for Patients With Rickets and Osteomalacia

Radiography or computed tomography of the bones show them to be thin in their cortices with indistinct structural characteristics for the medullary cavities (described as "fuzzy texture").[12,22,24-26,28,64,65] In children with rickets, bowing or knock-knee deformities are common in the lower extremities; the epiphyseal plates are enormously increased in axial height and, to a lesser extent, in width. The changes in the epiphyseal plates are dependent on the rate of growth, thus the findings are most marked in the distal femur, proximal tibia, proximal femur, and radius and less so in the hands and feet, particularly distally.[24-26,64] As noted in the discussion of the pathology, Looser's lines are common, most often in the tibia and femur as well as the ribs, and resemble incomplete fractures.[24] Fractures through the Looser's lines are common, as are fractures in other sites. Patients with osteomalacia do not ordinarily show the knock-knee or bow-leg deformities characteristic of rick-

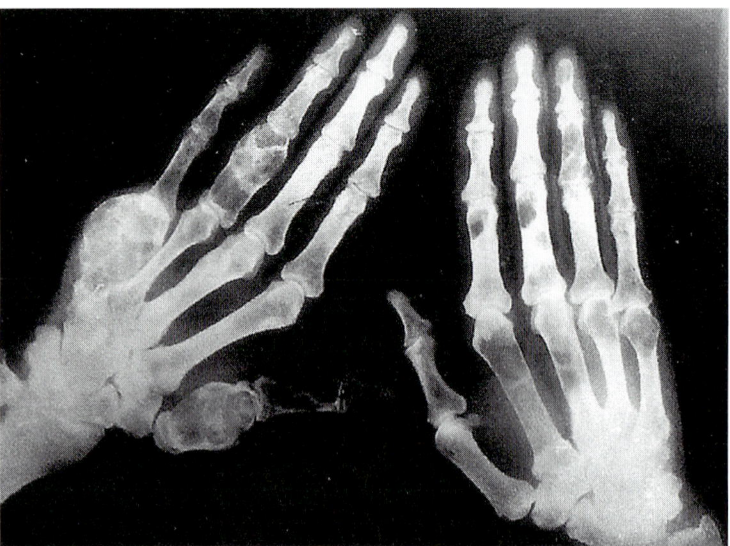

Figure 6
Radiographs of the hands of a patient with renal osteodystrophy and severe changes associated with hyperparathyroidism. The tufts are partially destroyed, there is subperiosteal resorption of the phalanges, and several sites of brown tumors can be noted in the digits.

ets. Examination of the bones usually show thin cortices and poorly structured medullary bone as well as many poorly healed and sometimes displaced fractures, particularly in the spine, pelvis, and ribs.[24,25,64]

Treatment of Rickets and Osteomalacia

The first approach to the treatment of rickets and osteomalacia is to be aware of the diseases and to use the dietary history, physical findings, and laboratory and imaging studies to make the diagnosis. Children who are apathetic and irritable, refuse to walk, and have bone tenderness and pain should be suspected of having rickets, especially if they come from a disadvantaged background. Adults with poor dietary habits who have defective bone structure and frequent fractures with a history of minimal trauma should be carefully studied.[22,23,25,26,28,29] As many as 15% to 20% of elderly patients with fractures of the hip allegedly related to osteoporosis have been estimated to have some osteomalacia as well.[24,87] Both of these groups should be examined carefully with imaging studies but also with laboratory tests, including calcium, phosphorus, 25 hydroxy and 1,25 dihydroxy vitamin D, PTH, and urinary phosphate levels.[24,25]

Children with nutritional rickets can be effectively treated with vitamin D at 400 units per day; the same dose in adults and children is very effective in preventing the disease.[25,28,29,50] Children and adults with resistant rickets should be carefully studied and then treated with alkalinization for renal tubular acidosis, 1,25 dihydroxy vitamin D for type 1 and type 2 dependent disease, and phosphate for Albright's syndrome.[21,22,24,67,68,73,75] Patients with oncologic osteomalacia should have their tumors completely removed, even if benign.[24,76,77] Patients with gastrointestinal causes of osteomalacia are much more difficult to treat and may require larger doses of vitamin D and other materials.[24,25]

Renal Osteodystrophy

Renal osteodystrophy represents a special form of rickets or osteomalacia in which the principal cause of the disorder is chronic renal failure. Although many of the characteristics are similar to those of nutritional or resistant rickets or osteomalacia, there are some special issues, particularly in terms of the cause of the syndrome, its nature, and some of the complications.[88-90]

The syndrome of renal osteodystrophy is caused by chronic renal failure with glomerular and tubular damage.[88,91-93] The renal failure causes a significant rise in blood urea nitrogen, creatinine, and phosphate, none of which can be excreted through the damaged kidney.[92-94] The injury to the renal tissue creates a reduced tubular mass, which makes it difficult or impossible for the kidney to synthesize 1,25 dihydroxy vitamin D.[24,88,93,94] This leads to a drop in the serum calcium, which causes a marked increase in PTH and a resultant sometimes severe hyperparathyroidism.[88,93] The bones show changes consistent with rickets and osteomalacia, but also show evidence of osteitis fibrosa cystica generalisata (the ancient term for hyperparathyroidism), with considerable destruction of bone and release of calcium.[24,92] The rise in calcium prevents the symptoms of hypocalcemia but is worrisome because of the high level of phosphate in the body fluids and the failure of the PTH to lower the level of TRP. Rising levels of calcium and phosphate lead to deposition of calcific material in a number of sites.[24,93,94] These locations include the conjunctivae (the "red eyes of renal failure"),[95] the peripheral arteries and aorta (Monckeberg's sclerosis), skin (the cause of itching in renal failure), and connective tissue sites.[24,88,93] Connective tissue sites are sometimes the most prominent problem. Calcification can occur in muscles (deltoid, quadriceps, or other sites), joints (knee, elbow, and small joints of the hands and feet), bursae, or cartilage (calcification in the knee joint).[24,93,94]

Histologic study of the bones show changes of osteomalacia but also show marked alterations consistent with hyperparathyroidism, including bone destruction, lytic areas filled with osteoclasts, and fractures through the Looser's lines (Figure 6). One other feature that is not clearly understood is the presence of areas of increased density within the bones.[24] These may affect the spine or the long bones. They do not represent healing, but rather an increase in the number of trabeculae, which show irregularity due to osteoclastic resorption and classic osteoid seams.[24,96]

Imaging studies show changes consistent with rickets or osteomalacia, but also show findings consistent with hyperparathyroidism, with a marked decrease in cortical structure and lytic areas that is described as "brown tumors."[90,97] The spinal segments frequently show marked loss of medullary bone, and multiple fractures are often present. Sites of increased density in the bones should not be interpreted as demonstrating healing. The most remarkable feature is the presence of calcification of the blood vessels, the muscles, cartilage, and sometimes tendons.[24]

The treatment of renal osteodystrophy is obviously dependent on the renal problem.[89,91,93] Dialysis helps by reducing the concentrations of phosphate and calcium, thus decreasing the risk of calcification.[89,91,93] Occasionally the hyperparathyroidism is so severe that one must consider parathyroidectomy[98] or use of the new agent cinacalcet, which blocks PTH actions in patients on dialysis.[99] Bisphosphonates may be useful for decreasing the osteoclastic bone destruction,[100] and recently bone morphogenetic protein-7 has shown some promise.[101]

References

1. Whistler D: Morbo puerili Anglorum, quem patrio idiomate indignae vocant The Rickets, in *Lugduni Batavorum*. 1645, vol 1-13.

2. Glisson F: De Rachitide, sive morbo puerili, qui vulgo The Rickets diciteur. London, England, G. Dugardi, 1650, pp 1-416.

3. Barlow T: On cases described as 'acute rickets' which are probably a combination of scurvy and rickets, the scurvy being essential and the rickets a variable element. *Med Surg Trans* 1883;66:159-219.

4. McCollum EV, Simmonds N, Parsons HT, et al: Studies on experimental rickets: I. The production of rachitis and similar diseases in the rat by deficient diets. *J Biol Chem* 1921;45:333-342.

5. McCollum EV, Simmonds N, Shipley PG, Park EA: Studies on experimental rickets: VIII. The production of rickets by diets low in phosphorus and fat soluble vitamin A. *J Biol Chem* 1921;47:507-527.

6. Erdheim J: Zur normalen and pathologischen histoligie der glandula thyreoidea, parathryreoidea and hypophysis. *Beit Path Anat* 1903;33:158-236.

7. Collip JB: The extraction of a parathyroid hormone which will prevent or control parathyroid tetany and which regulates the level of blood calcium. *J Biol Chem* 1925;63:395-438.

8. Bourdillon RB, Fischman C, Jenkins RGC, Webster TA: The absorption spectrum of vitamin D. *Proc R Soc Lond B Biol Sci* 1929;104:561-583.

9. Askew FA, Bourdillon RB, Bruce HM, et al: Crystalline vitamin D. *Proc R Soc Lond B Biol Sci* 1932;109:488-506.

10. Albright F, Butler AM, Bloomberg E: Rickets resistant to vitamin D therapy. *Am J Dis Child* 1937;54:529-547.

11. Reifenstein EC, Albright F, Wells SL: The accumulation, interpretation and presentation of data pertaining to metabolic balances, notably of calcium, phosphorus and nitrogen. *J Clin Endocrinol* 1945;5:367-395.

12. Albright F, Burnett CH, Parson W, et al: Osteomalacia and late rickets. *Medicine* 1946;25:399-479.

13. Albright F, Bloomberg E, Castleman B, Churchill ED: Hyperparathyroidism due to diffuse hyperplasia of all parathyroid glands rather than an adenoma of one. *AMA Arch Intern Med* 1934;54:315-329.

14. Albright F, Reifenstein C: *The Parathyroid Glands and Metabolic Bone Disease*. Baltimore, MD, Williams and Wilkins, 1948.

15. Albright F: Polyostotic fibrous dysplasia: A defense of the entity. *J Clin Endocrinol* 1947;7:307-324.

16. Albright F, Butler AM, Hampton AO, Smith P: Syndrome characterized by osteitis fibrosa disseminata, areas of pigmentation and endocrine dysfunction with precocious puberty in females: Report of five cases. *N Engl J Med* 1937;216:727-746.

17. Albright F, Bloomberg E, Smith PH: Postmenopausal osteoporosis. *Trans Assoc Am Physicians* 1940;55:298-305.

18. Albright F: Cushing's syndrome: Its pathological physiology, its relationship to the adreno-genital syndrome, and its connection with the problem of the reaction of the body to injurious agents. *Harvey Lect* 1943;38:123-186.

19. Albright F, Burnett CH, Smith PH, Parson W: Pseudo-hypoparathyroidism, an example of 'Seabright-Bantam' syndrome: Report of three cases. *Endocrinology* 1942;30:922-932.

20. Brautbar N, Levine BS, Walling MW, Coburn JW: Intestinal absorption of calcium: Role of dietary phosphate and vitamin D. *Am J Physiol* 1981;241:G49-G53.

21. Holick MF: Vitamin D, photobiology, metabolism, mechanism of action and clinical applications, in Favus MJ (ed): *Primer on the Metabolic Bone Diseases and Disorders of Mineral Metabolism*, ed 4. Philadelphia, PA, Lippincott Williams and Wilkins, 1999, pp 92-98.

22. Klein GL: Nutritional rickets and osteomalacia, in Favus MJ (ed): *Primer on the Metabolic Bone Diseases and Disorders of Mineral Metabolism*, ed 4. Philadelphia, PA, Lippincott Williams and Wilkins, 1999, pp 315-318.

23. Ladhani S, Srinivasan L, Buchanan C, Allgrove J: Presentation of vitamin D deficiency. *Arch Dis Child* 2004;89:781-784.

24. Mankin HJ: Metabolic bone disease. *Instr Course Lect* 1995;44:3-32.

25. Mundy GR: Osteomalacia and rickets, in *Bone Remodeling and Its Disorders*, ed 2. London, England, Martin Dunitz, 1999, pp 200-207.

26. Reginato AJ, Coquia JA: Musculoskeletal manifestations of osteomalacia and rickets. *Best Prac Res Clin Rheumatol* 2003;17:1063-1080.

27. Reichel H, Koeffler HP, Norman AW: The role of the vitamin D endocrine system in health and disease. *N Engl J Med* 1989;320:980-991.

28. Weisberg P, Scanlon KS, Li R, Cogswell ME: Nutritional rickets among children in the United States: Review of cases reported between 1996 and 2003. *Am J Clin Nutr* 2004;80:1697S-1705S.

29. Wharton B, Bishop N: Rickets. *Lancet* 2003;362:1389-1400.

30. Wu-Wong JR, Tian J, Goltzman D: Vitamin D analogs as therapeutic agents: A clinical study update. *Curr Opin Investig Drugs* 2004;5:320-326.

31. Birge SJ, Avioli LV: Pathophysiology of calcium and phosphate absorptive disorders, in Avioli LV, Krane SM (eds): *Metabolic Bone Disease*, ed 2. Philadelphia, PA, WB Saunders Co, 1990, pp 196-221.

32. Boskey AL: Mineral-matrix interactions in bone and cartilage. *Clin Orthop Relat Res* 1992;281:244-274.

33. Bronner F: Current concepts of calcium absorption: An overview. *J Nutr* 1992;122(3 Suppl):641-643.

34. Carmichael KA, Fallon MD, Dalinka M, Kaplan FS, Axel L, Haddad JG: Osteomalacia and osteitis fibrosa in a man ingesting aluminum hydroxide antacid. *Am J Med* 1984;76:1137-1143.

35. Charles P: Calcium absorption and calcium bioavailability. *J Intern Med* 1992;231:161-168.

36. Cross HS, Debiec H, Peterlik M: Mechanism and regulation of intestinal phosphate absorption. *Miner Electrolyte Metab* 1990;16:115-124.

37. Heaney RP, Weaver CM: Oxalate: Effect on calcium absorbability. *Am J Clin Nutr* 1989;50:830-832.

38. Karbach U: Mechanism of intestinal calcium transport and clinical aspects of disturbed calcium absorption. *Dig Dis* 1989;7:1-18.

39. Lemann J Jr, Favus M: The intestinal absorption of calcium, magnesium and phosphate, in Favus MJ (ed): *Primer on the Metabolic Bone Diseases and Disorders of Mineral Metabolism*, ed 4. Philadelphia, PA, Lippincott Williams and Wilkins, 1999, pp 63-66.

40. Lemann J Jr: Intestinal absorption of calcium, magnesium and phosphorus, in Favus ME (ed): *Primer on Metabolic Bone Diseases and Disorders of Mineral Metabolism*. Kelseyville, CA, American Society for Bone and Mineral Research, 1990, pp 37-41.

41. Ott SM, Maloney NA, Klein GL, et al: Aluminum is associated with low bone formation in patients receiving chronic parenteral nutrition. *Ann Intern Med* 1983;98:910-914.

42. Recker RR: Calcium absorption and achlorhydria. *N Engl J Med* 1985;313:70-73.

43. Bartos HR, Henneman PH: Parathyroid hyperplasia in osteomalacia. *J Clin Endocrinol Metab* 1965;25:1522-1523.

44. Boden SD, Kaplan FS: Calcium homeostasis. *Orthop Clin North Am* 1990;21:31-42.

45. Broadus AE: Physiologic functions of calcium, magnesium and phosphorus, in Favus ME (ed): *Primer on Metabolic Bone Diseases and Disorders of Mineral Metabolism*. Kelseyville, CA, American Society for Bone and Mineral Research, 1990, pp 29-30.

46. Bronner F: Intestinal calcium transport: The cellular pathway. *Miner Electrolyte Metab* 1990;16:94-100.

47. Bushinsky DA: Calcium, magnesium and phosphorus: Renal handling and urinary excretion, in Favus MJ (ed): *Primer on the Metabolic Bone Diseases and Disorders of Mineral Metabolism*, ed 4. Philadelphia, PA, Lippincott Williams and Wilkins, 1999, pp 67-73.

48. Jüppner H, Brown EM, Kronenburg HM: Parathyroid hormone, in Favus MJ (ed): *Primer on the Metabolic Bone Diseases and Disorders of Mineral Metabolism*, ed 4. Philadelphia, PA, Lippincott Williams and Wilkins, 1999, pp 80-87.

49. Kumar R: Vitamin D metabolism and mechanisms of transport. *J Am Soc Nephrol* 1990;1:30-42.

50. Wasserman RH, Brindak ME, Buddle MM, et al: Recent studies on the biological actions of vitamin D on intestinal transport and the electrophysiology of peripheral nerve and cardiac muscle. *Prog Clin Biol Res* 1990;332:99-126.

51. Wasserman RH, Chandler JS, Meyer SA, et al: Intestinal calcium transport and calcium extrusion processes at the basolateral membrane. *J Nutr* 1992;122(suppl):662-671.

52. Aub C, Tibbets DM, McLean R: The influence of parathyroid hormone, urea, sodium chloride, fat and intestinal activity upon calcium balance. *J Nutr* 1937;132:635-655.

53. Rizzoli R, Ferrari LS, Pizurki L, Caverzasio J, Bonjour JP: Actions of parathyroid hormone and parathyroid hormone-related protein. *J Endocrinol Invest* 1992;15(suppl 6):51-56.

54. Segre GV: Secretion, metabolism and circulating heterogeneity of parathyroid hormone, in Favus ME (ed): *Primer on Metabolic Bone Diseases and Disorders of Mineral Metabolism*. Kelseyville, CA, American Society for Bone and Mineral Research, 1990, pp 43-44.

55. Avioli LV, McDonald JE, Henneman PH, Lee SW: The relationship of parathyroid to pyrophosphate excretion. *J Clin Invest* 1966;45:1093-1102.

56. Bilezikian JP: Primary hyperparathyroidism, in Favus MJ (ed): *Primer on the Metabolic Bone Diseases and Disorders of Mineral Metabolism*, ed 4. Philadelphia, PA, Lippincott Williams and Wilkins, 1999, pp 187-191.

57. Jacobson H, Knochel JP: Renal handling of phosphate in health and disease, in Brenner BM, Rector EC Jr (eds): *The Kidney*, ed 3. Philadelphia, PA, WB Saunders, 1986, pp 340-388.

58. Lemann J Jr: The urinary excretion of calcium,

magnesium and phosphorus, in Favus ME (ed): *Primer on Metabolic Bone Diseases and Disorders of Mineral Metabolism*. Kelseyville, CA, American Society for Bone and Mineral Research, 1990, pp 32-36.

59. Silverberg SJ: The distribution and balance of calcium, magnesium and phosphorus, in Favus ME (ed): *Primer on Metabolic Bone Diseases and Disorders of Mineral Metabolism*. Kelseyville, CA, American Society for Bone and Mineral Research, 1990, pp 30-32.

60. Yanagawa N, Lee DBN: Renal handling of calcium and phosphorus, in Cole FL, Favus ME (ed): *Disorders of Bone and Mineral Metabolism*. New York, NY, Raven Press, 1992, pp 3-40.

61. Glimcher MJ: The nature of the mineral phase in bone, in Avioli LV, Krane SM (eds): *Metabolic Bone Diseases and Related Disorders*, ed 3. San Diego, CA, Academic Press, 1998, pp 23-95.

62. Mundy GR: Bone remodeling, in Favus MJ (ed): *Primer on the Metabolic Bone Diseases and Disorders of Mineral Metabolism*, ed 4. Philadelphia, PA, Lippincott Williams and Wilkins, 1999, pp 30-38.

63. Raisz LG: Mechanisms and regulation of bone resorption by osteoclastic cells, in Coe FL, Flavus ME (eds): *Disorders of Bone and Mineral Metabolism*. New York, NY, Raven Press, 1992, pp 287-311.

64. Rauch F: The rachitic bone. *Endocr Dev* 2003;6:69-79.

65. States LJ: Imaging of rachitic bone. *Endocr Dev* 2003;6:80-92.

66. Francis F, Rowe PS, Econs MJ, et al: A YAC contig spanning the hypophosphatemic rickets gene (HYP) candidate region. *Genomics* 1994;21:229-237.

67. Glorieux FH: Hypophosphatemic vitamin D resistant rickets, in Favus MJ (ed): *Primer on the Metabolic Bone Diseases and Disorders of Mineral Metabolism*, ed 4. Philadelphia, PA, Lippincott Williams and Wilkins, 1999, pp 328-330.

68. Balsan S, Garaedian M, Ligerman UA, et al: Rickets and alopecia with resistance to 1,25-dihydroxyvitamin D: Two different clinical courses with two different cellular defects. *J Clin Endocrinol Metab* 1983;57:803-811.

69. Friedman PA, Gesek FA: Calcium transport in renal epithelial cells. *Am J Physiol* 1993;264:F181-F198.

70. Gross M, Kumar R: Physiology and biochemistry of vitamin D-dependent calcium binding proteins. *Am J Physiol* 1990;259:F195-F209.

71. Hollis BW, Clemens TL, Adams JS: Vitamin D metabolites, in Favus MJ (ed): *Primer on the Metabolic Bone Diseases and Disorders of Mineral Metabolism*, ed 4. Philadelphia, PA, Lippincott Williams and Wilkins, 1999, pp 124-127.

72. Liberman UA, Marx SJ: Vitamin D dependent rickets, in Favus MJ (ed): *Primer on the Metabolic Bone Diseases and Disorders of Mineral Metabolism*, ed 4. Philadelphia, PA, Lippincott Williams and Wilkins, 1999, pp 323-327.

73. Rosen JF, Fleischman AR, Finberg L, Hamstra A, DeLuca HF: Rickets with alopecia: An inborn error of vitamin D metabolism. *J Pediatr* 1979;94:729-735.

74. Sultan Al-Khenaizan, Vitale P: Vitamin D-dependent rickets Type II with alopecia: Two case reports and review of the literature. *Int J Dermatol* 2003;42:682-685.

75. Chattophadhyay A, Bhansali A, Mohanty SK, Khandelwal N, Mathur SK, Dash RJ: Hypo-

76. Drezner MK: Tumor-induced osteomalacia, in Favus MJ (ed): *Primer on the Metabolic Bone Diseases and Disorders of Mineral Metabolism*, ed 4. Philadelphia, PA, Lippincott Williams and Wilkins, 1999, pp 331-336.

77. Shulman DI, Hahn G, Benator R, et al: Tumor-induced rickets: Usefulness of MR gradient echo recall imaging for tumor localization. *J Pediatr* 2004;144:381-385.

78. Fukumoto S, Yamashita T: Fibroblast growth factor-23 is the phosphaturic factor in tumor-induced osteomalacia and may be phosphatonin. *Curr Opin Nephrol Hypertens* 2002;11:385-389.

79. Kumar R: New insights into phosphate homeostasis: Fibroblast growth factor 23 and frizzled-related protein–4 are phosphaturic factors derived from tumors associated with osteomalacia. *Curr Opin Nephrol Hypertens* 2002;11:547-553.

80. Pack AM, Gidal B, Vazquez B: Bone disease associated with antiepileptic drugs. *Cleve Clin J Med* 2004;71(Suppl 2):S42-S48.

81. Wikvall K: Cytochrome P450 enzymes in the bioactivation of vitamin D to its hormonal form. *Int J Mol Med* 2001;7:201-209.

82. Brink F: The role of calcium ions in neural processes. *Pharmacol Rev* 1954;6:243-298.

83. Khosla S, Kleerekoper M: Biochemical markers of bone turnover, in Favus MJ (ed): *Primer on the Metabolic Bone Diseases and Disorders of Mineral Metabolism*, ed 4. Philadelphia, PA, Lippincott Williams and Wilkins, 1999, pp 128-133.

84. Lian JB, Stein GS, Canalis E, Gehron Robey P, Boskey AL: Bone formation: Osteoblast lineage cells, growth factors, matrix proteins and the mineralization process, in Favus MJ (ed): *Primer on the Metabolic Bone Diseases and Disorders of Mineral Metabolism*, ed 4. Philadelphia, PA, Lippincott Williams and Wilkins, 1999, pp 14-29.

85. Landis WJ, Glimcher MJ: Electron diffraction and electron probe micronanalysis of the mineral phase of bone tissue prepared by anhydrous techniques. *J Ultrastruct Res* 1978;63:188-223.

86. Broadus AE: Mineral balance and homeostasis, in Favus MJ (ed): *Primer on the Metabolic Bone Diseases and Disorders of Mineral Metabolism*, ed 4. Philadelphia, PA, Lippincott Williams and Wilkins, 1999, pp 74-80.

87. Hordon LD, Peacock M: Vitamin D metabolism in women with femoral neck fracture. *Bone Miner* 1987;2:413-426.

88. Goodman WG, Coburn JW, Slatopolsky E, Salusky IB: Renal osteodystrophy in adults and children, in Favus MJ (ed): *Primer on the Metabolic Bone Diseases and Disorders of Mineral Metabolism*, ed 4. Philadelphia, PA, Lippincott Williams and Wilkins, 1999, pp 347-366.

89. Moe SM: Management of renal osteodystrophy in peritoneal dialysis patients. *Perit Dial Int* 2004;24:209-216.

90. Roe S, Cassidy MJ: Diagnosis and monitoring of renal osteodystrophy. *Curr Opin Nephrol Hypertens* 2000;9:675-681.

91. Cushner HM, Adams ND: Review: Renal osteodystrophy. Pathogenesis and treatment. *Am J Med Sci* 1986;291:264-275.

92. Hoyland JA, Picton ML: Cellular mechanisms of

renal osteodystrophy. *Kidney Int Suppl* 1999;73:S8-S13.

93. Slatopolsky E, Gonzalez E, Martin K: Pathogenesis and treatment of renal osteodystrophy. *Blood Purif* 2003;21:318-326.

94. Sutton RA, Cameron EC: Renal osteodystrophy: Pathophysiology. *Semin Nephrol* 1992;12:91-100.

95. Cogan DG, Henneman PH: Diffuse calcification of the cornea in hypercalcemia. *N Engl J Med* 1957;257:451-453.

96. Brockman EP: Some observations on the bone changes in renal rickets. *Br J Surg* 1926;14:634-635.

97. Ambrosoni P, Olaizol I, Heuguerot C, et al: The role of imaging techniques in the study of renal osteodystrophy. *Am J Med Sci* 2000;320:90-95.

98. Olson JA Jr, Leight GS Jr: Surgical management of secondary hyperparathyroidism. *Adv Ren Replace Ther* 2002;9:209-218.

99. Peacock M, Bilezikian JP, Klassen PS, Guo MD, Turner SA, Shoback D: Cinacalcet hydrochloride maintains long-term normocalcemia in patients with primary hyperparathyroidism. *J Clin Endocrinol Metab* 2005;90:135-141.

100. Fan SL, Cunningham J: Bisphosphonates in renal osteodystrophy. *Curr Opin Nephrol Hypertens* 2001;10:581-588.

101. Li T, Surendran K, Zawaideh MA, Mathew S, Hruska KA: Bone morphogenetic protein 7: A novel treatment for chronic renal and bone disease. *Curr Opin Nephrol Hypertens* 2004;23:417-422.

Chapter 21

Primary Hyperparathyroidism

Hyperparathyroidism was for many years a mysterious entity of seemingly unknown cause that often resulted in severe renal, osseous, cardiac, and neural symptomatology and sometimes death.[1-5] The changes seen, particularly in the bones, often dominated the picture, but the cause of these sometimes quite severe alterations could not be identified. Without systems for assessing the body's stores of calcium and phosphorus and without knowledge of the amount of parathyroid hormone (PTH) present, physicians could only document the progressive deterioration of the patient and try to use nonspecific treatment systems in an effort to control the symptoms. The disease is an old one. Zink[6] described changes attributable to hyperparathyroidism in skeletons from 7,000 years ago. According to Cave,[7] Richard Owen first discovered the parathyroid glands in the latter part of the 19th century. In 1906, Askanazy[8] described a parathyroid adenoma, and shortly thereafter Jakob Erdheim[9] identified enlargement of the parathyroid glands in patients with rickets, thus establishing the relationship of these tissues to calcium metabolism. Mandl[10] described a mysterious bone disease in 1926 that he named "osteitis fibrosa cystica" but did not suspect the cause. In 1929, Wilder[11] described a patient who had a tumor of the parathyroid glands and also had rather striking bone deterioration that appeared to be osteitis fibrosa cystica, identical to that reported by Mandl. Based on these findings, Barr and Bulger[12] described a clinical syndrome associated with the now classic bone changes that they named "hyperparathyroidism." Jaffe[13,14] described the bone changes in association with parathyroid adenomas in 1933; in 1934, Albright, Aub, and Bauer[15] described 17 cases of clinical hyperparathyroidism seen at the Massachusetts General Hospital. They identified the syndrome as a rather frequently encountered but sometimes subtle cause of skeletal abnormality and disorders of other body systems. A remarkable review of the entire subject was presented in a book written by Albright and Reifenstein entitled *The Parathyroid Glands and Metabolic Bone Disease: Selected Studies* that was published in 1948, in which they stated that hyperparathyroidism is a "disease of bones and stones and abdominal groans, occasionally complicated by psychological moans."[1] Based on their work and with the assistance of many others, the entity became well recognized and various forms of treatment were begun. Because of these discoveries, the problems previously associated with hypercalcemia, sometimes severe bone disease, and systemic illness now occur far less frequently and can be dealt with by appropriate protocols that limit and sometimes eliminate the effects of the disease.

Actions of Parathyroid Hormone

PTH is a major player in the system of calcium and phosphorus metabolism.[16-18] The material is produced by the four small parathyroid glands attached to the posterior aspect of the thyroid gland. The glands produce PTH in response to a lowering of calcium ion concentration in the extracellular fluid. The PTH then acts to increase the calcium concentration in the following manner:

- Vitamins D2 and D3 are activated in the liver by microsomal p450 enzymes to form 25 hydroxy vitamin D.[19,20] This material then passes to the kidney, where it is further acted on by PTH.[19,21-23] In the presence of low serum calcium and low serum phosphorus in the serum, a high level of PTH appears to activate 25 hydroxy vitamin D hydrolase, oxygen, magnesium ion, and reduced pyridine nucleotide, all of which act to convert the 25 hydroxy vitamin D to 1,25 dihydroxy vitamin D.[21-24] The 1,25 dihydroxy vitamin D is a very potent agent in the transport of calcium from the lumen of the gastrointestinal tract into the body fluids and also in increasing tubular reabsorption of calcium from the renal tubule.[21,22,24-28]

- PTH acts on the gastrointestinal cells in the lower part of the duodenum and

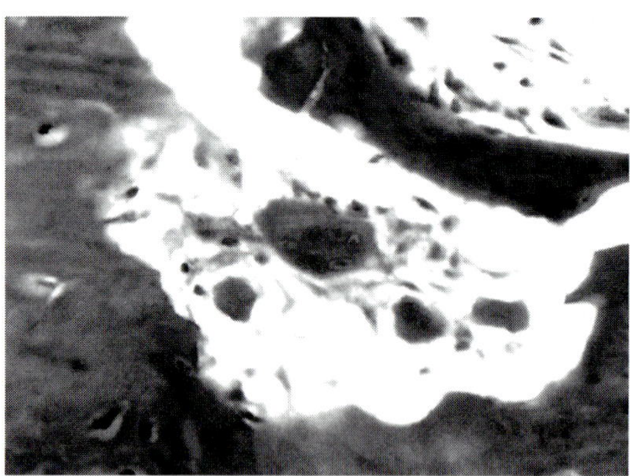

Figure 1

Classic histologic appearance of osteoclasts destroying bone and producing a Howship's lacuna. Hematoxylin and eosin × 400.

the upper jejunum to increase the absorption of calcium from the food material in the lumen.[29-31] PTH opens windows in the cell membrane through the mechanism of converting adenosine triphosphate to cyclic adenosine monophosphate; this not only allows calcium to enter the cell, but it stimulates the release of calcium ions from the cellular mitochondria.[19,30,31] The 1,25 dihydroxy vitamin D then activates the messenger RNA to stimulate the endoplasmic reticulum of the gut cells to synthesize calbindin, a calcium transport protein, which then carries the calcium from within the cell into the extracellular fluid.[19,26,27,30,31]

- Actions similar to those that take place in the gut cells are believe to occur in the renal tubule, increasing tubular reabsorption of calcium, which is filtered out of the blood by the glomerulus.[28,32-34] A similar action occurs in the bone that can be described as "crystal-lysis" of calcium hydroxyapatite crystals, which leads to a release of the calcium and phosphate ions into the serum.[19] All of these actions increase the calcium ion concentration in the extracellular fluids.
- Another major action of PTH is the stimulation and activation of osteoclasts to destroy bone and release calcium and phosphate from the hydroxyapatite crystals in much greater quantities than occurs with crystal-lysis.[3,13-15,17,19] This process is known as osteoclastic resorption and leads to an

irregular, partly destroyed bony structure with the osteoclasts sitting in Howship's lacunae[13,14,19] (Figure 1).

- Because the rising calcium ion concentration associated with the action of PTH may, in the presence of phosphate, exceed the critical solubility product for Ca HPO_4, PTH has one additional action that prevents the patient from "turning to stone." PTH acts on the renal tubule to decrease the percentage of tubular reabsorption of phosphate, which results in a hyperphosphaturia and a sometimes profound hypophosphatemia.[19,23,32,34,35] Thus as the level of calcium rises, the phosphate declines; this prevents deposition of calcific material in blood vessels, tendons, cartilage, and kidneys, as is frequently seen in patients with renal osteodystrophy.[3,4,19,36]

Etiology of Primary Hyperparathyroidism: Adenomas, Hyperplasia, and Carcinoma

Approximately 80% of patients with primary hyperparathyroidism have adenomas of a single gland.[3,4] These are composed of chief cells and less commonly of oxyphil cells. The tumors are light in weight (0.5 to 5.0 g) and are not locally symptomatic. Parathyroid hyperplasia is less common (approximately 20% of patients); it involves all four glands and histologically may look like adenomas.[3,4] Carcinomas are very rare (less than 1%), and may occur at any age. The hypercalcemia associated with carcinomas is more marked and is more often associated with nephrocalcinosis.[3,4,37] The tumors are locally invasive and may metastasize—usually to lymph nodes, but occasionally to lungs, liver, or bone.[3,4,37-39]

Primary hyperparathyroidism is rare in children and usually occurs in patients over 35 years of age.[40-42] The disease appears to be more common in women than men, and particularly in postmenopausal women.[43-45] True familial hyperparathyroidism is a rare event, but may be related to some genetic abnormalities.[41,46-51]

However, hyperparathyroidism may occur with two familial disorders known as multiple endocrine neoplasia (MEN).[46-49,52,53] MEN type I is associated with a growth factor similar to fibroblast growth factor and is possibly related to the INT-2 oncogene.[52] Half of the patients with MEN type I have an alteration in chromosome 11 that can drive the expression of a gene product PRAD-1, which is a D-cyclin protein that plays a role in cell division.[3,4,52-54] The other neoplasms associated with MEN type I occur in the pituitary and pancreas.[55] MEN type IIA includes medullary carcinoma of the thyroid gland, pheochromocytoma and adrenal tumors. Another less common form of the disease is MEN Type IIB, which not only includes thyroid, pheochromocytoma, and adrenal tumors but also a mucocutaneous syndrome known as ganglioneuromatosis, which presents as small polypoid neuromas of the eyelids and lips and sometimes marked thickening of the tongue.[3,4,38]

The Syndrome of Primary Hyperparathyroidism

Regardless of whether the patient has primary or genetic disease, or whether the lesion consists of an adenoma, hyperplasia, or carcinoma, the clinical result is a "runaway train in the neck," which ignores signals from the serum concentration of calcium or phosphorus.[3,4,19,38,39] The PTH is produced in excessive concentration and acts as described above to increase the calcium absorption in the gastrointestinal tract, the renal tubular reabsorption of calcium in the kidney, and the osteoclastic destruction of bone, all of which lead to an often extraordinary increase in the serum calcium.[2,4,5,38,56] In the presence of normal renal function, this is associated with a decrease in the serum phosphorus that is related to the marked diminution in the tubular reabsorption of phosphate.[3,4,19,32,36]

The hypercalcemia that occurs in this syndrome sometimes causes profound changes in neuromuscular status that are characterized by lethargy, confusion, impaired mentation, depression, memory loss, and muscular weakness.[3,4,57-59] The bone changes are sometimes striking, and consist of osteopenia observed on radiography with subperiosteal resorption of the tufts and digits of the hands and feet[3,13-15,19,60] (Figure 2). Fractures of long bones, clavicles, pelvis, and ribs are common[19,61] (Figure 3). Because the disease appears to be more common in postmenopausal women, the findings may be confused with osteoporosis except for the

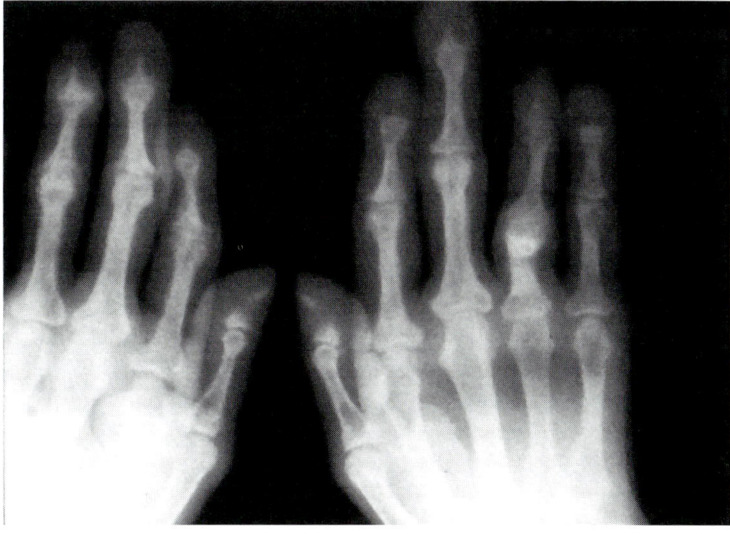

Figure 2

Typical changes in the hands of a patient with severe primary hyperparathyroidism. Note the destruction of the tufts and subperiosteal resorption of the remainder of the bones. A fracture is present in the right third proximal phalanx.

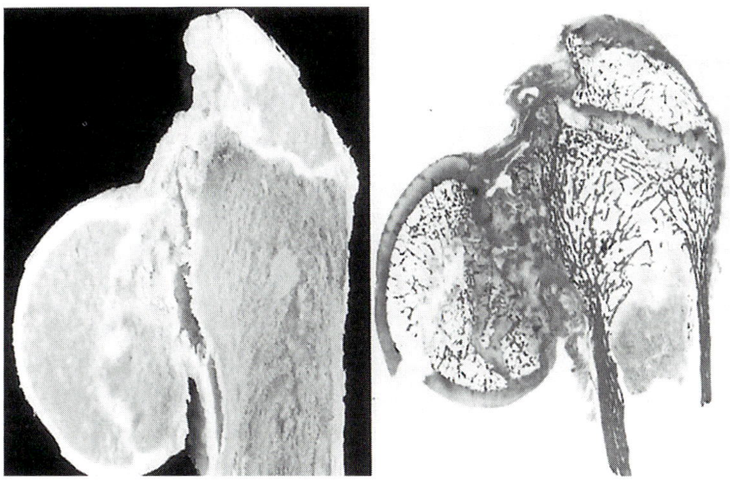

Figure 3

Fractures in a patient with primary hyperparathyroidism often displace and heal slowly (if at all). The fracture and deformity of the femoral neck are evident on both the gross and microscopic studies.

presence of erosions of the hand bones and the presence of a "salt and pepper skull" and especially "brown tumors," which consist of lytic areas within the bones, sometimes with expansion of the cortex and pathologic fractures[19,43,44,60-62] (Figure 4). These may be mistaken for metastatic tumor foci. In addition, there is occasionally a loss of the lamina dura in the teeth. Renal manifestations are common and may include a mild renal tubular acidosis, phosphaturia, aminoaci-

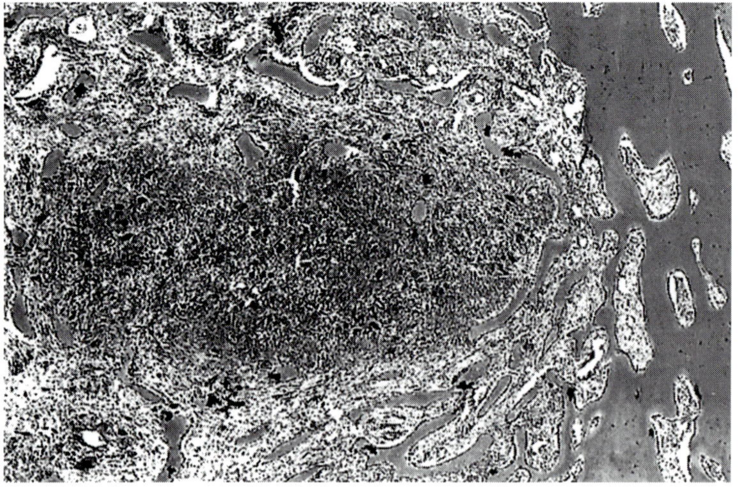

Figure 4
Histologic study of a brown tumor that shows a segment of bone with no osseous tissue that consists almost entirely of granulation tissue, hemorrhage, and osteoclasts. Hematoxylin and eosin × 20.

duria, and glycosuria. Calcification of meniscal and articular cartilage and renal calculi are frequently encountered and sometimes are the cause of the presenting complaint.[4,19,36,63,64]

Renal failure is a consequence of severe or prolonged disease in elderly patients and leads to the syndrome of renal osteodystrophy, which is at times very difficult to treat.[3,4,19] Patients with hyperparathyroidism often have gastrointestinal complaints and findings that include loss of appetite, anorexia, nausea and vomiting, constipation, and sometimes peptic ulceration and pancreatitis.[2-4,38,55] Occasionally the patients develop heart problems; in that group, death may be a consequence.[65,66]

Laboratory Diagnosis of Hyperparathyroidism

Some patients with hyperparathyroidism are asymptomatic; even the calcium level in the serum is at times either normal or only slightly elevated.[62,67-71] For these few patients, the only finding of note is the increase in the immunometric analysis for PTH and possibly hypophosphatemia. The majority of the patients, however, have hypercalcemia that can be as high as 16 mg/dL, often profound hypophospatemia, and usually an increase in alkaline phosphatase.[38,71-73] Urinary findings usually show hypercalcuria, hyperphosphaturia, and mild hyperchloremic acidosis.[2-4,19,39,68] The most

important studies to assess the presence of the disease are measurement of the PTH and the calcium concentration in the serum.[3,4,19,39] The tumor may be identified in the neck with ultrasound, magnetic resonance imaging, or most recently by sestamibi scan or positron emission tomography (PET) scan.[71,74-78]

Bone markers frequently disclose an increase in alkaline phosphatase and a positive bone scan.[3,4,19,73,74] Osteocalcin may be elevated, along with other markers suggestive of osteoporosis.[3,4] Bone densitometry will almost always show a low value on dual energy X-ray absorptiometry scan.[38,45,62,68,71,74,79-81]

Treatment of Primary Hyperparathyroidism

In sharp contrast to the original descriptions of the disease, it is now clear that not every patient with hyperparathyroidism needs treatment.[38,54,62,67-70] Unlike the early days of hyperparathyroidism, when all patients had marked and often severe disorders of bone and soft tissue, most of the patients seen today have mild disease.[38,41,51,67,69,70,82] Patients with very mild disease who have normal calcium levels, no overt bone lesions, and virtually no symptoms may be followed but should be reevaluated regularly. For patients suspected of having MEN type I or II, a thorough study of the body for evidence of tumors in other organs is essential. For the patients with symptomatic disease and high calcium levels, there are several treatment options:

- Maintenance of fluid balance and control of renal and central nervous system problems are essential. Patients with hyperparathyroidism should be encouraged to increase their fluid intake and take ample quantities of vitamins.[56,62,83,84] Chemistries should be requently evaluated to make sure that renal function is normal. Blood levels of calcium, phosphorus, blood urea nitrogen, creatinine, glucose, 25 hydroxy and 1,25 dihydroxy vitamin D, PTH, thyroid-stimulating hormone, and liver function studies should be measured regularly. Rest and particularly sleep are valuable, and appropriate medication may be useful in avoiding nervous system problems. An exercise and physiotherapy program will perhaps increase the strength of the bones, just as with elderly women who have postmenopausal osteoporosis.[38,41,44,51,61,67,69,70,74,82]

- Surgery. Removing a parathyroid adenoma can be curative.[79,85-89] Finding the affected gland by sestamibi or PET scanning may be necessary to be certain that all hyperplastic or multiple adenomatous sites are present in the site of the surgery, which some surgeons perform using minimally invasive techniques.[49,86,87,90-92] Occasionally in the past, a segment of a gland has been implanted in another site following resection of all four glands to provide a source of PTH if it becomes necessary.[49,86,88] If concern exists about the possibility of a recurrence after surgery or a carcinoma, a computed tomography or ultrasound-guided needle biopsy can be done prior to a wide resection and a PET scan performed to determine if nodal or pulmonary disease is present.[37,75-77,89,91] Bone lesions sometimes require surgery as well, particularly if a fracture has occurred or if some form of deformity interferes with function. Patients with longstanding hyperparathyroidism may have considerable osteoarthritic change in hips, knees, and shoulders; surgery may be required to restore the patient to useful function.[19,60,63]
- Medical agent therapy. The principal agent used in the past to reduce the potential damage from the hypercalcemic state and the osteitis fibrosa cystica has been calcitonin, which is very effective in interfering with the osteoclastic bone destruction.[72,93] Estrogen therapy may also be useful for postmenopausal women with bone density problems.[80] Bisphosphonates may be helpful in restoring strength to the bone structure and avoiding pathologic fracture.[72,94] Recently another group of drugs known as calcimimetics have been introduced.[84,95-97] The most experience with these to date is with a material known as cinacalcet, which can markedly reduce an increased serum level of calcium in either primary or secondary hyperparathyroidism.[96]

Summary

Primary hyperparathyroidism is a disease that was originally a major problem in severity of presentation, definition, and management because of our inability to diagnose it and our failure to recognize the changes associated with hypercalcemia, renal disease, neuromuscular problems, and osteitis fibrosa cystica. We owe a great deal to talented investigators such as Albright, Reifenstein, and Jaffe, and more recently Potts, Mundy, Silverberg, Bilezikian, Favus, and many others who have defined the disease, devised methods of following patients with laboratory studies, and developed effective treatment protocols. Nevertheless, hyperparathyroidism remains a problem, particularly if the syndrome is subtle in presentation and confused with other disorders such as osteoporosis.

References

1. Albright F, Reifenstein EC Jr: *The Parathyroid Glands and Metabolic Bone Disease: Selected Studies.* Baltimore, MD, Williams and Wilkins, 1948.

2. Bilezikian JP: Primary hyperparathyroidism, in Favus M (ed): *Primer on the Metabolic Bone Disease and Disorders of Mineral Metabolism*, ed 4. Philadelphia, PA, Lippincott Williams and Wilkins, 1999, pp 187-199.

3. Mundy GR: *Bone Remodeling and Its Disorders*, ed 2. London, England, Martin Dunitz Ltd, 1999.

4. Potts JT Jr: Primary hyperparathyroidism, in Avioli LV, Krane SM (eds): *Metabolic Bone Disease.* San Diego, CA, Academic Press, 1998, pp 411-442.

5. Silverberg SJ: Natural history of primary hyperparathyroidism. *Endocrinol Metab Clin North Am* 2000;29:451-464.

6. Zink AR, Panzer S, Fesq-Martin M, Burger-Heinrich E, Wahl J, Nerlich AG: Evidence for a 7000-year-old case of primary hyperparathyroidism. *JAMA* 2005;293:40-42.

7. Cave AJE: Richard Owen and the discovery of the parathyroid glands, in Underwood EA (ed): *Science, Medicine and History.* Oxford, England, Oxford University Press, 1953, vol 2, 217-222.

8. Askanazy M: Ueber ein adenom der glandula parathyroidea. *Verh Dtsch Ges Pathol* 1906;10:85-88.

9. Erdheim J: Uber epithelkorperbefunde bei osteomalacie. *Akad Wiss Wien Math Naturwiss Kl* 1907;116:311-370.

10. Mandl F: Klinisches und experimentelles zur frage der lokalisierten ostitis fibrosa. B: Die generalisierte form der ostitis fibrosa. *Arch Klin Chir* 1926;143:1-26.

11. Wilder RM: Hyperparathyroidism: Tumor of the parathyroid glands associated with osteitis fibrosa. *Endocrinology* 1929;13:231-238.

12. Barr DP, Bulger HA: The clinical syndrome of hyperparathyroidism. *Am J Med Sci* 1930;179:449-476.

13. Jaffe HL: Hyperparathyroidism (Recklinghausen's disease of bone). *Arch Pathol* 1933;16:63-112.

14. Jaffe HL: Hyperparathyroidism (Recklinghausen's disease of bone). *Arch Pathol* 1933;16:236-258.

15. Albright F, Aub JC, Bauer W: Hyperparathyroidism: A common and polymorphic condition as illustrated by 17 proved cases from one clinic. *JAMA* 1934;102:1276-1287.

16. Boden SD, Kaplan FS: Calcium homeostasis. *Orthop Clin North Am* 1990;21:31-42.

17. Broadus AE: Mineral balance and homeostasis, in Favus M (ed): *Primer on the Metabolic Bone Diseases and Disorders of Mineral Metabolism*, ed 4. Philadelphia, PA, Lippincott Williams and Wilkins, 1999, pp 74-80.

18. Segre GV: Secretion, metabolism and circulating heterogeneity of parathyroid hormone, in Favus MJ (ed): *Primer on Metabolic Bone Diseases and Disorders of Mineral Metabolism*. Kelseyville, CA, American Society for Bone and Mineral Research, 1990, pp 43-44.

19. Mankin HJ: Metabolic bone disease. *Instr Course Lect* 1995;44:3-32.

20. Wikvall K: Cytochrome P450 enzymes in the bioactivation of vitamin D to its hormonal form. *Int J Mol Med* 2001;7:201-209.

21. Holick MF: Vitamin D: Photobiology, metabolism, mechanism of action, and clinical applications, in Favus MJ (ed): *Primer on the Metabolic Bone Diseases and Disorders of Mineral Metabolism*, ed 4. Philadelphia, PA, Lippincott Williams and Wilkins, 1999, pp 92-98.

22. Hollis BW, Clemens TL, Adams JS: Vitamin D metabolites, in Favus MJ (ed): *Primer on the Metabolic Bone Diseases and Disorders of Mineral Metabolism*, ed 4. Philadelphia, PA, Lippincott Williams and Wilkins, 1999, pp 124-127.

23. Jüppner H, Brown EM, Kronenburg HM: Parathyroid hormone, in Favus MJ (ed): *Primer on the Metabolic Bone Diseases and Disorders of Mineral Metabolism*, ed 4. Philadelphia, PA, Lippincott Williams and Wilkins, 1999, pp 80-87.

24. Reichel H, Koeffler HP, Norman AW: The role of the vitamin D endocrine system in health and disease. *N Engl J Med* 1989;320:980-991.

25. Kumar R: Vitamin D metabolism and mechanisms of transport. *J Am Soc Nephrol* 1990;1:30-42.

26. Lemann J Jr, Favus M: The intestinal absorption of calcium, magnesium and phosphate, in Favus MJ (ed): *Primer on the Metabolic Bone Diseases and Disorders of Mineral Metabolism*, ed 4. Philadelphia, PA, Lippincott Williams and Wilkins, 1999, pp 63-66.

27. Wasserman RH, Brindak ME, Buddle MM, et al: Recent studies on the biological actions of vitamin D on intestinal transport and the electrophysiology of peripheral nerve and cardiac muscle. *Prog Clin Biol Res* 1990;332:99-126.

28. Wright FS, Bromsztyk K: Calcium transport by the proximal tubule. *Adv Exp Med Biol* 1986;208:165-170.

29. Brautbar N, Levine BS, Walling MW, Coburn JW: Intestinal absorption of calcium: Role of dietary phosphate and Vitamin D. *Am J Physiol* 1981;241:G49-G53.

30. Bronner F: Intestinal calcium transport: The cellular pathway. *Miner Electrolyte Metab* 1990;16:94-100.

31. Bronner F: Current concepts of calcium absorption: An overview. *J Nutr* 1992;122(3 Suppl):641-643.

32. Bushinsky DA: Calcium, magnesium and phosphorus: Renal handling and urinary excretion, in Favus M (ed): *Primer on the Metabolic Bone Diseases and Disorders of Mineral Metabolism*, ed 4. Philadelphia, PA, Lippincott Williams and Wilkins, 1999, pp 67-73.

33. Friedman PA, Gesek FA: Calcium transport in renal epithelial cells. *Am J Physiol* 1993;264:F181-F198.

34. Yanagawa N, Lee DBN: Renal handling of calcium and phosphorus, in Coe FL, Favus ME (eds): *Disorders of Bone and Mineral Metabolism*. New York, NY, Raven Press, 1992, pp 3-40.

35. Cross HS, Debiec H, Peterlik M: Mechanism and regulation of intestinal phosphate absorption. *Miner Electrolyte Metab* 1990;16:115-124.

36. Grahame R, Sutor DJ, Metchener MB: Crystal deposition in hyperparathyroidism. *Ann Rheum Dis* 1971;30:597-604.

37. Shane E: Clinical review 122: Parathyroid carcinoma. *J Clin Endocrinol Metab* 2001;86:485-493.

38. Bilezikian JP, Silverberg SJ: Clinical spectrum of primary hyperparathyroidism. *Rev Endocr Metab Disord* 2000;1:237-245.

39. Silverberg SJ, Bilezikian JP: Primary hyperparathyroidism, in Becker KL, Bilezikian JP, Bremmer W (eds): *Principles and Practice of Endocrinology and Metabolism*, ed 3. Philadelphia, PA, Lippincott Williams and Wilkins, 2001, pp 564-573.

40. Girard RM, Belanger A, Hazel B: Primary hyperparathyroidism in children. *Can J Surg* 1982;25:11-13.

41. Heath H III, Hodgson SF, Kennedy MA: Primary hyperparathyroidism: Incidence, morbidity and potential economic impact in a community. *N Engl J Med* 1980;302:189-193.

42. Joshua B, Feinmesser R, Ulanovski D, et al: Primary hyperparathyroidism in young adults. *Otolaryngol Head Neck Surg* 2004;131:628-632.

43. Adami S, Marcocci C, Gatti D: Epidemiology of primary hyperparthyroidism in Europe. *J Bone Miner Res* 2002;17(suppl 2):18-23.

44. Albertazzi P, Steel SA, Purdie DW, Gurney E, Atkin SL, Robertson WS: Hyperparathyroidism in elderly osteopenic women. *Maturitas* 2002;43:245-249.

45. Sitges-Serra A, Girvent M, Pereira JA, et al: Bone mineral density in menopausal women with primary hyperparathyroidism before and after parathyroidectomy. *World J Surg* 2004;28:1148-1152.

46. Arnold A, Brown M, Urena P, Gaz RD, Sarfati E, Drueke TB: Monoclonality of parathyroid tumors in chronic renal failure and in primary parathyroid hyperplasia. *J Clin Invest* 1995;95:2047-2053.

47. Arnold A, Kim HG: Clonal loss of one chromosome 11 in a parathyroid adenoma. *J Clin Endocrinol Metab* 1989;69:496-499.

48. Brandi ML, Falchetti A: Genetics of primary hyperparathyroidism. *Urol Int* 2004;72(suppl 1):11-16.

49. Carling T, Udelsman R: Parathyroid surgery in familial hyperparathyroid disorders. *J Intern Med* 2005;257:27-37.

50. Friedman E, Bale AE, Marx SJ, et al: Genetic abnormalities in sporadic parathyroid adenomas. *J Clin Endocrinol Metab* 1990;71:293-297.

51. Melton LJ III: The epidemiology of primary hyperparathyroidism in North America. *J Bone Miner Res* 2002;17(suppl 2):N12-N17.

52. Brandi ML, Aurbach GD, Fitzpatrick LA, et al: Parathyroid mitogenic activity in plasma from patients with familial multiiple endocrine neoplasia Type 1. *N Engl J Med* 1986;314:1287-1293.

53. Miedlich S, Krohn K, Lamesch P: Frequency of somatic MEN1 gene mutations in monoclonal parathyroid tumours of patients with primary hyperparathyroidism. *Eur J Endocrinol* 2000;143:47-54.

54. Mundy GR, Cove DH, Fisken R: Primary hyperparathyroidism: Changes in the pattern of clinical presentation. *Lancet* 1980;1:1317-1320.

55. Bess MA, Edis AJ, van Heerden JA: Hyperparathyroidsm and pancreatitis: Chance or causal association? *JAMA* 1980;243:246-247.

56. Stenstrom G, Heedman PA: Clinical findings in patients with hypercalcaemia: A final investigation based on biochemical screening. *Acta Med Scand* 1974;195:473-477.

57. Joborn C, Hetta J, Johansson H, et al: Psychiatric morbidity in primary hyperparathyroidism. *World J Surg* 1988;12:476-481.

58. Solomon BL, Schaaf M, Smallridge RC: Psychologic symptoms before and after parathyroid surgery. *Am J Med* 1994;96:101-106.

59. Turken SA, Cafferty M, al Silverberg SJ: Neuromuscular involvement in mild, asymptomatic primary hyperparathyroidism. *Am J Med* 1989;87:553-557.

60. Silverberg SJ, Shane E, de la Cruz L, et al: Skeletal disease in primary hyperparathyroidism. *J Bone Miner Res* 1989;4:283-291.

61. Katagiri T, Takahashi N: Regulatory mechanisms of osteoblast and osteoclast differentiation. *Oral Dis* 2002;8:147-159.

62. Potts JT Jr: Clinical review 9: Management of asymptomatic hyperparathyroidism. *J Clin Endocrinol Metab* 1990;70:1489-1493.

63. Dodds WJ, Steinbach HL: Primary hyperparathyroidism and articular cartilage calcification. *Am J Roentgenol Radium Ther Nucl Med* 1968;104:884-892.

64. Rodman JS, Mahler RJ: Kidney stones as a manifestation of hypercalcemic disorders: Hyperparathyroidism and sarcoidosis. *Urol Clin North Am* 2000;27:275-285.

65. Andersson P, Rydberg E, Willenheimer R: Primary hyperparathyroidism and heart disease: A review. *Eur Heart J* 2004;25:1776-1787.

66. Vestergaard P, Mollerup CL, Frokjaer VG, Christiansen P, Blichert-Toft M, Mosekilde L: Cardiovascular events before and after surgery for primary hyperparathyroidism. *World J Surg* 2003;27:216-222.

67. Bilezikian JP, Potts JT Jr: Asymptomatic primary hyperparathyroidism: New issues and new questions. Bridging the past with the future. *J Bone Miner Res* 2002;17(suppl 2):N57-N67.

68. Bilezikian JP, Silverberg SJ, Shane E, Parisien M, Dempster DW: Characterization and evaluation of asymptomatic primary hyperparathyroidism. *J Bone Miner Res* 1991;6(suppl 2):S85-S89.

69. Bilezikian JP: Primary hyperparathyroidism: When to observe and when to operate. *Endocrinol Metab Clin North Am* 2000;29:465-478.

70. Clark OH, Wilkes W, Siperstein AE, Duh Q-Y: Diagnosis and management of asymptomatic hyperparathyroidism: Safety, efficacy and deficiencies in our knowledge. *J Bone Miner Res* 1991;6(suppl 2):S135-S142.

71. Valdemarsson S, Lindergaard B, Tibblen S, Bergenfelz A: Increased biochemical markers of bone formation and resorption in primary hyerparathyroidism, with special reference to patients with mild disease. *J Intern Med* 1998;243:115-122.

72. Bilezikian JP: Management of acute hypercalcemia. *N Engl J Med* 1992;326:1196-1203.

73. Bodansky A, Jaffe HL: Phosphatase studies: III. Serum phosphatase in diseases of bone. *Arch Intern Med* 1934;54:88-110.

74. Adami S, Braga V, Squaranti R, Rossini M, Gatti D, Zamberlan N: Bone measurements in asymptomatic primary hyperparathyroidism. *Bone* 1998;22:565-570.

75. Catargi B, Raymond JM, Lafarge-Gense V, Leccia F, Roger P, Tabarin A: Localization of parathyroid tumors using endoscopic ultrasonography in primary hyperparathyroidism. *J Endocrinol Invest* 1999;22:688-692.

76. Dackiw AP, Sussman JJ, Fritsche HA Jr, et al: Relative contributions of technetium Tc 99m sestamibi scintigraphy, interoperative gamma probe detection, and the rapid parathyroid hormone assay to the surgical management of hyperparathyroidism. *Arch Surg* 2000;135:550-555.

77. De Feo ML, Colagrande S, Biagini C, et al: Parathyroid glands: Combination of (99m)Tc MIBI scintigraphy and US for demonstration of parathyroid glands and nodules. *Radiology* 2000;214:393-402.

78. Gotway MB, Higgins CB: MR imaging of the thyroid and parathyroid glands. *Magn Reson Imaging Clin N Am* 2000;8:163-182.

79. Gonnelli S, Montagnani A, Cepollaro C, et al: Quantitative ultrasound and bone mineral density in patients with primary hyperparathyroidism before and after surgical treatment. *Osteoporos Int* 2000;3:255-260.

80. Orr-Walker BJ, Evans MC, Clearwater JM, Horne A, Grey AB, Reid IR: Effects of hormone replacement therapy on bone mineral density in postmenopausal women with primary hyperparathyroidism: Four-year follow-up and comparison with healthy postmenopausal women. *Arch Intern Med* 2000;160:2161-2166.

81. Silverberg SJ, Gartenberg F, Jacobs TP, et al: Increased bone mineral density after parathyroidectomy in primary hyperparathyroidism. *J Clin Endocrinol Metab* 1995;80:729-734.

82. Mitlak BH, Daly M, Potts JT Jr: Asymptomatic primary hyperparathyroidism. *J Bone Miner Res* 1991;6(suppl 2):S103-S110.

83. Locker FG, Silverberg SJ, Bilezikian JP: Optimal dietary calcium intake in primary hyperparathyroidism. *Am J Med* 1997;102:543-550.

84. Strewler GJ: Medical approaches to primary hyperparathyroidism. *Endocrinol Metab Clin North Am* 2000;29:523-539.

85. Cope O, Barnes BA, Castleman B, Mueller GC, Roth SI: Vicissitudes of parathyroid surgery: Trail of diagnosis and management in 51 patients with a variety of disorders. *Ann Surg* 1961;154:491-508.

86. Eigelberger MS, Clark OH: Surgical approaches to primary hyperparathyroidism. *Endocrinol Metab Clin North Am* 2000;29:479-502.

87. Martin RC, Greenwell D, Flynn MB: Initial neck exploration for untreated hyperparathyroidism. *Am Surg* 2000;66:269-272.

88. Organ CH Jr: The history of parathyroid surgery 1850-1996: The Excelsior Surgical Society 1998

Edward D Churchill Lecture. *J Am Coll Surg* 2000;191:284-299.

89. Walgenbach S, Hommel G, Junginger T: Outcome after surgery for primary hyperparathyroidism: Ten-year prospective follow-up study. *World J Surg* 2000;24:564-569.

90. Chen H, Sokoll LJ, Udelsman R: Outpatient minimally invasive parathyroidectomy: A combination of sestamibi-SPECT localization, cervical block anesthesia, and intraoperative parathyroid hormone assay. *Surgery* 1999;126:1016-1021.

91. Hedback G, Oden A: Recurrence of hyperparathyroidism: A long–term follow-up after surgery for primary hyperparathyroidism. *Eur J Endocrinol* 2003;148:413-421.

92. Reeve TS, Babidge WJ, Parkyn RF, et al: Minimally invasive surgery for primary hyperparathyroidism: Systematic review. *Arch Surg* 2000;135:481-487.

93. Deftos LJ, Roos BA, Oates EL: Calcitonin, in Favus M (ed): *Primer on the Metabolic Bone Diseases and Disorders of Mineral Metabolism*, ed 4. Philadelphia, PA, Lippincott Williams and Wilkins, 1999, pp 99-103.

94. Gallacher SJ, Ralson SH, Fraser WD, et al: A comparison of low versus high dose pamidronate in cancer-associated hypercalcemia. *Bone Miner* 1991;15:249-256.

95. Joy MS, Kshirsagar A, Franceschini N: Calcimimetics and the treatment of primary and secondary hyperparathyroidism. *Ann Pharmacother* 2004;38:1871-1880.

96. Peacock M, Bilezikian JP, Klassen PS, Guo MD, Turner SA, Shoback D: Cinacalcet hydrochloride maintains long term normocalcemia in patients with primary hyperparathyroidism. *J Clin Endocrinol Metab* 2005;90:135-141.

97. Silverberg SJ, Thys-Jacobs S, Locker FG, et al: The effect of calcimimetic drug NPS R568 on parathyroid hormone secretion in primary hyperparathyroidism. *J Bone Miner Res* 1996;11(suppl):87.

Chapter 22

Osteoporosis

Osteoporosis is a major orthopaedic problem of our time. It involves more patients, hospital and rehabilitation beds, and health care professionals than many other disorders. In 1903, the average lifespan in the US was 47 years. There is no doubt that people suffered with poliomyelitis, tuberculosis, scurvy, many types of infections, and a host of other afflictions; however, there was no acquired immunodeficiency syndrome, not nearly as much cancer, and almost no osteoporosis. By 2003, the average lifespan had increased to 77 years. Although many of the diseases from the past are far less common, with longer lives we now have to deal with Alzheimer's; sociologic and psychological issues; considerable increases in cancer, strokes, and heart disease and resultant chronic disability; and postmenopausal and senile osteoporosis.

The physician's role in caring for patients has likely had significant impact on this trend. Our success in controlling the diseases of the 20th century has allowed our patients to survive long enough for these other disorders to occur. Some even speculate that we have possibly allowed people to live too long, and that they have now exceeded their physical and emotional capacity to live as productive citizens!

Osteoporosis represents a decrease in the density of the bones. In 1824, Sir Astley Cooper remarked that "the regular decay of nature which is called old age is attended with changes. One of the principal of these is found in the bones, for they become thin in their shell and spongy in their texture".[1] In 1940, Fuller Albright noted how this disease differed from osteomalacia or hyperparathyroidism, writing "there is less bone, but what bone there is, is normal"[2] (Figure 1). Over the years since the disease was characterized, it became clear to clinicians and investigators that the synthesis of bone is diminished and there is likely excessive destruction of bone as well; the two together cause the bones to be thinner and more likely to fracture.[3-9] Loss of bone structure in this fashion is asymptomatic. Because the patients have no complaints of pain or even disability until a fracture occurs, they are less likely to limit their activities or seek medical care, and physicians are less likely to consider their status to be potentially serious bone disorders.[3,5,6,9-13]

Causes of Osteoporosis

There are many causes of osteoporosis. Because family history clearly plays a role, physicians should ask about parents and grandparents in reviewing the patient's his-

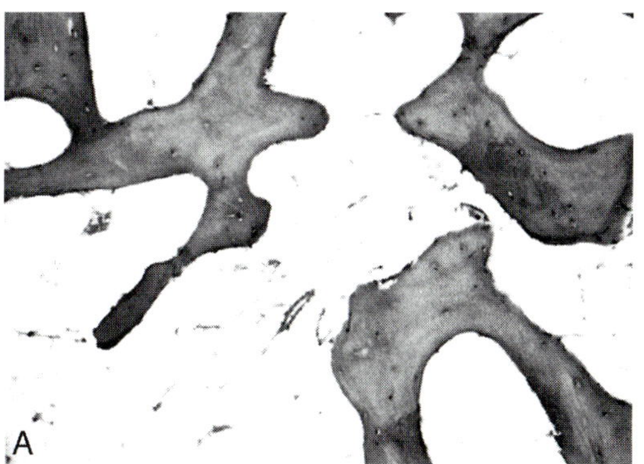
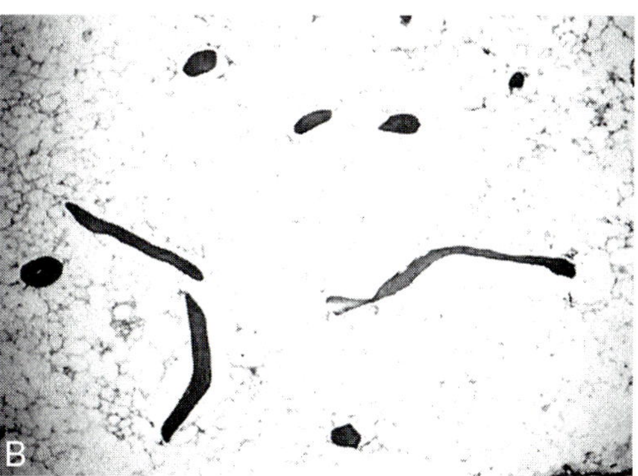

Figure 1
A, Histologic section of the normal bone structure in a 65-year-old woman showing the size and structure of the trabeculae. **B,** Section of the same enlargement of the trabecular architecture in a patient with severe osteoporosis. What bone there is, is normal, but they become "thin in their shell and spongy in their texture".[1] Hematoxylin and eosin × 20.

tory.[3,5,6,11,14] Studies are currently underway to assess the changes in bone density associated with alterations in chromosome 11; the possibility exists for candidate genes where some polymorphism has been identified.[5,8,15-17] These candidates include the vitamin D receptor gene and genes coded for type I collagen and insulin growth factor; however, to date any association with the syndrome of osteoporosis has not been clearly defined.[16-18] Generally low body weight is more likely to be associated with osteoporosis than normal or increased weight.[4,9,12,19] Several studies have demonstrated that osteoporosis is less likely to occur in patients who have osteoarthritis in multiple sites.[20] Osteoporosis occurs frequently in patients with eating disorders or smoking or alcohol abuse; the frequency of fractures in anorectic and alcoholic patients is alarmingly high.[3-6,12,19,21,22] Chronic physical disuse is a cause in patients with extreme disability or long-term dietary calcium deficiency; chronic renal disease, diabetes mellitus, metastatic cancer, chronic hyper- or hypothyroidism, hypogonadism, corticosteroid administration, rheumatoid arthritis, Gaucher disease, Marfan's syndrome, Turner's disease, osteogenesis imperfecta, homocystinuria, and many other disorders are characterized by the presence of progressive and at times severe osteopenia.[2-7,19,23-29] However, all of the above account for less than 2% of patients who present with osteoporosis. The vast majority of patients with the classic disease have what is now termed postmenopausal or senile osteoporosis.[6]

Mechanism and Effect of Postmenopausal or Senile Osteoporosis

An understanding of the process of bone loss in patients with postmenopausal or senile osteoporosis is essential. Bone continues to accrete in the skeleton until 30 years of age. For a 10-year period, bones remain stable in that bone destruction and bone production are equivalent. At 40 years of age, however, both males and females begin a cortical and medullary bone loss of approximately 0.3% per year, which remains constant throughout life and accounts for loss of 3% of the bony tissue every 10 years. In addition, women have a postmenopausal

bone loss of 10 times that amount, another 3% per year, for the first 10 years after menopause. After losing 30% of their bone during those terrible 10 years, they return to the standard rate of 0.3% per year[3-8,12,22,30,31]

Fractures in Osteoporosis

The decline in bone structure leads to fractures that are now known as fragility fractures or low-energy fractures.[3-6,8,11,12,21,26,31-34] Most of these are located in the spine, wrist, hip, proximal humerus, and ankle and may be associated with alterations in physical stability either from neurologic disease or muscle wasting. Patients state that they lose balance, and report frequent falling as an issue in their lives.[28,35,36] Each year in the US, 1.5 million osteoporotic fractures occur. Of these, 700,000 are in the spine, 300,000 in the hip, and 200,000 in the wrist.[3-8,21,37] The cost of these problems is enormous, amounting to over $30 billion per year. Of greater concern is the fact that people with one fracture are five times more likely to have a second fracture in the same year; of highest concern is that people with a hip fracture have a 20% chance of dying within a year.[3,6,21,26,31,32,38-42]

Definition of Osteoporosis

Osteoporosis is best defined by determination of bone mineral density (BMD) usually by a technique using dual energy X-ray absorptiometry (DEXA).[5,8,10,28,37,43,44] The World Health Organization has defined normal as equal to or no more than 1 standard deviation (SD) below the mean for young healthy individuals with no bone disease. A DEXA score of greater than 1 SD but still no more than 2.5 SD below the normal is considered diagnostic of osteoporosis, while a score of greater than 2.5 SD below the normal represents severe osteoporosis with a very high risk of fracture.[5,37] Recently an ultrasound technology has been introduced; however, there are limitations on how this can be applied, and concern exists as to the correlation with the gold standard BMD technologies.[45,46]

Laboratory Studies of Osteoporosis

Laboratory studies for identification of the syndrome are more helpful in ruling out other disorders than in identifying postmeno-

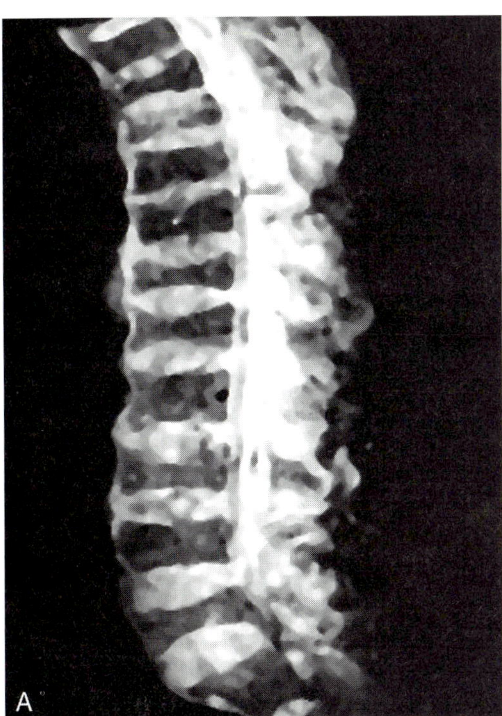 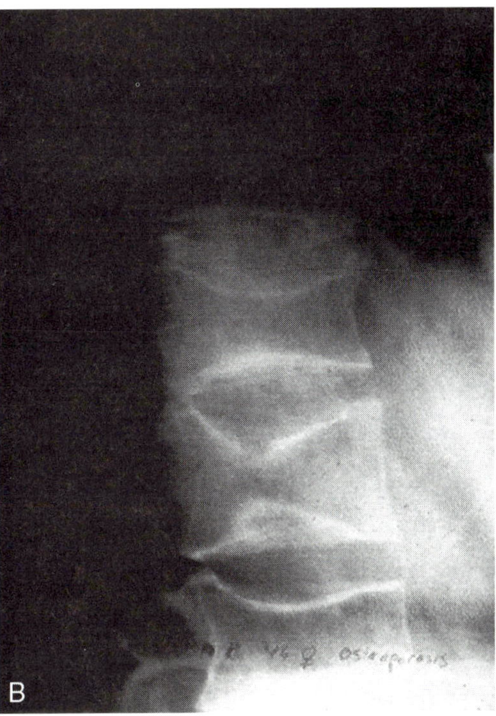

Figure 2
A, Photograph of a section of the spine of a 75-year-old patient with severe osteoporosis showing the extraordinary collapse of almost all the vertebral segments. **B,** Radiographic study that shows a similar finding for two segments in a 56-year-old woman who had an oophorectomy at 36 years of age.

pausal or senile osteoporosis. Calcium, phosphorus, alkaline phosphatase, 25 hydroxy and 1,25 dihydroxy vitamin D, and parathyroid hormone (PTH) levels are usually normal; if abnormal, osteomalacia or hyperparathyroidism should be suspected.[6] Thyroid function should also be normal; if abnormal, either hyper- or hypothyroidism may be the cause.[24] Serum immunoelectrophoresis, hematocrit, and sedimentation rate are usually normal; if abnormal, one should rule out myeloma, which occasionally presents as diffuse osteopenia.[6] There are some tests that are helpful in assessing the extent of the disease. Homocysteine levels may be useful in defining patients with high risk for fracture.[5] Bone-specific alkaline phosphatase, osteocalcin, and amino-terminal and carboxyterminal propeptides of type 1 collagen may serve as indicators of reduced bone formation.[6,8,15,43] Tartrate-resistant acid phosphatase may be indicative of bone resorption.[15] Urinary hydroxyproline and pyridine nucleotides may represent evidence of bone resorption, as may N and C telopeptides of collagen crosslinks.[6,15,43] These markers are of less value as diagnostic tools than they

may be to assess the effectiveness of treatment.[6]

Imaging studies are sometimes helpful in defining the extent of the disease, identifying sites of stress fractures, and perhaps most importantly in ruling out other diseases such as other metabolic bone diseases, myeloma, lymphoma, or metastatic carcinoma.[4-6,8,11,13,22,27,28,30,31] Radiographs show thin cortices and poorly defined medullary bone based on the sometimes tiny size of the trabecular structures. Vertebral segments are frequently affected and may show not only thin cortices, but also mild compression fractures of the anterior aspects of the segments that lead to a thoracic kyphotic appearance with a minimal lumbar lordosis (called a "dowager's hump" in the past) (Figure 2). The presence of a clearly displayed Ward's triangle on radiographs of the hip may be indicative of osteoporosis and, even more importantly, an impending fracture. Bone scans may be useful to indicate the presence of impending or stress fractures. Stress fractures are sometimes easier to identify on computed tomography or magnetic resonance imaging (MRI) scans; certainly MRI of the spine is very useful in assessing the presence of nerve or cord compression.

Several studies have shown that elderly patients with fragility fractures and what appears to be osteoporosis on imaging studies are not studied more extensively to determine if osteomalacia or hyperparathyroidism may be associated causations. More importantly, a large percentage of patients with hip or spine fractures who clearly have osteoporosis do not receive BMD studies, laboratory tests, or appropriate drug treatments for their osteoporosis.[3,26,34,37,38,40,41,47-49]

Treatment of Osteoporosis

The treatment of osteoporosis will in large measure depend on the age of the patient; the extent of the disease; and the need for surgery, physiotherapy, or bracing to treat or prevent fractures.

Prevention

Exercise is very valuable for patients at risk for osteoporosis.[19,23,25,26,48] Young patients at risk or elderly patients with osteopenia should be encouraged to exercise daily by walking outdoors or on treadmills or even using stationary bicycles. Swimming is helpful, but as a non–weight-bearing activity it is less likely to help the patient regain bone structure. Bracing of the spine or sometimes lower extremities can be helpful.[5] Calcium and vitamin D administration are essential even at a very young age.[5,7,19,48,50-53] Adults should take at least 1,200 mg of calcium daily and a minimum of 800 units of vitamin D. Higher doses of both can be given to elderly patients who have little exposure to sunlight.

The use of estrogen and/or progesterone for pre- or postmenopausal women is theoretically an excellent approach to the problem but has some serious potential side effects. The drugs probably stimulate osteoblastic activity and may decrease osteoclastic bone loss.[5,6,26,54] The incidence of heart disease, stroke, and breast and uterine cancer is considerably higher for patients who take estrogen; the risk, especially for breast cancer, is far too great to warrant the use of this type of therapy. Reloxifene is a material that has estrogen-like activity but is less likely to have the side effects of the hormone; unfortunately, however, it is less effective than many of the other agents now available.[5,55,56] Calcitonin, which acts to almost completely impede osteoclastic activity, may be valuable in the treatment of osteoporosis but it is more successful with spinal disease than with hip disease; ideally, it should be injected, which makes it more of a problem.[5,7,52,57,58] It is now possible to take calcitonin by nasal administration, which may make it more tolerable.[57]

Drugs That Decrease Bone Destruction

The bisphosphonates are drugs that interfere with bone resorption by altering the action of the osteoclast on the adjacent bone. The materials are thought to induce caspase cleavage of mst-1 kinase during apoptosis.[59] Although a number of drugs are currently available, the four that seem to be most useful in preventing bone from being resorbed are alendronate, risedronate, pamidronate, and zolendronate.

Alendronate is the drug most frequently used. Several studies have demonstrated increased BMD and decreased fracture risk with use of 10 mg of alendronate daily or, more recently, 70 mg weekly.[5,39,60,61] The difficulty with alendronate is the possible gastrointestinal complications, in particular esophagitis and gastritis.[62] The drug must be taken with water while standing, and the patient should not eat for about an hour. For these reasons, an increasing number of patients are finding the drug difficult to take. In addition, central nervous system problems related to hearing and vision have been reported; fortunately, they are easily reversible with discontinuation of the drug.[61] Of some value under these circumstances is the introduction of risedronate, which has a moderately diminished risk of side effects.[63-65] Although it must be taken in a similar manner and is not quite as effective as alendronate in reducing fractures or increasing BMD, risedronate is sometimes a better choice for older women. A recent report suggests that osteonecrosis of the jaw may occur on rare occasions in patients who take either of these oral bisphosphonates.[66]

Two other drugs can be given intravenously, thus reducing the possible effect on the gastrointestinal tract. Pamidronate is administered intravenously at approximately 2- to 3-month intervals and appears to be effective not only for osteoporosis but for metastatic cancer and myeloma.[67,68] In a study of this agent, BMD was increased and the number of fractures reduced.[67] Perhaps the most unusual of the bisphosphonates in terms of protocol is zolendronate, which is very aggressive in controlling for osteoclastic resorption of bone and has the greatest effect on BMD.[68,69] This material is administered only once a year. Its effect on fracture frequency is still being investigated.

Drugs That Increase Bone Formation

Recombinant PTH (1-34) seems to be of value in the management of osteoporosis by increasing bone formation. The material is believed to activate adenyl cyclase and a number of phospholipases, thus increasing the levels of cyclic adenosine monophosphate and calcium transport and reducing osteoblast apoptosis.[70-74] The number of osteoclasts is also slightly increased but the principal action is on bone production, which causes a marked increase in BMD at the doses administered. The drug is given subcutaneously daily and seems very effective in preventing fractures. Some investigators have suggested that the use of PTH with bisphosphonates may be more effective than PTH alone, particularly for increasing the BMD; however, this issue remains a subject of controversy.[75-77]

Two other agents are currently in trials. Strontium ranelate appears to stimulate bone formation, and patients have been shown to have a lower fracture rate and an increased BMD.[52,78] Another agent is low-dose recombinant human growth hormone administered nasally, which possibly acts through the stimulation of production of insulin-like growth factor-1.[17,56,74,79,80] The agent appears to be very effective in Turner's syndrome, Prader-Willi disease, and other low-growth hormone disorders.[81] The response of menopausal or senile osteoporosis is much less clearly defined. Several studies have suggested that BMD is increased in patients who receive the drug, but it is more effective when combined with alendronate therapy.[79]

Some issues that remain problematic with all of these agents are how long one should continue to use them and what side effects might be associated with prolonged use, particularly with elderly patients.[63] Oral bisphosphonates may cause significant esophageal difficulties, and recent reports suggest that patients may develop osteone-crosis of the jaw[82] or temporary auditory or visual problems.[66] PTH (1-34) and the recombinant PTH may enhance the growth of malignant cells in tumors. Estrogen should be avoided; reloxifene may be safe initially, but may over time have some estrogenic effects on breast and uterine disease.[5-7,54,55]

Surgical Treatment of Patients With Osteoporosis

Fractures of the wrist can usually be treated with immobilization, or sometimes insertion of bone substitute agents such as calcium sulfate, bone morphogenetic (BMP)-7, or demineralized bone matrix with glycerol (Grafton).[28] Fractures of the spine are much more difficult to treat. Unless the patient develops root or cord problems, bracing may be all that can be done. It is possible to perform percutaneous kyphoplasty and use a balloon to expand a collapsed segment. Insertion of methylmethacrylate with coralline or recombinant human BMP-2, or even a titanium mesh, may help correct the collapse and diminish the symptoms.[83-88]

Fractures of the hip should almost always be reduced and either fixed with appropriate hardware or, if sufficient destruction has occurred, a total hip procedure may be indicated.[4,21,22,32,33,39,40] The proximal humerus is generally less of a problem but may require immobilization, open reduction, or even prosthetic replacement.

Summary

Osteoporosis remains a major problem for the elderly and especially for postmenopausal women. The disorder can occur silently and patients and their physicians may not be aware of the extent of the bone loss and the relative risk of very disabling fragility fractures. Once fractures occur, the patients often require surgery and may lose their ability to care for themselves or continue in a productive life. They may become psychologically or sociologically impaired. Rehabilitation is helpful, as is protected living in a retirement community, but it is still not the life that many of these people would like to live. With the likelihood of an even greater increase in the average age of the population over the next 10 years, many of our citizens are at risk for spending their last years in pain, functionally impaired, and living in a difficult social setting.

It is the responsibility of the patient, the patient's family, and particularly the caring physician to institute preventive measures in the form of exercise, appropriate diets, and medications. The physician must study the patients at regular intervals with densitometry, physical examination, and laboratory tests and institute appropriate measures to improve the quality of their bones, prevent the fragility fractures, and if they do occur restore the patient as rapidly as possible to an acceptable lifestyle. That is the challenge for elderly patients, their families, and especially their physicians.

References

1. Cooper AP: *A Treatise on Dislocation of Joints*, ed 4. London, England, Longman, Hearst, Reese, Ormy, Brown and Green, 1824.

2. Albright F, Bloomberg E, Smith PH: Postmenopausal osteoporosis. *Trans Assoc Am Physicians* 1940;55:298-305.

3. Arden N, Cooper C: Present and future of osteoporosis: Epidemiology, in Meunier PJ (ed): *Osteoporosis: Diagnosis and Management*. St. Louis, MO, Mosby, 1998, pp 1-16.

4. Elliott ME: Osteoporotic fractures in older women. *Curr Womens Health Rep* 2002;2:356-365.

5. Lin JT, Lane JM: Osteoporosis: A review. *Clin Orthop Relat Res* 2004;425:126-134.

6. Mankin HJ: Metabolic bone disease. *Instr Course Lect* 1995;44:3-32.

7. Mundy GR: Bone remodeling and mechanisms of bone loss in osteoporosis, in Meunier PJ (ed): *Osteoporosis: Diagnosis and Management*. St. Louis, MO, Mosby, 1998, pp 17-36.

8. Mundy GR: *Bone Remodeling and Its Disorders*, ed 2. London, England, Martin Dunitz Ltd, 1999.

9. Pacifici R, Avioli LV: Effect of aging on bone structure and metabolism, in Avioli LV (ed): *The Osteoporotic Syndrome: Detection, Prevention and Treatment*, ed 4. San Diego, CA, Academic Press, 2000, pp 25-34.

10. Grampp S, Jergas M, Lang P, Genant H, Gluer C: Quantitative assessment of osteoporosis: Current and future status, in Sartoris DJ (ed):*Osteoporosis Diagnosis and Treatment*. New York, NY, Marcel Dekker, Inc, 1996, pp 233-266.

11. Olszynski WP, Shawn Davison K, Adachi JD, et al: Osteoporosis in men: Epidemiology, diagnosis, prevention and treatment. *Clin Ther* 2004;26:15-28.

12. Repa-Eschen L: The necessity of a managed care approach for osteoporosis, in Avioli LV (ed): *The Osteoporotic Syndrome: Detection, Prevention and Treatment*, ed 4. San Diego, CA, Academic Press, 2000, pp 1-24.

13. Stock H, Schneider A, Strauss E: Osteoporosis: A disease in men. *Clin Orthop Relat Res* 2004;425:143-151.

14. Seeman E, Hopper JL, Bach LA, et al: Reduced bone mass in daughters of women with osteoporosis. *N Engl J Med* 1989;320:554-558.

15. Civatelli R: Biochemical markers of bone turnover, in Avioli LV (ed): *The Osteoporotic Syndrome: Detection, Prevention and Treatment*, ed 4. San Diego, CA, Academic Press, 2000, pp 67-89.

16. Rosen EJ: The genetics of osteoporosis, in Avioli LV (ed): *The Osteoporotic Syndrome: Detection, Prevention and Treatment*, ed 4. San Diego, CA, Academic Press, 2000, pp 37-44.

17. Zofkova I: Pathophysiological and clinical importance of insulin-like growth factor-I with respect to bone metabolism. *Physiol Res* 2003;52:657-679.

18. Yakar S, Rosen SJ, Beamer WG, et al: Circulating levels of IGF-1 directly regulate bone growth and density. *J Clin Invest* 2002;110:771-781.

19. Heaney RP: Non-pharmacological prevention of osteoporosis: Nutrition and exercise, in Meunier PJ (ed): *Osteoporosis: Diagnosis and Management*. St. Louis, MO, Mosby, 1998, pp 161-164.

20. Dequeker J, Aerssens J, Luyten FP: Osteoarthritis and osteoporosis: Clinical and research evidence of inverse relationship. *Aging Clin Exp Res* 2003;15:426-439.

21. Cummings SR, Melton LJ: Epidemiology and outcomes of osteoporotic fractures. *Lancet* 2002;359:1761-1767.

22. Koval KJ, Chen AL, Aharonoff GB, Egol KA, Zuckerman JD: Clinical pathway for hip fractures in the elderly: The Hospital for Joint Diseases experience. *Clin Orthop Relat Res* 2004;425:72-81.

23. Bassey EJ: Exercise in primary prevention of osteoporosis in women. *Ann Rheum Dis* 1995;54:861-862.

24. Greenspan SL, Greenspan FS: The effect of thyroid hormone on skeletal integrity. *Ann Intern Med* 1999;130:750-758.

25. Kemmler W, Lauber D, Weineck J, Hensen J, Kalender W, Engelke K: Benefits of 2 years of intense exercise on bone density, physical fitness, and blood lipids in early postmenopausal osteopenic women: Results of the Erlangen Fitness Osteoporosis Prevention Study (EFOPS). *Arch Intern Med* 2004;164:1084-1091.

26. Kessel B: Hip fracture prevention in postmenopausal women. *Obstet Gynecol Surv* 2004;59:446-455.

27. Taylor JAM, Resnick DL, Sartoris DJ: Radiographic-pathologic correlation, in Sartoris DJ (ed): *Osteoporosis Diagnosis and Treatment*. New York, NY, Marcel Dekker, Inc, 1996, pp 147-200.

28. Vogt MT, Cauley JA, Tomaino MM, Stone K, Williams JR, Hendon JH: Distal radius fractures in older women: A 10-year follow-up study of descriptive characteristics and risk factors. The study of osteoporotic fractures. *J Am Geriatr Soc* 2002;50:97-103.

29. Wallace BA, Cumming RG: Systematic review of randomized trials of the effect of exercise on bone mass in pre- and postmenopausal women. *Calcif Tissue Int* 2000;67:10-18.

30. Jeong GK, Bendo JA: Spinal disorders in the elderly. *Clin Orthop Relat Res* 2004;425:110-125.

31. Kado DM, Browner WS, Palermo L, Nevitt MC, Genant HK, Cummings SF: Vertebral fractures and mortality in older women: A prospective study. Study of Osteoporotic Fractures Research Group. *Arch Intern Med* 1999;159:1215-1220.

32. Chao EYS, Inoue N, Koo TKK, Kim YH: Biomechanical considerations of fracture treatment and

bone quality maintenance in elderly patients and patients with osteoporosis. *Clin Orthop Relat Res* 2004;425:12-25.

33. Cummings SR, Black DM, Nevitt MC, et al: Bone density at various sites for prediction of hip fractures: The Study of Osteoporotic Fractures Research Group. *Lancet* 1993;341:72-75.

34. Kiebzak GM, Beinart GM, Perser K, Ambrose CG, Siff SJ, Heggeness MH: Undertreatment of osteoporosis in men with hip fracture. *Arch Intern Med* 2002;162:2217-2222.

35. Stevens JA, Olson S: Reducing falls and resulting hip fractures among older women. *MMWR Recomm Rep* 2000;49:3-12.

36. Westfall G, Littlefield R, Heaton A, Martin S: Methodology for identifying patients at high risk for osteoporotic fracture. *Clin Ther* 2001;23:1570-1588.

37. World Health Organization: Assessment of fracture risk and its application to screening for postmenopausal osteoporosis: Report of a WHO study group. *World Health Organ Tech Rep Ser* 1994;843:1-129.

38. Andrade SE, Majumdar SR, Chan KA, et al: Low frequency of treatment of osteoporosis among postmenopausal women following a fracture. *Arch Intern Med* 2003;163:2052-2057.

39. Black DM, Thompson DE, Bauer DC, et al: Fracture risk reduction with alendronate in women with osteoporosis: The Fracture Intervention Trial. FIT Research Group. *J Clin Endocrinol Metab* 2000;85:4118-4124.

40. Harrington JT, Broy SB, Derosa AM, Licata AA, Shewmon DA: Hip fracture patients are not treated for osteoporosis: A call to action. *Arthritis Rheum* 2002;47:651-654.

41. Johnell O, Oden A, Caulin F, Kanis JA: Acute and long-term increase in fracture risk after hospitalization for vertebral fracture. *Osteoporos Int* 2001;12:207-214.

42. Taillandier J, Langue F, Alemanni M, Taillandier-Heriche E: Mortality and functional outcomes of pelvic insufficiency fractures in older patients. *Joint Bone Spine* 2003;70:287-289.

43. Ebeling PR, Atley LM, Guthrie JR, et al: Bone turnover markers and bone density across the menopausal transition. *J Clin Endocrinol Metab* 1996;81:3366-3371.

44. Jergas M, Genant HK: Contributions of bone mass measurements by densitometry in the definition and diagnosis of osteoporosis, in Meunier PJ (ed): *Osteoporosis: Diagnosis and Management*. St. Louis, MO, Mosby, 1998, pp 37-58.

45. Bauer DC, Palermo L, Black D, Cauley JA: Quantitative ultrasound and mortality: A prospective study. *Osteoporos Int* 2002;13:606-612.

46. Hans D, Gluer CC, Njeh CF: Ultrasonic evaluation of osteoporosis, in Meunier PJ (ed): *Osteoporosis: Diagnosis and Management*. St. Louis, MO, Mosby, 1998, pp 59-78.

47. Follin SL, Black JN, McDermott MT: Lack of diagnosis and treatment of osteoporosis in men and women after hip fracture. *Pharmacotherapy* 2003;23:190-198.

48. Gardner MJ, Brophy RH, Dematrakopoulos D, et al: Interventions to improve osteoporosis treatment following hip fracture: A prospective randomized trial. *J Bone Joint Surg Am* 2005;87:3-7.

49. Siris ES, Chen Y-T, Abbott TA, et al: Bone mineral density thresholds for pharmacological intervention to prevent fractures. *Arch Intern Med* 2004;164:1108-1112.

50. Chapuy MC, Arlot ME, Duboeuf F, et al: Vitamin D3 and calcium to prevent hip fractures in the elderly women. *N Engl J Med* 1992;327:1637-1642.

51. Dawson-Hughes B: Calcium, vitamin D and bone metabolism, in Avioli LV (ed): *The Osteoporotic Sysndrome: Detection, Prevention and Treatment*, ed 4. San Diego, CA, Academic Press, 2000, pp 91-99.

52. Doggrell SA: Present and future pharmacotherapy for osteoporosis. *Drugs Today (Barc)* 2003;39:633-657.

53. Reid IR, Ames RW, Evans MC, Gamble GD, Sharpe SJ: Long-term effects of calcium supplementation on bone loss and fractures in postmenopausal women: A randomized controlled trial. *Am J Med* 1995;98:331-335.

54. Roussouw JE, Anderson GL, Prentice RL, et al: Risks and benefits of estrogen plus progestin in healthy postmenopausal women: Principal results from the Women's Health Initiative randomized controlled trial. *JAMA* 2002;288:321-333.

55. Maricic M, Adachi JD, Sarkar S, Wu W, Wong M, Harper KD: Early effects of raloxifene on clinical vertebral fractures at 12 months in postmenopausal women with osteoporosis. *Arch Intern Med* 2002;162:1140-1143.

56. Rubin MR, Bilezikian JP: New anabolic therapies in osteoporosis. *Endocrinol Metab Clin North Am* 2003;32:285-307.

57. Chesnut CH III, Silverman S, Andriano K, et al: A randomized trial of nasal spray salmon calcitonin in post-menopausal women with established osteoporosis: The Prevent Recurrence of Osteopenic Fractures Study. PROOF Study Group. *Am J Med* 2000;109:267-276.

58. Silverman SL: Calcitonin. *Endocrinol Metab Clin North Am* 2003;32:273-284.

59. Reszka AA, Halasy-Nagy JM, Masarachia PH, Rodan GA: Bisphosphonates act directly on the osteoclast to induce caspase cleavage of mst1 kinase during apoptosis: A link between inhibition of the mevalonate pathway and regulation of an apoptosis-promoting kinase. *J Biol Chem* 1999;274:34967-34973.

60. Black DM, Cummings SR, Karpf DB, et al: Randomized trial of effect of alendronate on risk of fracture in women with existing vertebral fractures: Fracture Intervention Trial Research Group. *Lancet* 1996;348:1535-1541.

61. Rodan GA, Reszka AA: Osteoporosis and bisphosphonates. *J Bone Joint Surg Am* 2003;85(Suppl 3):8-12.

62. Rodan G, Reszka AA, Golub E, Rizzoli R: Bone safety of long-term bisphosphonate treatment. *Curr Med Res Opin* 2004;20:1291-1300.

63. Boonen S, McClung MR, Eastell R, El-Hajj Fuleihan G, Barton IP, Delmas P: Safety and efficacy of risedronate in reducing fracture risk in osteoporotic women age 80 and older: Implications for the use of antiresorptive agents in the old and the oldest old. *J Am Geriatr Soc* 2004;52:1832-1839.

64. Cranney A, Waldegger L, Zytaruk N, et al: Risedronate for the prevention and treatment of postmenopausal osteoporosis. *Cochrane Database Syst Rev* 2003;4:CD004523.

65. Harris ST, Watts NF, Genant HK, et al: Effects of risedronate treatment on vertebral and nonvertebral fractures in women with postmenopausal

osteoporosis: A randomized controlled trial. *JAMA* 1999;282:1344-1352.

66. Coleman CI, Perkerson KA, Lewis A: Alendronate-induced auditory hallucinations and visual disturbances. *Pharmacotherapy* 2004;24:799-802.

67. Chan SS, Nery LM, McElduff A, et al: Intravenous pamidronate in the treatment and prevention of ostoporosis. *Intern Med J* 2004;34:162-166.

68. Sartori L, Adami S, Filipponi P, Crepaldi G: Injectable bisphosphonates in the treatment of postmenopausal osteoporosis. *Aging Clin Exp Res* 2003;15:271-283.

69. Reid IR, Brown JP, Burckhardt P, et al: Intravenous zoledronic acid in postmenopausal women with low bone mineral density. *N Engl J Med* 2002;346:653-661.

70. Brixen K, Christensen PM, Ejersted C, Langdahl BL: Teriparatide (biosynthetic human parathyroid hormone 1-34): A new paradigm in the treatment of osteoporosis. *Basic Clin Pharmacol Toxicol* 2004;94:260-270.

71. Dempster DW, Cosman F, Kurland ES, et al: Effects of daily treatment with parathyroid hormone on bone microarchitecture and turnover in patients with osteoporosis: A paired biopsy study. *J Bone Miner Res* 2001;16:1846-1853.

72. Jilka RL, Weinstein RS, Bellido T, Roberson P, Parfitt AM, Manolagas SC: Increased bone formation by prevention of osteoblast apoptosis with parathyroid hormone. *J Clin Invest* 1999;104:439-446.

73. Neer RM, Arnaud CD, Zanchetta JR, et al: Effect of parathyroid hormone (1-34) on fractures and bone mineral density in postmenopausal women with osteoporosis. *N Engl J Med* 2001;344:1434-1441.

74. Ueland T: Bone metabolism in relation to alterations in systemic growth hormone. *Growth Horm IGF Res* 2004;14:404-417.

75. Black DM, Greenspan XL, Ensrud KE, et al: The effects of parathyroid hormone and alendronate alone or in combination in postmenopausal osteoporosis. *N Engl J Med* 2003;349:1207-1215.

76. Body JJ, Gaich GA, Scheele WH, et al: A randomized double-blind trial to compare the efficacy of teriparatide (recombinant human parathyroid hormone (1-34)) with alendronate in postmenopausal women with osteoporosis. *J Clin Endocrinol Metab* 2002;87:4528-4535.

77. Finkelstein JS, Hayes A, Hunzelman JL, Wyland JJ, Lee H, Neer RM: The effect of parathyroid hormone, alendronate or both in men with osteoporosis. *N Engl J Med* 2003;349:1216-1226.

78. Meunier PJ, Roux C, Seeman E, et al: The effect of strontium ranelate on the risk of vertebral fracture in women with postmenopausal osteoporosis. *N Engl J Med* 2004;350:459-468.

79. Biermasz NR, Hamdy NA, Pereira AM, Romijn JA, Roelfsema F: Long-term skeletal effects of recombinant human growth hormone (rhGH) alone and rhGH combined with alendronate in GH deficient adults: A seven-year follow-up study. *Clin Endocrinol (Oxf)* 2004;60:568-575.

80. Landin-Wilhelmsen K, Nilsson A, Bosaeus I, Bengtsson B: Growth hormone increases bone mineral content in postmenopausal osteoporosis: A randomized placebo-controlled trial. *J Bone Miner Res* 2003;18:393-405.

81. Allen DB, Carrel AL: Growth hormone therapy for Prader-Willi syndrome: A critical appraisal. *J Pediatr Endocrinol Metab* 2004;17(Suppl 4):1297-1306.

82. Ruggiero SL, Mehrotra B, Rosenberg TJ, Engroff SL: Osteonecrosis of the jaws associated with the use of bisphosphonates: A review of 63 cases. *J Oral Maxillofac Surg* 2004;62:527-534.

83. Boden SD, Kang J, Sandhu H, Heller JG: Use of recombinant human bone morphogenetic protein-2 to achieve posterolateral lumbar spine fusion in humans: A prospective, randomized clinical pilot trial. *Spine* 2002;27:2662-2673.

84. Dudeney S, Lieberman IH, Reinhardt MK, Hussein M: Kyphoplasty in the treatment of osteolytic vertebral compression as a result of multiple myeloma. *J Clin Oncol* 2002;20:2382-2387.

85. Glazer PA, Spencer UM, Alkalay RN, Schwardt J: In vivo evaluation of calcium sulfate as a bone graft substitute for lumbar spinal fusion. *Spine J* 2001;1:395-401.

86. Lieberman IH, Dudeney S, Reinhardt MK, Bell G: Initial outcome and efficacy of "kyphoplasty" in the treatment of painful osteoporotic vertebral compression fractures. *Spine* 2001;26:1631-1638.

87. Thalgott JS, Giuffre JM, Fritts K, Timlin M, Klezl Z: Instrumented posterolateral lumbar fusion using coralline hydroxyapatite with or without demineralized bone matrix, as an adjunct to autologous bone. *Spine J* 2001;1:131-137.

88. Theodorou DJ, Theodorou SJ, Duncan TD, Garfin SR, Wong WH: Percutaneous balloon kyphoplasty for the correction of spinal deformity in painful vertebral body compression fractures. *Clin Imaging* 2002;26:1-5.

Chapter 23

Giant Cell Tumor of Bone

Giant cell tumor of bone is one of the more common benign tumors of the skeletal system but also one of the most enigmatic. The tumor is well defined in terms of its appearance on imaging, its rather striking histology, and its location in special anatomic sites. What has puzzled investigators and clinicians for centuries are the unpredictability of its clinical behavior, the origin of the giant cells, and the occasional appearance of the disease in multicentric sites at varying intervals after discovery. Perhaps the most alarming aspect of this "benign" disorder is its occurrence as a malignant disease that may cause the death of the patient.

History

Although descriptions of malignant tumors of bone first appeared in the medical literature in the early 1800s, they were not well defined and probably represented osteosarcomas or malignant soft-tissue tumors. The term "sarcoma" was introduced by Abernethy in 1803,[1] but histology was not really available to further define the entities until the middle of the century. An illustration in the 1818 surgical essay by Astley Cooper and Travers,[2] however, shows a lesion that appears to be a giant cell tumor of the proximal tibia. In his volume on pathologic physiology published in 1845, Hermann Lebert stressed the fact that tumors could not be identified or classified without histologic studies.[3] In his review, he separated a tumor from the osteosarcomas; he noted that it was fibrous in nature, containing numerous giant cells, and called it "tumeur fibroplastique."[3] He indicated that the lesion was curable by amputation, unlike other more malignant lesions. In 1860, Eugene Nelaton published a monograph on giant cell-containing tumors of bone and included many types of lesions, some of them infectious; he stated that these were generally benign.[4] Rudolf Virchow, considered by many to be the father of modern pathology, not only defined the nature of the various tumors based on their histologic pattern but identified a "benign" tumor characterized by the presence of multinucleated giant cells that he called a "giant cell tumor."[5,6] In 1879, Samuel Gross[7] wrote an extensive survey of the malignant tumors of bone but also included the giant cell tumor as a benign variant. One of Sir James Paget's lectures on the pathology of bone tumors at the Royal Society of Medicine was a presentation devoted to the benign giant cell tumor in which he showed both gross and histologic studies.[8] Terminology for the tumors became an issue because the terms osteoclastoma, myeloid sarcoma, hemorrhagic osteomyelitis, and giant cell sarcoma were all introduced to describe the relatively benign tumor now known as giant cell tumor of bone.[9-15] In 1898, when roentgenograms of the giant cell tumor were produced, the diagnosis became accepted as a sometimes aggressive but nonmetastasizing primary tumor of bone.[14] In 1923, Bloodgood[16] described a surgical procedure for the treatment of giant cell tumor. Subsequent reports by Coley and Higinbotham[17] in 1938, and by Myerding[18] in 1941 supported the concept that the tumor was curable and did not require ablative surgery.

In 1940, Jaffe, Lichtenstein, and Portis[19] authored the seminal article that described the imaging and gross and histologic pattern for the tumor, named it definitively as giant cell tumor of bone, and further indicated the occasional relationship to Paget's disease as well as its sometimes malignant behavior pattern. These features are supported by other investigators who have reported large numbers of cases followed over many years.[20-31] Some of these presentations have emphasized the multiple metachronous nature of some of the tumors and their unpredictable potential for metastasis.

Clinical Presentation of Giant Cell Tumor

Giant cell tumors are relatively common and are one of the more frequent primary tumors of bone; approximately 1,000 cases occur annually in the US. The disease occurs most frequently in Chinese people, and

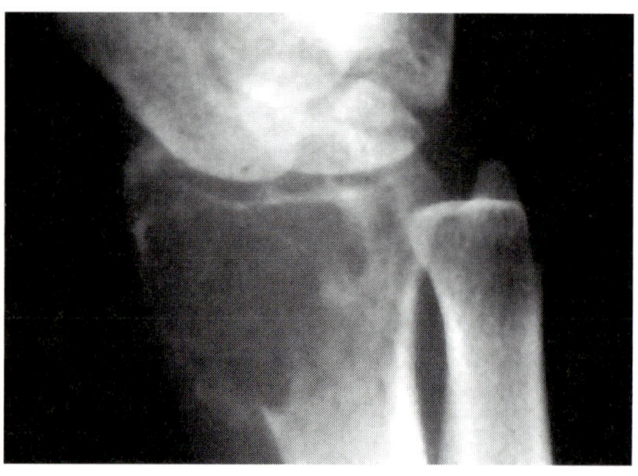

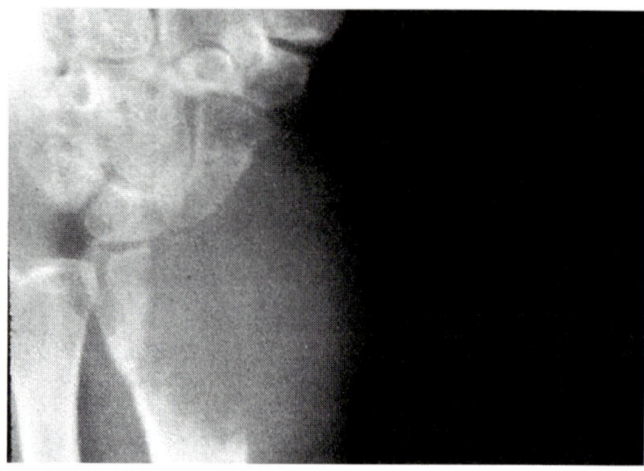

Figure 1

Radiograph of a giant cell tumor of the distal radius that shows the characteristic features of a stage 1 or stage 2 tumor. The lesion is located in the epiphyseometaphyseal region and shows expansion and marked thinning of the cortex, but no soft-tissue extension. The tumor does not invade the joint.

Figure 2

This radiograph shows a much more aggressive stage 3 tumor at the same site as the patient in Figure 1. This lesion shows destruction of the cortex and a large soft-tissue mass that has invaded the joint. The tumor has features that suggest malignancy.

less frequently in African-Americans.[32] The gender distribution shows that approximately 60% of the patients are women; the age distribution is in the middle years, 20 to 50 years of age.[10,19,23,31] Giant cell tumors are infrequent in children with open epiphyses and even less frequently seen in elderly individuals, except when the tumor occurs in association with Paget's disease of bone.[10,19,23,31,33-36]

The anatomic locations in which the tumors occur are principally in the epiphyseal portion of the bone and extend to the metaphysis and to the subchondral bony endplate. The most frequent sites are the distal femur and proximal tibia.[10,23,31] The distal radius is the third most frequent site,[26,37] followed by the proximal femur and proximal humerus.[10,23] The tumors occur with less frequency in the pelvis, proximal fibula, and the bones of the hands and feet; they are even less common in the vertebral bodies or the sacrum.[10,21-24,29,31,38]

Imaging studies most frequently show giant cell tumors to be eccentric and to deform the bony structure by expanding the bone with marked thinning of the cortex[10,21-25] (Figure 1). Portions of the cortex may be dense, which is particularly noted on computed tomography.[26] The central portion of the tumor is almost always lytic unless pathologic fractures have occurred.[10,23,26] The bone scan is almost always positive; edema can be noted on magnetic resonance imaging (MRI), with a pattern of

low intensity on T1 and high intensity on T2.[10,31,39] Gadolinium enhancement is almost always increased for the tumors.[39] Campanacci and associates[10,21,22] and Enneking[40] described the aggressiveness of the benign lesions in a three-stage system. Stage 1 tumors show a lytic lesion on imaging with thinning of the cortex but only minimal deformity of the bony structure. Stage 2 shows marked expansion of the bone with deformity, but no cortical breaks or soft-tissue extension of the tumor. Stage 3 is characterized by marked expansion, cortical destruction, and an often large soft-tissue mass (Figure 2). Fractures are common in stage 3 tumors and are less common in stage 2. Serum acid phosphatase has been shown to be a good tumor marker for giant cell tumors and probably correlates well with the extent and stage of the disease.[41,42] Expressions of vascular endothelial growth factor (VEGF) and tumor necrosis factor-α in the tissues have been thought to correlate with the stage of the disease and the extent of destruction.[43]

Gross and Histologic Patterns

Although the lesions look "clear" on imaging studies, the gross appearance shows irregular soft-tissue linear folds, with intervening spaces filled with a thickened jelly-like material.[10,23] The cortices are thin, expanded, irregular, and at times quite dense. Histologically, the principal cellular element is the mesenchymal monocyte that fills the spaces

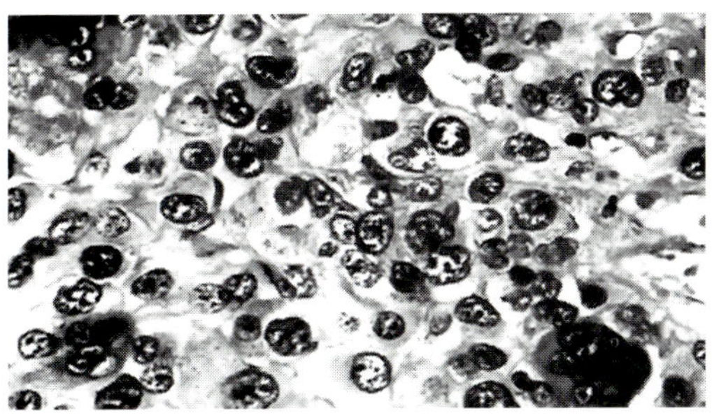

Figure 3
The principal neoplastic cell in the giant cell tumor is the monocyte, which does not show major atypism and has only limited findings suggesting active DNA synthesis. Hematoxylin and eosin × 400.

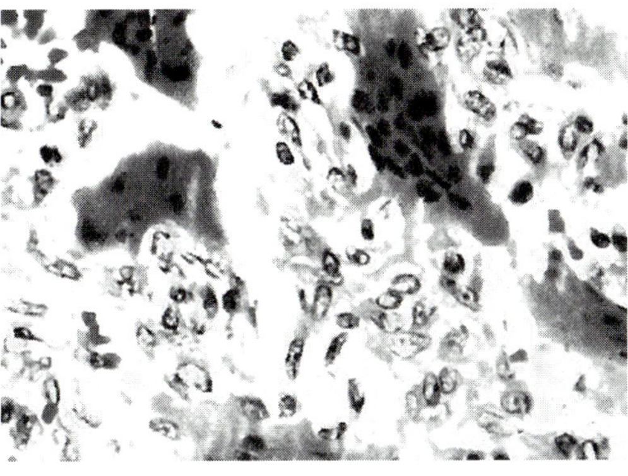

Figure 4
The giant cell in these tumors shows a sometimes irregular cellular contour, with multiple, centripetally located nuclei. Hematoxylin and eosin × 350.

and sometimes will be replaced by small numbers of fibrous cells, which serve to extend and support the structure of the linear folds[10,22,23,25,31,44] (Figure 3). The most impressive aspect of the histology are the giant cells. The nuclei in the giant cells number as many as 50 or more and are centripetally placed[10,21-23,31] (Figure 4). The nuclei are similar in appearance to the nuclei of the monocytic mesenchymal cellular element of the tumor.[45] Mitotic figures are rare, and cellular atypism is even less common.[10,22,23,45]

The origin of the giant cells is a subject of continuing debate. Are they osteoclasts and, as some investigators have proposed, are the tumors "osteoclastomas"? Despite efforts including special stains and electron microscopy, there is no agreement as to the "clastic" nature of the giant cells; indeed, they are not found at the margins of the tumor where the bone is being destroyed.[10,23,31,44,45] The cells are quite unique in appearance; the number of nuclei and their central placement help to distinguish them from giant cells seen in hyperparathyroidism, Langerhans cell histiocytosis, chondroblastoma, malignant fibrous histiocytoma, sarcoidosis, and Paget's disease.[23] Furthermore, they are considerably different in structure and size from the Langhans giant cells seen in tuberculous granulomas and the Reed-Sternberg cells seen in Hodgkin's disease. The origin of the tumor remains enigmatic, and the origin of the giant cell itself is still a mystery.[10,23,30,44,45]

Biologic Markers for Giant Cell Tumors

In a study performed in 1986, Goldring and associates[44] were able to establish three types of cells in the giant cell tumors—some macrophages that were not related to osseous activities; another group of monocytes that were; and the giant cell, which had some characteristics of an osteoclast but did not seem to function as one. Since then, numerous attempts have been made to discover the agents or factors that are responsible for the development of the atypical giant cells from the monocytic mesenchymal cells that make up the structure of the tumor.[32,43,46-53] The concept of a virus infection has been eliminated by appropriate studies.[10] True genetics appear to play some role in terms of the excessive numbers of cases that occur in Chinese people, but no specific error has been identified.[31,32,50] The presence of HLA DRB-1 alleles appears to increase the risk of developing the disease, and fibroblast growth factor-3-positive mesenchymal stem cells seem to serve as precursors in the development of the production of the giant cells.[48,52] A recent study showed that stromal cell-derived factor-1 (SDF-1) appears to be responsible for recruiting the precursor cells.[54] Another study supports the concept that some gene errors are possibly present and that tartrate-resistant acid phosphatase and osteoprotegrin ligand are overexpressed in the tumors.[55] Another report presents the concept that although the giant cells of the tumor are not "true" osteoclasts, they could be activated to osteoclastic activity by exposure to bone morphogenetic proteins and SDF-1.[54,56] Cathepsin K was defined in a 2004 study as the principal protease in giant cell tumors of bone.[57] Interleukin-6 has been found in some tumors and appears to correlate with the aggressiveness of the lesion.[58]

In another study, progesterone receptors were found in five of ten tumors.[46] Three forms of VEGF and matrix metalloproteinase-9 have been found in giant cell tumors, and these materials seem to correlate well with the destructive nature of the tumors.[43] Another study showed low levels of cyclin D1 gene amplification in 60% of giant cell tumors, and Ki-67 (MIB-1) was present in all of the tumors.[59] Roux and colleagues[49] propose that RANK and RANKL are expressed in giant cell tumors and may be related to the development of the giant cells.

Although many of these studies are suggestive, two things are apparent. They do not provide a clear definition of a genetic or in fact any type of cause for the giant cell tumor of bone. Further, only limited evidence is available to support the concept that the giant cell in the tumor is in fact a true functioning osteoclast.

Strange Behavior Patterns of Giant Cell Tumors

In addition to the three-stage disease pattern described above, four other unusual forms of giant cell tumors may be present.

- Metachronous multicentric disease.[10,23,31,60-64] Some patients who present with a single classical site of stage 1 or 2 disease are treated effectively and have no recurrence, but at some point several months or years later develop another tumor in another site. The new tumor resembles the first in histologic pattern but does not appear to be a metastasis. The same patient may develop several more such lesions at intervals and could require a considerable number of operative procedures and possibly radiation. There is no explanation for this type of tumor behavior for a lesion, which ordinarily does not metastasize; however, it does suggest some type of genetic or biochemical abnormality in the patient.
- Metastasizing "benign" giant cell tumors.[10,13,15,18,31,65-72] Some patients with benign giant cell tumors that show no evidence of malignant change in the primary lesion will develop pulmonary metastases. The pulmonary lesions are often limited in number and in size and do not grow rapidly. De-

spite the evidence of malignant behavior, the patients do not become ill and in fact have a very high rate of survival; however, they will require pulmonary resective surgery and/or radiation.

- Malignant form of giant cell tumor.[10,15,23,31,65-67,73-75] The malignant form of the tumor is much more aggressive; despite surgical, chemotherapeutic, and radiation therapies, patients may die of disease on the basis of extensive bilateral aggressive and histologically malignant tumor masses in the lungs.
- Giant cell tumor in patients with Paget's disease.[10,23,31,33-36] Patients with extensive Paget's disease sometimes develop a highly malignant Paget's sarcoma that resembles an osteosarcoma and is very likely to cause the patient's death in a short time. Occasionally, however, instead of the sarcoma, the destructive and quite aggressive lesion occurring in a focus of Paget's disease proves to be a giant cell tumor. Patients respond to surgical or radiation therapy for the lesions and can be restored to good health. There is no evidence to support the likelihood that the next tumor will be a Paget's sarcoma, but the local damage as a result of the combined Pagetoid and giant cell tumor destruction often requires ablative surgery.

Treatment of Giant Cell Tumors

In the early history of orthopaedic oncology, amputation was the only type of surgery deemed reasonable for what were thought to be malignant lesions.[10,12,16,25,28,66] These lesions included osteosarcomas, Ewing's tumors, soft-tissue sarcomas, and chondrosarcomas; aside from those with low-grade cartilage tumors, patients frequently died of disease a short period of time after surgery.[7,28] The notable exceptions were patients with giant cell tumors, the majority of whom survived.[12,16] In the late 1900s, it became apparent that the surgical procedures for giant cell tumors could be less aggressive and that limbs could be spared.[28] Many giant cell tumors at various sites were treated with resection and insertion of autograft bone and, for the tumors about the knee, an autograft arthrodesis.[76] The use of allograft implants began in the early 1920s with efforts by Lexer,[77] who used them principally for low-grade tumors. Multiple procedures performed by Frank Parrish[78] and Carlos Ottolenghi[79] demonstrated that the procedure could be successful if the donor bone was sterile, of good quality, and had been frozen.[28,80] Most of the allograft replacements for giant cell tumors have a reasonable success rate in that the local recurrence rate is very low. Allograft complications including infection, nonunion, and fracture reduce the success rate for the procedure to approximately 75%.[26,37,80] Marcove and associates[81] introduced the use of liquid nitrogen treatment of the tumor bed after curettage and had some success, although the complication rate was high. In later years, it became apparent that curettage and implantation of either bone graft or polymethylmethacrylate has a high success rate, particularly if the site of the tumor is treated by high-speed burring or with phenol. These methods are in use today and have a very low recurrence rate.[10,22,24-26,28,82-84] Resection of some parts such as the proximal fibula, distal ulna, or clavicle is also a reasonable approach.[10,24,26]

Radiation has been used for giant cell tumors for many years with considerable success.[85-88] The tumors are sensitive to a relatively low dose of radiation, which reduces the likelihood of complications. This treatment protocol is particularly useful for tumors in the spine and sacrum or in other sites where surgery seems complex or inappropriate.[10,85-87]

In recent years, particularly for recurrent tumors in sites that are difficult to treat, several investigators have introduced bisphosphonates, which seem to reduce the local recurrence rate by increasing the apoptotic rates of the monocytes. It is reasonable to suggest that this treatment may be useful for patients with metachronous disease by reducing the likelihood of new foci.[89,90]

Summary

Giant cell tumor of bone remains a pathologic and orthopaedic puzzle. We do not know what causes it, nor do we understand the role and character of the giant cell. We have no idea why some patients develop metachronous or malignant disease, or why the tumor appears in patients with Paget's disease. Fortunately, most of the tumors are relatively benign and the current success rate for conservative surgical procedures is high enough so that patients, their families, and their physicians can be pleased with the results.

References

1. Abernethy J: *Surgical Observations on Tumors.* London, England, Longman and Rees, 1804.

2. Cooper A, Travers B: *Surgical Essays.* London, England, Cox and Son and Longman and Co, 1818, vol 1, pp 186-208.

3. Lebert H: *Physiologic Pathologique.* Paris, France, JB Balliere, 1845, vol 2.

4. Nelaton E: *D'une Nouvelle Espèce de Tumeurs Bénignes des Os, ou Tumeurs à Myéloplaxes.* Paris, France, Adrien Delahaye, 1860.

5. Virchow R: *Die Krankhaften Gewulste.* Berlin, Germany, Hirschwald, vol 2, 1867.

6. Wilson JW: Virchow's contribution to the cell theory. *J Hist Med* 1947;2:163-178.

7. Gross SA: Sarcoma of the long bone: Based upon a study of one hundred and seventy-five cases. *Am J Med Sci* 1879;155:2-57.

8. Paget J: *Lectures in Surgical Pathology.* London, England, Brown, Green and Longman, 1853, p 446.

9. Barrie GL: Haemorrhagic osteomyelitis. *Surg Gynecol Obstet* 1914;1:42-52.

10. Campanacci M: *Bone and Soft Tissue Tumors.* New York, Springer Verlag, 1999, pp 99-142.

11. Ewing J: A review and classification of bone sarcomas. *Arch Surg* 1922;4:485-533.

12. Ewing J: *The Classification and Treatment of Bone Sarcomas.* New York, NY, Cancer Wood, 1928, p 365.

13. Finch GF, Gleave HH: A case of osteoclastoma (myeloid sarcoma, benign giant cell tumor) with pulmonary metastases. *J Pathol Bacteriol* 1926;29:339.

14. McCarthy EF: Giant-cell tumor of bone: An historical perspective. *Clin Orthop Relat Res* 1980;153:14-25.

15. Murphy WR, Ackerman LV: Benign and malignant giant-cell tumors of bone: A clinical-pathological study of thirty-one cases. *Cancer* 1956;9:317-339.

16. Bloodgood JC: Benign giant-cell tumor of bone: Its diagnosis and conservative treatment. *Am J Surg* 1923;37:105-116.

17. Coley BL, Higinbotham NL: Giant cell tumor of bone. *J Bone Joint Surg* 1938;20:870-884.

18. Myerding HW: Benign and malignant giant cell tumor of bone: Diagnosis and results of treatment. *JAMA* 1941;117:1849-1855.

19. Jaffe HL, Lichtenstein L, Portis RB: Giant cell tumor of bone: Its pathologic appearance, grading, supposed variants and treatments. *Arch Pathol* 1940;30:993-1031.

20. Aegerter EE: Giant cell tumors of bone: A critical survey. *Am J Pathol* 1947;23:283-297.

21. Campanacci M, Giunti A, Olmi R: Giant-cell

tumors of bone: A study of 209 cases with long term follow-up in 130. *Ital J Orthop Traumatol* 1975;1:249-277.

22. Campanacci M, Baldini N, Boriani S, Sudanese A: Giant-cell tumor of bone. *J Bone Joint Surg Am* 1987;69:106-114.

23. Dorfman HD, Czerniak B: Giant cell lesions, in *Bone Tumors*, St. Louis, MO, Mosby, 1998, pp 559-606.

24. Eckardt J, Grogan TJ: Giant cell tumor of bone. *Clin Orthop Relat Res* 1986;204:45-58.

25. Goldenberg RR, Campbell CJ, Bonfiglio M: Giant-cell tumor of bone. An analysis of two-hundred and eighteen cases. *J Bone Joint Surg Am* 1970;52:619-663.

26. Harness NG, Mankin HJ: Giant-cell tumor of the distal forearm. *J Hand Surg [Am]* 2004;29:188-193.

27. Johnson EW Jr, Dahlin DC: Treatment of giant-cell tumor of bone. *J Bone Joint Surg Am* 1959;41:895-904.

28. Mankin HJ: History of the treatment of musculo-skeletal tumours, in Klenerman L (ed): *The Evolution of Orthopaedic Surgery*, London, England, Royal Society of Medicine Press, 2002, pp 191-210.

29. Scaglietti O, Mondolfo S: Sulla varieta xantomatosa die tumor gigantocellulari. *Chir Organ Mov* 1938;23:435-459.

30. Schajowicz F, Mondolfo S: Aproposito de la llamada variedad xantomatosa de los tumors gigantocellulari. *Rev Ortop Traumatol* 1947;17:34-35.

31. Schajowicz F: Giant cell tumor (osteoclastoma), in *Tumor and Tumorlike Lesions of Bone and Joints*. New York, NY, Springer Verlag, 1981, pp 205-242.

32. Guo W, Xu W, Huvos AG, Healey JH, Feng C: Comparative frequency of bone sarcomas among different racial groups. *Chin Med J (Engl)* 1999;112:1101-1104.

33. Haibach H, Farrell C, Dittrich FJ: Neoplasms arising in Paget's disease of bone: A study of 82 cases. *Am J Clin Pathol* 1985;83:594-600.

34. Jacobs TP, Michelsen J, Polay JS, D'Adamo AC, Canfield RE: Giant cell tumor in Paget's disease of bone: Familial and geographic clustering. *Cancer* 1979;44:742-747.

35. Potter HG, Schneider R, Ghelman B, Healey JH, Lane JM: Multiple giant cell tumors and Paget's disease of bone: Radiographic and clinical correlations. *Radiology* 1991;180:261-264.

36. Russell DS: Malignant osteoclastoma and the association of malignant osteoclastoma with Paget's osteitis deformans. *J Bone Joint Surg Br* 1949;31:281-290.

37. Smith RJ, Mankin HJ: Allograft replacement of distal radius for giant cell tumor. *J Hand Surg [Am]* 1977;2:299-308.

38. Randall RL: Giant cell tumor of the sacrum. *Neurosurg Focus* 2003;15:E13.

39. Herman SD, Mesgarzadeh M, Bonakdarpur A, Dalinka MK: The role of magnetic resonance imaging in giant cell tumor of bone. *Skeletal Radiol* 1987;16:635-643.

40. Enneking WF: Staging benign lesions, in *Musculoskeletal Tumor Surgery*. New York, NY, Churchill Livingstone, 1983, p 87.

41. Gamberi G, Serra M, Ragazzini P, et al: Identification of markers of possible prognostic value in 57 giant cell tumors of bone. *Oncol Rep* 2003;10:351-356.

42. Goto T, Iijima T, Kawano H, et al: Serum acid phosphatase as a tumour marker in giant cell tumour of bone. *Arch Orthop Trauma Surg* 2001;121:411-413.

43. Kumta SM, Huang L, Cheng YY, Chow LT, Lee KM, Zheng MH: Expression of VEGF and MMP-9 in giant cell tumor of bone and other osteolytic lesions. *Life Sci* 2003;73:1427-1436.

44. Goldring SR, Schiller AL, Mankin HJ, Dayer JM, Krane SM: Characterization of cells from human giant cell tumors of bone. *Clin Orthop Relat Res* 1986;204:59-85.

45. Schajowicz F: Giant cell tumors of bone (osteoclastoma): A pathological and biochemical study. *J Bone Joint Surg Am* 1961;43:1-29.

46. Demertzis N, Kotsiandri F, Giotis I, Apostolikas N: Giant cell tumors of bone and progesterone receptors. *Orthopedics* 2003;26:1209-1212.

47. Komiya S, Sasaguri Y, Inoue A, et al: Characterization of cells cultured from human giant cell tumors of bone: Phenotypic relationship to the monocyte macrophage and osteoclast. *Clin Orthop Relat Res* 1990;258:304-309.

48. Robinson D, Segal M, Nevo Z: Giant cell tumor of bone: The role of fibroblast growth factor 3 positive mesenchymal stem cells in its pathogenesis. *Pathobiology* 2002-2003;70:333-342.

49. Roux S, Arnazit L, Meduri G, Guiochon-Mantel A, Milgrom E, Mariette X: RANK (receptor activator of nuclear factor kappa B) and RANK ligand are expressed in giant cell tumors of bone. *Am J Clin Pathol* 2002;117:210-216.

50. Skubitz KM, Chang EY, Clohisy DR, Thompson RC, Skubitz AP: Gene expression in giant-cell tumors. *J Lab Clin Med* 2004;144:193-200.

51. Tian BL, Wen JM, Zhang M, Xie D, Xu RB, Luo CJ: The expression of ADAM12 (meltrin alpha) in human giant cell tumours of bone. *Mol Pathol* 2002;55:394-397.

52. Varanasi SS, Athanasou NA, Briceno I, Papiha SS, Datta HK: Association of HLA-DRB1 alleles with giant cell tumour of bone. *J Clin Pathol* 1999;52:782-784.

53. Zheng MH, Xu J, Robbins P, et al: Gene expression of vascular endothelial growth factor in giant cell tumors of bone. *Hum Pathol* 2000;31:804-812.

54. Atkins GJ, Haynes DR, Graves SE, et al: Expression of osteoclast differentiation signals by stromal elements of giant cell tumors. *J Bone Miner Res* 2000;15:640-649.

55. Hu Y, Yu S: Gene expression of osteoprotegerin and osteoclast differentiation factor in giant cell tumor. *Zhonghua Bing Li Xue Za Zhi* 2002;31:128-131.

56. Liao TS, Yurgelun MB, Chang SS, et al: Recruitment of osteoclast precursors by stromal cell derived factor-1 (SDF-1) in giant cell tumor of bone. *J Orthop Res* 2005;23:203-209.

57. Lindeman JH, Hanemaaijer R, Mulder A, et al: Cathepsin K is the principal protease in giant cell tumor of bone. *Am J Pathol* 2004;165:593-600.

58. Gamberi G, Benassi MS, Ragazzini P, et al: Proteases and interleukin-6 gene analysis in 92 giant cell tumors of bone. *Ann Oncol* 2004;15:498-503.

59. Kauzman A, Li SQ, Bradley G, Bell RS, Wunder JS, Kandel R: Cyclin alterations in giant cell tumor of bone. *Mod Pathol* 2003;16:210-218.

60. Haskell A, Wodowoz O, Johnston JO: Metachronous multicentric giant cell tumor: A case report and literature review. *Clin Orthop Relat Res* 2003;412:162-168.

61. Lausten GS, Jensen PK, Schiodt T, Lind BJ: Local recurrences in giant cell tumour of bone: Long term followup of 31 cases. *Int Orthop* 1996;20:172-176.

62. Peimer CA, Schiller AL, Mankin HJ, Smith RJ: Multicentric giant-cell tumor of bone. *J Bone Joint Surg Am* 1980;62:652-656.

63. Rousseau MA, Handra-Luca A, Lazennec JY, Catonne Y, Saillant G: Metachronous multicentric giant-cell tumor of the bone in the lower limb: Case report and Ki-67 immunohistochemistry study. *Virchows Arch* 2004;445:79-82.

64. Scully SP, Mott MP, Temple HT, O'Keefe RJ, O'Donnell RJ, Mankin HJ: Late recurrence of giant-cell tumor of bone: A report of four cases. *J Bone Joint Surg Am* 1994;76:1231-1233.

65. Bertoni F, Bacchini P, Staals EL: Malignancy in giant cell tumor of bone. *Cancer* 2003;97:2520-2529.

66. Bloodgood JC: The giant cell tumor of bone and the specter of the metastasizing giant cell tumor. *Surg Gynecol Obstet* 1924;38:784-789.

67. Cheng JC, Johnston JO: Giant cell tumor of bone: Prognosis and treatment of pulmonary metastases. *Clin Orthop Relat Res* 1997;338:205-214.

68. Dyke SC: Metastases of the "benign" giant cell tumor of bone (osteoclastoma). *J Pathol Bacteriol* 1931;34:259-262.

69. Kay RM, Eckardt JJ, Seeger LL, Mirra JM, Hak DJ: Pulmonary metastasis for benign giant cell tumor of bone: Six histologically confirmed cases, including one of spontaneous regression. *Clin Orthop Relat Res* 1994;302:219-230.

70. Lasser EC, Tetewsky H: Metastasizing giant cell tumors: Report of an unusual case with indolent bone and pulmonary metastases. *AJR Am J Roentgenol* 1957;78:804-811.

71. Maloney WJ, Vaughan LM, Jones HH, Ross J, Nagel DA: Benign metastasizing giant-cell tumor of bone: Report of three cases and review of the literature. *Clin Orthop Relat Res* 1989;243:208-215.

72. Rock MG, Pritchard DJ, Unni KK: Metastases from histologically benign giant-cell tumor of bone. *J Bone Joint Surg Am* 1984;66:269-274.

73. Bertoni F, Present D, Sudanese A, Baldini N, Bacchini P, Campanacci M: Giant cell tumor of bone with pulmonary metastases: Six case reports and a review of the literature. *Clin Orthop Relat Res* 1988;237:275-285.

74. Brien EW, Mirra JM, Kessler S, Suen M, Ho JK, Yang WT: Benign giant cell tumor of bone with osteosarcomatous transformation ("dedifferentiated" primary malignant GCT): Report of two cases. *Skeletal Radiol* 1997;26:246-255.

75. Gitelis S, Wang JW, Quast M, Schajowicz F, Templeton A: Recurrence of a giant-cell tumor with malignant transformation to a fibrosarcoma twenty-five years after primary treatment: A case report. *J Bone Joint Surg Am* 1989;71:757-761.

76. Enneking WF, Eady JL, Burchardt H: Autogenous cortical bone grafts in the reconstruction of segmental skeletal defects. *J Bone Joint Surg Am* 1980;62:1039-1058.

77. Lexer E: Joint transplantation and arthroplasty. *Surg Gynecol Obstet* 1925;40:782-809.

78. Parrish F: Treatment of bone tumors by total excision and replacement with massive autologous and homologous grafts. *J Bone Joint Surg Am* 1966;48:968-990.

79. Ottolenghi CE: Massive osteoarticular bone grafts. *J Bone Joint Surg Br* 1966;48:646-659.

80. Mankin HJ, Hornicek FJ: The use of massive allografts in the treatment of knee tumors, in Wickiewicz TL, Windsor RE, Simonian PT, Lonner JH (eds): *Techniques in Knee Surgery*. Philadelphia, PA, Lippincott, Williams and Wilkins, 2004.

81. Marcove RC, Weis LD, Vaghaiwalla MR, Pearson R: Cryosurgery in the treatment of giant cell tumors of bone. *Clin Orthop Relat Res* 1978;134:275-279.

82. Durr HR, Maier M, Jansson V, Baur A, Refior HJ: Phenol as an adjuvant for local control in the treatment of giant cell tumour of the bone. *Eur J Surg Oncol* 1999;25:610-618.

83. O'Donnell RJ, Springfield DS, Motwani HK, Ready JE, Gebhardt MC, Mankin HJ: Recurrence of giant cell tumors on the long bones after curettage and packing with cement. *J Bone Joint Surg Am* 1994;76:1827-1833.

84. Saiz P, Virkus W, Piasecki P, Templeton A, Shott S, Gitelis S: Results of giant cell tumor treated with intralesional excision. *Clin Orthop Relat Res* 2004;424:221-226.

85. Caudell JJ, Ballo MT, Zagars GK: Radiotherapy in the management of giant cell tumor of bone. *Int J Radiat Oncol Biol Phys* 2003;57:158-165.

86. Chakravarti A, Spiro I, Hug EB, Mankin HJ, Efird JT, Suit HD: Megavoltage radiation therapy for axial and inoperable giant-cell tumor of bone. *J Bone Joint Surg Am* 1999;81:1566-1573.

87. Feigenberg SJ, Marcus RB Jr, Zlotecki RA: Radiation therapy for giant cell tumors of bone. *Clin Orthop Relat Res* 2003;411:207-216.

88. Seider MJ, Rich TA, Ayala AG, Murray JA: Giant cell tumors of bone: Treatment with radiation therapy. *Radiology* 1986;161:537-540.

89. Chang SS, Suratwal SJ, Jung KM: Bisphosphonates may reduce recurrence in giant cell tumor by inducing apoptosis. *Clin Orthop Relat Res* 2004;426:103-109.

90. Cheng YY, Huang L, Lee KM, et al: Bisphosphonates induce apoptosis of stromal tumor cells in giant cell tumor of bone. *Calcif Tissue Int* 2004;75:71-77.

Chapter 24

Extra-Abdominal Desmoid Tumor

Desmoid tumors arising in the soft tissue of the extremities are quite rare—probably under 400 cases per year in the US. The lesions can be aggressive. They can recur after surgical excision or appear in multiple parts of the body, but do not metastasize or cause death. Histologically, the tumors consist of fibroblastic or myofibroblastic tissue and are sometimes quite cellular, but usually show no evidence of either rapid growth or atypism. Desmoid tumors may be a part of the syndrome of colonic polyposis known as Gardner's disease, which suggests that extra-abdominal desmoids may result from a genetic abnormality; however, limited information exists to support such an assumption. The tumors may have a relationship to estrogen production. They occur with greater frequency in young women and seem to become less aggressive at the time of menopause. This presentation only applies to extra-abdominal tumors; it does not include those arising from the uterus, viscera, colon, or other sites within the abdomen or even those that occur in the abdominal wall. Those lesions have similar histologic findings but a different pattern of presentation and frequently a different outcome.

History and Nomenclature

The first reported case of a fibrous tumor in the soft tissues was McFarlane's 1832 description of a patient with a prominent lesion occurring in the anterior abdominal wall.[1] In 1838, Müller[2] identified another such tumor, which he named a "desmoid" because the appearance of the gross structure seemed similar to fibrous or tendinous tissue known in Greek as "desmos." Most of the reported tumors in the earlier days seemed to be in relation to the abdominal wall, such as the descriptions by Bennett[3] in 1849 and Sanger[4] in 1884. Sir James Paget described the first case of a desmoid tumor that occurred in peripheral parts.[5] Although

Rokitansky[6] initially suggested that the desmoid tumors were histologically benign, in 1849 Wilks[7] described the tumors as low-grade fibrosarcomas. In 1923, Nichols[8] established the extra-abdominal desmoid tumors as distinct and separate entities from those in the abdomen or in the abdominal wall. Although Ewing[9] felt that that these lesions should continue to be considered low-grade fibrosarcomas, in 1948 Musgrove and McDonald[10] declared the tumor to be "benign," based on the absence of metastases or patient death in most series. This view was further reinforced by the study reported in 1954 by Stout,[11] who described the tumor as "desmoid fibromatosis."

In the early 1950s, Elton J. Gardner[12,13] described an autosomal dominant hereditary syndrome that is now known by his name. According to the original description, Gardner's syndrome consisted of polyposis of the colon, intra-abdominal fibrous tumors, osteomas of bone, and multiple subcutaneous nodules. In 1958, Smith[14] identified the histology of the subcutaneous and subfascial nodular masses as desmoid tumors. Some patients with Gardner's syndrome also have supernumerary teeth, gastric polyps, papillary carcinomas of the thyroid gland, adrenal adenomas, and multiple pigmented ocular fundus lesions.[15-22] The incidence of malignancy in the intestinal lesions is quite high, but not in the desmoid tumors or osteomas that accompany them.[17-19,23,24]

Incidence and Clinical Presentation

Extra-abdominal desmoids are quite rare. If those occurring in the abdominal or chest wall or those associated with Gardner's syndrome are excluded, the number of reported cases is small indeed. The three largest series reported include one from Weiss and Goldblum,[24] who reported 367 cases; another by Rock and his colleagues[25] from the Mayo Clinic, who described 194 patients

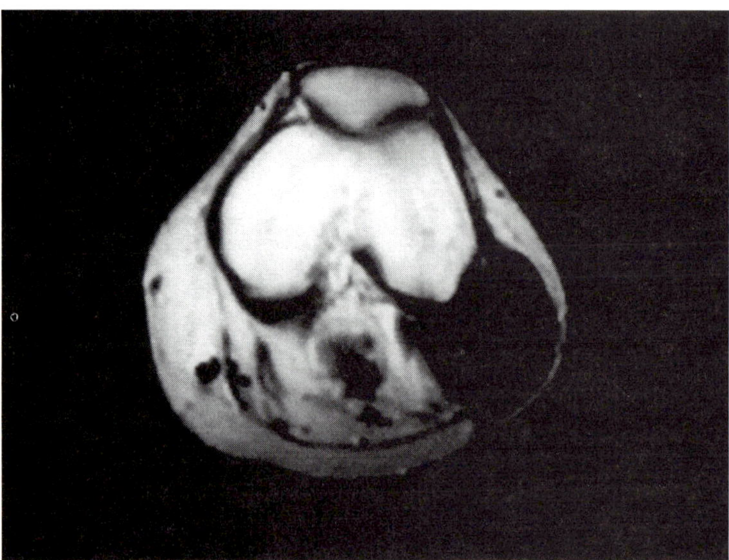

Figure 1

Classic appearance of a desmoid tumor of the distal femur, attached to the posterior aspect of the medial femoral condyle. The tumor is usually dark on both T1 and T2.

seen between 1908 and 1980; and one from Posner and associates,[26] who cited 144 cases seen at Memorial Sloan-Kettering Hospital between 1965 and 1984. The incidence is believed to be very low for the general population, but it is markedly increased for patients with Gardner's syndrome (approximately 17% of them have desmoid tumors).[18,19,24] Most investigators report greater frequency in females than in males.[18,24,25,27-33] The disease is one of younger individuals, with the mean age in most series approximately 25 years.[18,25,29,31-34] Young children seem to have a particularly aggressive form of the disease.[11,19,34,35] Although desmoids are rarely reported in infants, these are sometimes the most difficult lesions to treat.[19,24,35]

Many of the extremity desmoids are located in the soft tissues of the lower and upper extremity; they are most frequently found in the region of the midthigh or proximal arm, shoulder, or scapula.[18,19,24] The tumors are firm and somewhat rubbery to palpation, and they seem to be tightly bound to the fibrous membranes that surround the muscles.[18] The lesions are ordinarily not tender to touch, but sometimes produce expansion and discoloration of the overlying skin. They occasionally involve the tendons of the underlying muscles or even the periosteum of the adjacent bone. Of greater concern, the

tumors may involve the blood vessels and nerves of the proximal upper or lower extremities; this may cause tingling, numbness, or a stabbing pain, and sometimes motor weakness.[25,30-33] Of particular concern are those desmoids that occur in the head and neck, which may cause nerve damage and paralysis.[36] A special form of the desmoid type of lesion, sometimes known as fibromatosis, occurs in the sole of the foot or, much less commonly, the palmar aspect of the hand.[18,19,24,37,38] These may be painful, and can sometimes cause deformity and a profound limitation of function.

Desmoids are not easily seen on standard radiographs, but are more readily defined with computed tomography.[19,39] Magnetic resonance imaging is very useful in defining the nature and extent of the tumors; most of the lesions are dark on both T1 and T2 and do not ordinarily become bright with the introduction of gadolinium[32,40-42] (Figure 1). Those tumors that have excessive vascularity or are limited in the extent of the fibrous tissue may be bright on T2.[40,42] Dissemination and extension of the tumor can sometimes be detected with thallium-201 scintigraphy.[43]

One issue of great concern regarding desmoid tumors of the extremities is their seemingly relentless and aggressive progression.[18,24-27,29,31-34,36-38,44,45] They may start as a solitary mass and then extend over time, most often proximally. A tumor in the midthigh may over time progress to the proximal portion of the lower extremity, sometimes as a separate tumor rather than an extension of the original lesion. Even with resection or treatment with radiation, recurrence and proximal migration may occur. Even less common, but very disconcerting, is the occurrence of new tumors in other anatomic sites, such as the opposite extremity or even in an arm when the primary site is in the thigh.

Etiology and Genetic Characteristics

The data related to the origin of extra-abdominal desmoid tumors are confusing. The disease is more common in women and may have an association with pregnancy and estrogen therapy.[18,24,25,27-33] The disease tends to diminish in severity at menopause or when treated with raloxifene or tamoxifen.[28,46,47] Immunostaining with vimentin, alpha smooth muscle actin, muscle actin, and desmin are often positive.[24] A genetic finding is that of the presence of trisomy 8 and trisomy 20 in tumor specimens of desmoids,[19,48-50] but these have also been noted in other forms of fibrous tumors. Fletcher and associates[51] suggested that trisomy 8 may be a predictor of recurrence. The relationship to Gardner's syndrome has been extensively studied; for these patients, a genetic defect in chromosome 5 or 20 is reported, but these defects are only rarely present in patients who do not have familial polyposis.[12,17,19,24,52-54] Immunohistochemistry studies of tumors from patients with Gardner's syndrome, and to a lesser extent those who do not have polyposis, often disclose an involvement of beta-catenin, which may be a factor in the growth of the tumors.[55-57]

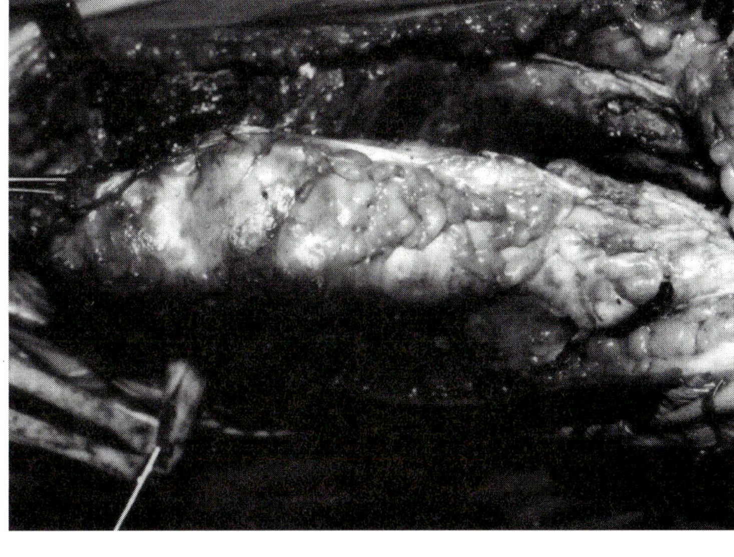

Figure 2

Examination of the gross structure of a desmoid tumor demonstrates irregularity of the surface and invasion of the adjacent muscle and soft tissues.

Histologic Features

The histologic appearance of extra-abdominal desmoids is well documented in the pathology literature.[18,19,24,26,29,31,32] The tumors are generally poorly circumscribed, and infiltrate adjacent muscle or fibrous capsule[24] (Figure 2). The tumors consist of elongated, slender, spindle-shaped cells of quite uniform appearance that are separated from each other by abundant collagen fibers[18] (Figure 3). The cells rarely contact one another and are almost never atypical.[24] The nuclei are sometimes vesicular, with minute nucleoli and indistinct cytoplasm.[18] Occasional cells are multinuclear, suggesting DNA synthetic activity.[19] Some of the cells adjacent to the muscle being invaded may appear as multinucleated giant cells, but this is uncommon.[24] Cells from desmoids routinely stain with vimentin, smooth muscle actin, and muscle-specific actin.[24] They often exhibit a response to cytokines such as transforming growth factor-β, interleukin-1, interleukin-7, and COX-2.[19,49]

Desmoid tumors are sometimes difficult to distinguish from reactive fibroblasts in a reparative site after muscle rupture. They may also be called low-grade fibrosarcomas by some pathologists, but rarely have a sufficient mitotic activity to justify such a definition.[18,19,24]

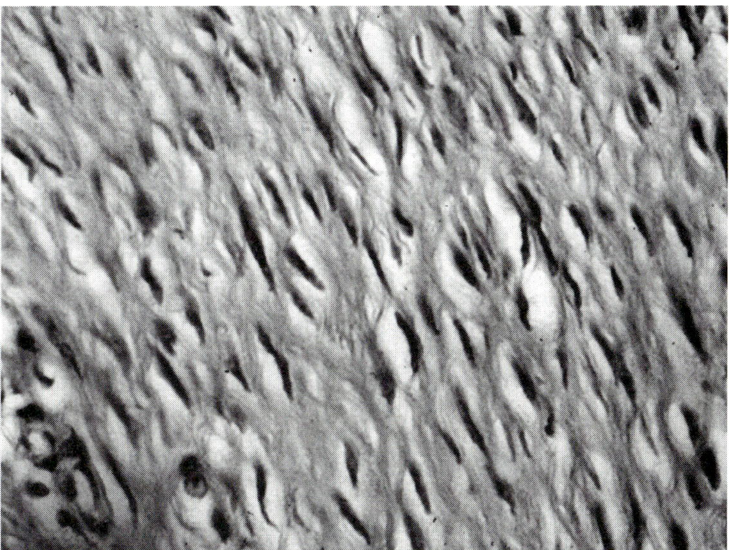

Figure 3

The histologic appearance of desmoid tumors shows fibroblast-like cells with little atypism and only occasional evidence of synthetic activity of giant cells. Hematoxylin and eosin × 100.

Treatment of Extra-Abdominal Desmoids

The earliest approaches to desmoid tumors of the extremities were surgical.[4,10,18,25,30-33,58] Surgical excision with a marginal or wide margin seems to be a logical approach for a tumor that is unlikely to metastasize or cause death. However, there are several problems with this approach. The tumors may be close to nerves or blood vessels or even muscles and tendons and thus may be difficult to resect with an appropriate margin.[25,27,33,59] Despite adequate resections the recurrence rate is extremely high, ranging from 15% to 65%.[18,19,25,27,29-34,36,37,44,45] Finally, even with wide resection and without a local recurrence, another lesion may appear adjacent or even distant to the site of the surgery, sometimes months or years after the resective surgery. For this reason, numerous attempts have been made to add sequential or sometimes even alternative approaches to the treatment of these difficult tumors.

Radiation has been introduced both as the primary treatment and as an adjunct to surgical excision.[27,44,45,59-66] The radiation dosage is lower than that used for malignant tumors but is still almost always over 50 Gy and must be given over a 5- to 8-week period. This seems to be successful in reducing the likelihood of recurrence and sometimes in decreasing the size of the tumor and limiting its growth.[27,33,44,59-61,63,64] Chemotherapeutic agents of various types have been introduced; some are declared successful, particularly for extensive or aggressive disease. The agents include tamoxifen, doxorubicin, dacarbazine, carboplatin, vinblastine and methotrexate, cyclo-oxygenase-2 agents, raloxifene, imatinib mesylate, and interferon alpha with or without tretinoin.[35,46,47,67-73]

Tumors in certain sites often require special treatment.[29] Lesions of the sole of the foot should be principally treated with surgery and, if necessary, radiation because the recurrence rate is relatively high but the likelihood of extension to other sites is low.[18,37] The same may be said for the rare lesions that occur in the palm.[38] The most distressing sites for tumors are in the axilla or the pelvic region, and especially those tumors close to the mandible or maxilla.[19,36] These are difficult to treat without neurologic or vascular damage or disfigurement and sometimes severe limitation of function. Tumors in patients with Gardner's syndrome probably respond less well to the chemotherapeutic agents, which also may interfere with management of polyposis or the resultant colonic cancers.[13,17,19,21,23,47]

Summary

Extra-abdominal desmoid tumors cause significant and often serious problems for the patient, the orthopaedist, and the oncologist. The tumors may involve vital areas, be difficult to resect, and have a high recurrence rate. Following what seems to be adequate treatment, they may appear in other adjacent or distal sites. We have only limited knowledge as to the cause and nature of these lesions, except for their appearance in patients with Gardner's syndrome, who sometimes have very widespread disorders in the colon, thyroid gland, bones, teeth, eyes, and skin. The relationship to estrogen is evident, but the other genetic and biochemical features are not clear. This leaves us with very limited information on improved methods of approaching the disease. The fortunate aspect of the entity is that although the patients may have a prolonged and troublesome course, they are not at risk for death.

References

1. Robertson D (ed): *Clinical Reports of the Surgical Practice of the Glasgow Royal Infirmary*, ed 63. Glasgow, Scotland, 1832.

2. Müller J: *Uber den Finern Bau und die Formen der Krankhafte Greschwulste*, ed 80. Berlin, Germany, 1838.

3. Bennett JH: *On Cancerous and Canceroid Growths.* Edinburgh, Scotland, S and Knox, 1849.

4. Sanger M: Uber desmoide greschwulste der bauchwand und deren operation mit resection des peritoneum parietale. *Arch Gynekol* 1884;24:1-8.

5. Paget J: Fibronucleated tumor of the abdomen of 14 years growth: Removal. *Lancet* 1856;1:625-635.

6. Rokitansky C: *Handbuch der Pathologischen Anatome.* Vienna, Austria, Braumuller und Seidel, 1846.

7. Wilks S: *Lectures on Pathological Anatomy.* London, England, Longman, 1849.

8. Nichols RW: Desmoid tumors: A report of 31 cases. *Arch Surg* 1923;7:277-282.

9. Ewing J: Fascial sarcoma and intermuscular myxoliposarcoma. *Arch Surg* 1935;31:507-511.

10. Musgrove JE, McDonald JR: Extra-abdominal desmoid tumors: Their differential diagnosis and treatment. *Arch Pathol* 1948;5:513-540.

11. Stout AP: Juvenile fibromatosis. *Cancer* 1954;7:953-958.

12. Gardner EJ: A genetic and clinical study of intestinal polyposis: A predisposing factor for carcinoma of the colon and rectum. *Am J Hum Genet* 1951;3:167-176.

13. Gardner EJ: Multiple cutanenous and subcutaneous lesions occurring simultaneously with hereditary polyposis and osteomatosis. *Am J Hum Genet* 1953;5:139-147.

14. Smith WG: Multiple polyposis, Gardner's syndrome and desmoid tumors. *Dis Colon Rectum* 1958;1:323-332.

15. Camiel MR, Mule JE, Alexander LL, Benninghoff DL: Association of thyroid carcinoma with Gardner's syndrome in siblings. *N Engl J Med* 1968;278:1056-1058.

16. Chang CH, Piatt ED, Thomas KE, Watne AL: Bone abnormalities in Gardner's syndrome. *Am J Roentgenol Radium Ther Nucl Med* 1968;103:645-652.

17. Gardner EJ, Burt RW, Freston JW: Gastrointestinal polyposis: Syndromes and genetic mechanisms. *West J Med* 1980;132:488-499.

18. Hajdu SI: *Pathology of Soft Tissue Tumors.* Philadelphia, PA, Lea and Febiger, 1979, pp 122-164.

19. McAnena OJ, Daly JM: Desmoid fibrosarcoma: Gardner's syndrome, in Raaf JR (ed): *Soft Tissue Sarcomas: Diagnosis and Treatment.* St. Louis, MO, Mosby, 1993, pp 151-163.

20. Naylor EW, Gardner EJ: Adrenal adenomas in a patient with Gardner's syndrome. *Clin Genet* 1981;20:67-73.

21. Naylor EW, Gardner EJ, Richards RC: Desmoid tumors and mesenteric fibromatosis and Gardner's syndrome. *Arch Surg* 1979;114:1181-1185.

22. Traboulsi EI, Krush AJ, Gardner EJ, et al: Prevalence and importance of pigmented ocular fundus lesions in Gardner's syndrome. *N Engl J Med* 1987;316:661-667.

23. Simpson RD, Harrison EG, Mayo CW: Mesenteric fibromatosis in familial polyposis: A variant of Gardner's syndrome. *Cancer* 1964;17:526-534.

24. Weiss SW, Goldblum JR: *Enzinger and Weiss's Soft Tissue Tumors,* ed 4. St. Louis, MO, Mosby, 2001, pp 320-346.

25. Rock MG, Pritchard DJ, Reiman HM, Soule EH, Brewster RC: Extra-abdominal desmoid tumors. *J Bone Joint Surg Am* 1984;66:1369-1374.

26. Posner MC, Shiu MH, Newsome JL, Hajdu SI, Gaynor JJ, Brennan MF: The desmoid tumor: Not a benign disease. *Arch Surg* 1989;124:191-196.

27. Ballo MT, Zagars GK, Pollack A, Pisters PW, Pollack RA: Desmoid tumor: Prognostic factors and outcome after surgery, radiation therapy, or combined surgery and radiation therapy. *J Clin Oncol* 1999;17:158-167.

28. Camiel MR, Solish GI: Desmoid tumors during pregnancy. *Am J Obstet Gynecol* 1982;144:988-989.

29. Fong Y, Rosen PP, Brennan MF: Multifocal desmoids. *Surgery* 1993;114:902-906.

30. Khorsand J, Karkousis CP: Desmoid tumors and their management. *Am J Surg* 1985;149:215-218.

31. Markhede G, Lundgren L, Bjurstam N, Berlin O, Stener B: Extra-abdominal desmoid tumors. *Acta Orthop Scand* 1986;57:1-7.

32. Pignatti G, Baranti-Brodano G, Ferrari D, et al: Extraabdominal desmoid tumor: A study of 83 cases. *Clin Orthop Relat Res* 2000;375:207-213.

33. Pritchard DJ, Nascimento AG, Petersen IA: Local control of extra-abdominal desmoid tumors. *J Bone Joint Surg Am* 1996;78:848-854.

34. Faulkner LB, Hajdu SI, Kher U, et al: Pediatric desmoid tumor: Retrospective analysis of 63 cases. *J Clin Oncol* 1995;13:2813-2818.

35. Skapek SX, Hawk BJ, Hoffer FA, et al: Combination chemotherapy using vinblastine and methotrexate for the treatment of progressive desmoid tumor in children. *J Clin Oncol* 1998;16:3021-3027.

36. Fasching MC, Saleh J, Woods JE: Desmoid tumors of the head and neck. *Am J Surg* 1988;156:327-333.

37. Barbella R, Fox IM: Recurring desmoid tumor of the foot: A case study. *Foot Ankle Int* 1996;17:221-225.

38. Karacaoglan N, Akbas H, Eroglu L, Kandemir B: Desmoid tumor of the hand. *Plast Reconstr Surg* 2000;106:954-955.

39. Magid D, Fishman EK, Jones B, Hoover HC, Feinstein R, Siegelman SS: Desmoid tumors in Gardner's syndrome: Use of computerized tomography. *AJR Am J Roentgenol* 1984;142:1141-1145.

40. Feld R, Burk DL Jr, McCue P, Mitchell DG, Lackman R, Rifkin MD: MRI of aggressive fibromatosis: Frequent appearance of high signal intensity on T2-weighted images. *Magn Reson Imaging* 1990;8:583-588.

41. O'Keefe F, Kim EE, Wallace S: Magnetic resonance imaging in aggressive fibromatosis. *Clin Radiol* 1990;42:170-173.

42. Robbin MR, Murphey MD, Temple HT, Kransdorf MJ, Choi JJ: Imaging of musculoskeletal fibromatosis. *Radiographics* 2001;21:585-600.

43. Murata H, Kusuzaki K, Hirata M, Hashiguchi S, Hirasawa Y: Extraabdominal desmoid tumor with dissemination detected by thallium-201 scintigraphy. *Anticancer Res* 2000;20:3963-3966.

44. Leibel SA, Wara WM, Hill DR, et al: Desmoid tumors: Local control and patterns of relapse following radiation therapy. *Int J Radiat Oncol Biol Phys* 1983;9:1167-1171.

45. Spear MA, Jennings LC, Mankin HJ, et al: Individualizing management of aggressive fibromatosis. *Int J Radiat Oncol Biol Phys* 1998;40:637-645.

46. Kinzbrunner B, Seymour R, Domingo J, Rosenthal CJ: Remission of rapidly growing desmoid tumors after tamoxifen therapy. *Cancer* 1983;52:2201-2204.

47. Tonelli F, Ficari F, Valanzano R, Brandi ML: Treatment of desmoids and mesenteric fibromatosis in familial adenomatous polyposis with raloxifene. *Tumori* 2003;89:391-396.

48. Bridge JA, Swarts SJ, Buresh C, et al: Trisomies 8 and 20 characterize a subgroup of benign fibrous lesions arising in both soft tissue and bone. *Am J Pathol* 1999;154:729-733.

49. Mills BG, Frausto A, Brien E: Cytokines associated with the pathophysiology of aggressive fibromatosis. *J Orthop Res* 2000;18:655-662.

50. Qi H, Dal Cin P, Hernandez JM, et al: Trisomies 8 and 29 in desmoid tumors. *Cancer Genet Cytogenet* 1996;92:147-149.

51. Fletcher JA, Naeem R, Xioao S, Corson JM: Chromosome aberrations in desmoid tumors: Trisomy 8 may be a predictor of recurrence. *Cancer Genet Cytogenet* 1995;79:139-143.

52. Bodmer WF, Bailey CJ, Bodmer FJ, et al: Localization for the gene for familial polyposis on chromosome 5. *Nature* 1987;328:614-616.

53. Hayry P, Reitam JJ, Vihko R, et al: The desmoid tumor: III. A biochemical and genetic analysis. *Am J Clin Pathol* 1982;77:681-685.

54. Leppert M, Dobbs M, Scambler P, et al: The gene for familial polyposis coli maps to the long arm of chromosome 5. *Science* 1987;238:1411-1423.

55. Alman BA, Pajersky ME, Diaz-Cano S, Corboy K, Wolfe HJ: Aggressive fibromatosis (desmoid

tumor) is a monoclonal disorder. *Diagn Mol Pathol* 1997;6:98-101.

56. Alman BA, Li C, Pajerski ME, Diaz-Cano S, Wolfe HJ: Increased beta-catenin protein and somatic APC mutations in sporadic aggressive fibromatoses (desmoid tumors). *Am J Pathol* 1997;151:329-334.

57. Couture J, Mitri A, Lagace R, et al: A germline mutation at the extreme 3′ end of the APC gene results in a severe desmoid phenotype and is associated with overexpression of beta catenin in the desmoid tumor. *Clin Genet* 2000;57:205-212.

58. Strode JE: Desmoid tumors particularly as related to their surgical removal. *Ann Surg* 1954;139:335-340.

59. Miralbell R, Suit HD, Mankin HJ, Zuckerberg LR, Stracher MA, Rosenberg AE: Fibromatoses: From postsurgical surveillance to combined surgery and radiation therapy. *Int J Radiat Oncol Biol Phys* 1990;18:535-540.

60. Goy BW, Lee SP, Eilber F, et al: The role of adjuvant radiotherapy in the treatment of resectable desmoid tumors. *Int J Radiat Oncol Biol Phys* 1997;39:659-665.

61. Kamath SS, Parsons JT, Marcus RB, Zlotecki RA, Scarborough MT: Radiotherapy for local control of aggressive fibromatosis. *Int J Radiat Oncol Biol Phys* 1996;36:325-328.

62. Kiel KD, Suit HD: Radiation therapy in the treatment of aggressive fibromatoses (desmoid tumors). *Cancer* 1984;54:2051-2055.

63. Merchant TE, Nguyen D, Walter AW, Pappo AS, Kun LE, Rao BN: Long-term results with radiation therapy for pediatric desmoid tumors. *Int J Radiat Oncol Biol Phys* 2000;47:1267-1271.

64. McCollough WM, Parson JT, Van Der Griend R, Enneking WF, Heare T: Radiation therapy for aggressive fibomatosi:. The experience at the University of Florida. *J Bone Joint Surg Am* 1991;73:717-725.

65. Sherman NE, Romsdahl M, Evans H, Zagars G, Oswald MJ: Desmoid tumors: A 20-year radiotherapy experience. *Int J Radiat Oncol Biol Phys* 1990;19:37-40.

66. Zelefsky MJ, Harrison LB, Shiu MH, Armstrong JG, Hajdu SI, Brennan MF: Combined surgical resection and iridium 192 implantation for locally advanced and recurrent desmoid tumors. *Cancer* 1991;67:380-384.

67. Hardell L, Breivald M, Henerdal S: Shrinkage of desmoid tumor with interferon alfa treatment. *Cytokines Cell Mol Ther* 2000;6:155-156.

68. Leithner A, Schnack B, Katterschafka T, et al: Treatment of extra-abdominal desmoid tumors with interferon-alpha with or without tretinoin. *J Surg Oncol* 2000;73:21-25.

69. Mace J, Sybil Biermann J, Sondak V, et al: Response of extraabdominal desmoid tumors to therapy with imatinib mesylate. *Cancer* 2002;95:2373-2379.

70. Okuno SH, Edmonson JH: Combination chemotherapy for desmoid tumors. *Cancer* 2003;97:1134-1135.

71. Patel SR, Evans HL, Benjamin RS: Combination chemotherapy in adult desmoid tumors. *Cancer* 1993;72:3244-3247.

72. Seiter K, Kemeny N: Successful treatment of a desmoid tumor with doxorubicin. *Cancer* 1993;71:2242-2244.

73. Weiss AJ, Lackman RD: Low dose chemotherapy of desmoid tumors. *Cancer* 1989;64:1192-1194.

Index